Cancer: Causes and Metastasis

Cancer: Causes and Metastasis

Editor: Davian Henderson

MURPHY & MOORE
www.murphy-moorepublishing.com

www.murphy-moorepublishing.com

MURPHY & MOORE

Cataloging-in-Publication Data

Cancer : causes and metastasis / edited by Davian Henderson.
p. cm.
Includes bibliographical references and index.
ISBN 978-1-63987-092-9
1. Cancer. 2. Cancer--Etiology. 3. Metastasis. I. Henderson, Davian.
RC261 .C36 2022
616.994--dc23

Murphy & Moore Publishing,
1 Rockefeller Plaza,
New York City, NY 10020, USA

ISBN 978-1-63987-092-9 (Hardback)

Contents

Preface

The substances which can cause cancer are known as carcinogens. They can cause damage to the genome or disturb the cellular metabolic processes. A few examples of cancer-causing substances are tobacco smoke, asbestos and dioxins. Carcinogens act by changing the metabolism of the cell or damaging their DNA. This in turn leads to the formation of tumors. The condition wherein the cancer cells move away from the original tumor and enter the lymphatic stream or the blood stream is known as metastasis. It involves the spread of cancer from one part of the body to another. Metastasis can be either treated through systemic therapy or through local therapy. Systemic therapy targets the entire body while local therapy focuses on the part of the body which is affected by cancer. This book discusses the fundamentals as well as modern approaches to the research on cancer-causing substances. Also included herein is a detailed explanation of their relationship to metastasis. This book will prove to be immensely beneficial to students and researchers in this field.

This book is a comprehensive compilation of works of different researchers from varied parts of the world. It includes valuable experiences of the researchers with the sole objective of providing the readers (learners) with a proper knowledge of the concerned field. This book will be beneficial in evoking inspiration and enhancing the knowledge of the interested readers.

In the end, I would like to extend my heartiest thanks to the authors who worked with great determination on their chapters. I also appreciate the publisher's support in the course of the book. I would also like to deeply acknowledge my family who stood by me as a source of inspiration during the project.

Editor

1

GWAS in Breast Cancer

Paulo C.M. Lyra-Junior, Nayara G. Tessarollo, Isabella S. Guimarães, Taciane B. Henriques, Diandra Z. dos Santos, Marcele L.M. de Souza, Victor Hugo M. Marques, Laura F.R.L. de Oliveira, Krislayne V. Siqueira, Ian V. Silva, Leticia B.A. Rangel and Alan T. Branco

Abstract

related deaths among women worldwide. It is expected that more than 240,000 new cases and 40,450 deaths related to the disease will occur in 2016. It is well known that inherited genetic variants are drivers for breast cancer development. There are many mechanisms through which germline genetic variation affects prognosis, such as BRCA1 and BRCA2 genes, which account for approximately 20% of the increased hereditary risks. Therefore, it is evident that the genetic pathways that underlie cancer development are complex in which networks of multiple alleles confer disease susceptibility and risks. Global analyses through genome-wide association studies (GWAS) have revealed several *loci* across the genome are associated with the breast cancer. This chapter compiles all breast GWAS released since 2007, year of the first article published in this area, and discuss the future directions of this field. Currently, hundreds of genetic markers are linked to breast cancer, and understanding the underlying mechanisms of these variants might lead to the discover of biomarkers and targets for therapy in patients.

Keywords: breast cancer, genome-wide association studies (GWAS), susceptibility, *Loci*, SNPs

1. Introduction

One of the main goals of human genetics is to understand genetic pathways underlying traits. It has been highly successful the gene mapping of disorders with a Mendelian pattern of inheritance using the tendency of genes and other genetic markers to be inherited together. It is well known that genetic variants underlying these single-gene Mendelian disorders are rare in the population and tend to be highly penetrant, which means that a high percentage of carriers of the genotype will manifest the phenotype. On the other hand, mapping of non-Mendelian (or complex) traits, cases in which variants in multiple genes contribute to the phenotype, was only possible after sequencing and study of the human genome. Inherited variants underlying complex diseases, opposing the Mendelian disorders, have modest penetrance but higher frequency in the population [1–4] (**Figure 1**). Thus, efforts have been made to identify genes and pathways that control human traits, and, in the future, predict illness and establish more appropriated methods of treatment.

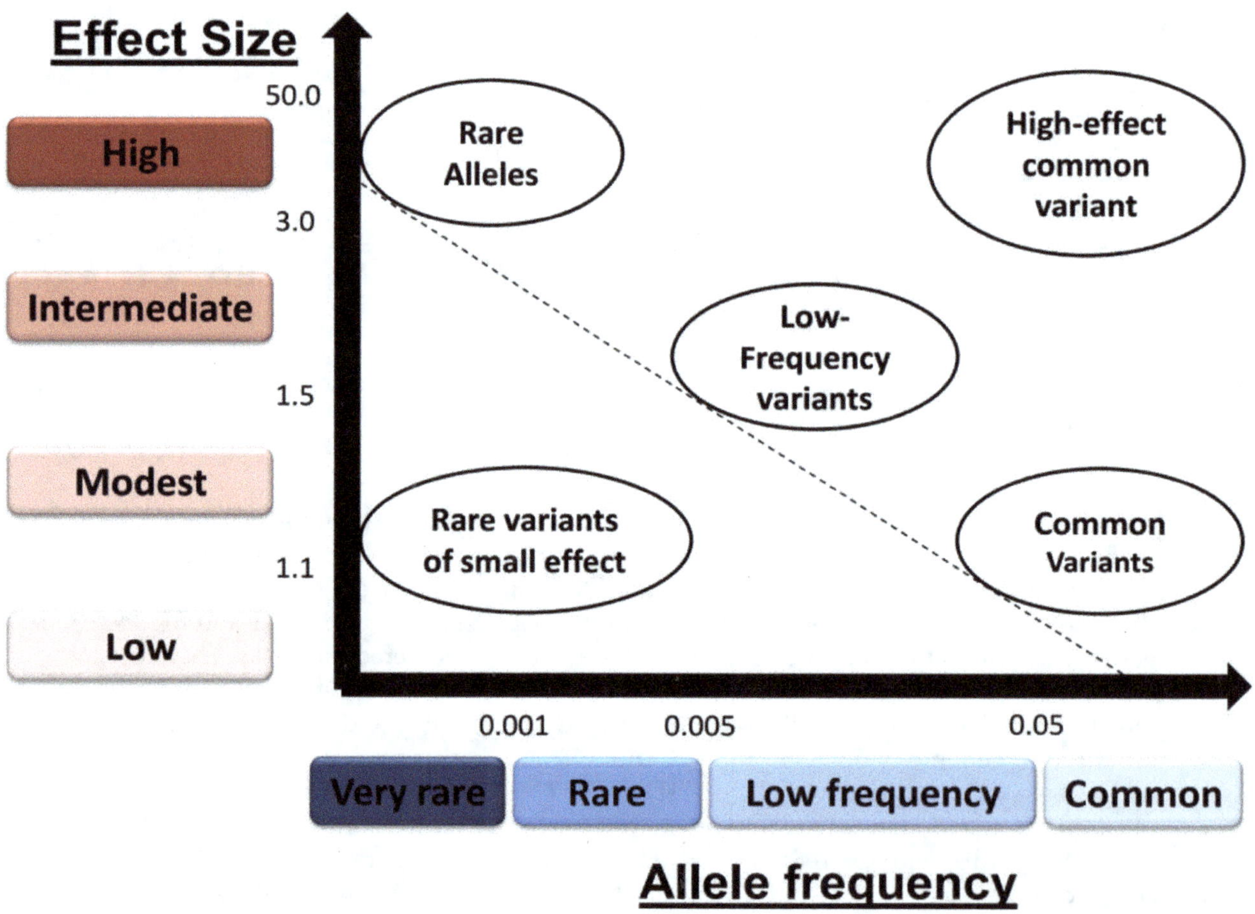

Figure 1. Features of genetic variants and correlation with disease severity. The panel shows the correlation between the frequency of alleles and the severity of the disease (odds ratio). Accordingly, Mendelian diseases (top left circle) have high effect on the individual, but the frequency of such mutations in the population is very rare. On the other hand, very rare variants with small effect (bottom left circle) are also found in the population, these features restrain the establishment of a reliable correlation between phenotype and genotype. GWAS have focused on identifying a massive number of genetic variants, which can be separated as (i) common variants associated with high effect size (top right circle) and (ii) abundant common alleles with apparent very low impact on human health (bottom right circle). Adapted from Manolio et al. [95].

A reflection of the urgency to unveil this research field is notable when looking through breast cancer numbers. Worldwide, the scenario is dramatic, with more than one million new cases of breast cancer diagnosed yearly (cancer genome atlas network 2012), and the fifth cause of death from cancer overall. In developing countries, breast cancer is the second cause of death from cancer and accounts for 15.4% of overall cancer-related deaths in women [5]. Moreover, it corresponds to the most common cancer-related death in women in the less developed regions (14.3%). In the United States, breast cancer is the second cause of cancer-related deaths among women, and it is estimated that one of eight American women will develop invasive breast cancer over the course of her lifetime. Accordingly, in the year of 2016, only in the United States, more than 240,000 new cases of the disease and 40,450 related deaths are expected [6].

Breast cancer comprises multiple diseases harbouring different genetic alterations; each subtype responds differently to treatments, and this feature leads to distinct clinical outcomes [7, 8]. Based on tumour histological biomarkers, breast cancer can be separated into three basic clinical types, such as HR positive (estrogen receptor and progesterone receptor), HER2+ (human epidermal growth factor receptor 2 positive), and triple-negative breast cancer, which are an essential part of the diagnostic workup of all breast cancer patients [9]. Approximately, 85% of all breast cancers are HR positive, about 20% are HER2+ and nearly 15% are triple-negative.

It is well understood that breast cancer is a complex and heterogeneous disease with a multi-factorial etiology involving genetic, dietary, hormonal and reproductive factors. Among these, genetic is of particular importance. Epidemiological studies estimate that women with history of breast cancer in a first-degree relative show nearly twofold higher risk to develop breast cancer than women without a family history, indicating that the genetic factors are important determinants of disease risk [10]. At least 10–15% of all breast cancer cases may be due to the inheritance of a single gene mutation or multiple genetic variants [10, 11]. In the 1990s, two major susceptibility genes for breast cancer, breast cancer 1 (BRCA1) and breast cancer 2 (BRCA2), were the first ones to be identified on the long arm of chromosome 17 and the short arm of chromosome 13, respectively [12–14]. These genes are responsible for 20–30% of hereditary breast cancer cases worldwide. BRCA1 and BRCA2 are important on the maintenance of genome stability by playing a critical role in the regulation of different cellular processes, such as transcription, cell cycle, DNA repair, cell proliferation and differentiation, in response to DNA damage [15]. Indeed, woman carrying such pathogenic variants have an increased risk of 60–80% of breast cancer [16, 17]. Moreover, inherited BRCA1/2 gene mutations are associated with a 39–80% lifetime risk of female breast cancer [18–21]. It is also well established that BRCA1/2 carriers with breast cancer have a strong lifetime risk of developing contralateral breast cancer range from 10 to 40% and are 2–6 times higher than the risk for non-carriers [22–27].

The identification of mutations in BRCA, considered as a critical factor for the development of breast cancer in some women, has boosted the interest of scientists to discover more mutations that drive tumour development. In this context, advances in DNA sequencing technologies empowered massive parallel sequencing, and, as a consequence, it has led to a fantastic discovery and assignment of other hereditary pre-disposition genes to high (TP53, PALB2, PTEN), moderated (CHEK2, ATM, NF1, NBN) and elevated, but imprecise, breast cancer risk (CDH1, STK11) [28–34]. Altogether, high and moderate penetrance breast cancer susceptibility mutations in these genes account for just over 30% of familial breast cancer cases, because linkage studies are not amenable to the identification of common alleles with small effects.

However, the major advance over the several years has led by genome-wide association studies (GWAS). This approach is based on genome-wide genotyping for thousands to millions of single-nucleotide polymorphisms (SNPs) in a large number of individuals and contrast between the groups with and without a specific phenotype. Therefore, this approach has successfully identified thousands of *loci* associated with hundreds of traits (National Human Genome Research Institute GWAS catalogue) [35]. Hence, this recent technology opens a new way to understand the underlying genetic causes of common diseases [1].

2. Genome-wide association studies

In the past, studying polymorphisms were limited by the technologies that only permitted analysis of one or a few *loci* at time, hence limiting the aims to particular genes or pathways. The selection for candidate genes or pathways to be studied were based on the potential relation with carcinogenesis, metabolism, cell cycle control and hormone synthesis. Therefore, the initial studies focused on single nucleotide polymorphisms which were associated with a crucial role in the cell functionality. With the advancement of techniques, sets of tagged SNPs included 'known common variants' across a gene. However, even though the number of candidates being analysed have increased, the number of well-validated association in those studies did not increase as expected. Association studies, involving direct testing of genetic polymorphisms in large series of cases versus controls, provide a powerful approach to identify lower penetrance alleles that cannot be detected by genetic linkage studies [36, 37]. However, additional susceptibility genes in which rare coding variants are associated with a moderate cancer risk have emerged through candidate gene re-sequencing [38].

GWAS have emerged as a powerful new approach that has the capacity of analysing the whole human genome in order to identify common variations in the population possibly associated with genetic factors of a specific disease. In other words, the intent of GWAS is to predict who is at the risk and develop new strategies for prevention and treatments of genetic diseases [39]. One of the initial successes of GWAS was the identification of the *complement factor* H gene as a major risk factor for age-related macular degeneration [40–42].

The GWAS technology is based on genotyping platforms (chip-based microarray technology) that can evaluate hundreds to thousands of SNPs simultaneously. The two primary platforms that have been used for most GWAS were developed by Illumina (San Diego, CA) and Affymetrix (Santa Clara, CA). These two competing technologies use different approaches to detect SNP variation. Accordingly, the Affymetrix platform prints short DNA sequences on a chip that recognizes a specific SNP allele. Alleles (i.e. nucleotides) are detected by a differential

DNA hybridization between the samples. Illumina, on the other hand, uses a bead-based technology with slightly longer DNA sequences to detect alleles. The Illumina technology is more expensive, but provides better specificity. Hence, it is possible to conduct association studies using sets of SNPs that tag most known common variants in the genome, and therefore, scan for the associations without prior knowledge of function or position [39, 43].

GWAS arrays have identified SNPs that are associated with many complex diseases or traits [44]; although they do not contain all mapped SNPs, rather they contain only index SNPs that represent SNPs in the same linkage disequilibrium (LD) block. The SNPs identified by GWAS are significantly correlated with a disease (or case) and are called as risk-associated SNPs, and the genomic regions containing the SNPs are called as risk *loci* for that particular disease [45, 46]. One common trend of the SNPs associated with the trait is that they are not frequently found in coding regions of the genome. Instead, most of them are located in non-coding regions of the genome and are equally distributed between intronic and intergenic compartments [47, 48]. This might initially reduce the potential of the index, SNPs being the causal, but it is important to keep in mind that all the SNPs in the same haplotype block with the index SNP could possibly play the role of a causal SNP. A commonly used approach to investigate SNPs other than the index SNPs present on the standard GWAS array has been to use an LD calculation [49–51] together with the 1000 Genomes Project reference panels from different populations [52, 53].

To move from the index SNP to a more refined list of putative causal SNPs located within the identified region, another approach called fine-mapping has also been used. Fine-mapping studies employ dense genotyping arrays that contain all common SNPs within the previously identified risk *loci*, which together with imputation [49–51] allow investigators to perform a more complete analysis of the risk regions. The most fine-mapping analyses have been done by international consortia with the shared interests for specific diseases or traits; examples include: the immunochip [54], the metabochip [55], the iCOGs array [56] and the Oncoarray [57].

3. GWAS in breast cancer

Over the past years, the results from GWAS have been published for breast cancer reporting well-validated novel associations. In total, these scans have identified approximately 100 common genetic susceptibility *loci* for breast cancer risk, and as additional scans are ongoing at some point, the number of cancer susceptibility *loci* is likely to change rapidly over the next years. This is only possible because there are many worldwide consortium groups, for example Asia Breast Cancer Consortium (ABCC) and Breast Cancer Association Consortium (BCAC), and it is through them that has been possible identifying the susceptibility of SNPs in large-scale and different populations.

The first GWAS for breast cancer was published in 2007 and identified novel susceptibility *loci* associated with this illness. Accordingly, as in reference [58], they studied 4398 breast cancer cases and 4316 controls, followed by a third stage in which 30 SNPs were tested for confirmation in 21860 cases and 22578 controls from 22 studies. In total 227876 SNPs were analyzed, which represented a coverage of approximately 77% of known common SNPs in Europeans at $r^2 > 0.5$. As a result, they found five novel independent *loci* associated with the breast cancer ($P < 10^{-7}$ using a stratified Cochran-Armitage trend test). The genes found around four *loci* are plausible causative genes (FGFR2, TNRC9, MP3K1 and LSP1). The most strongly associated SNP was in the intron 2 of the FGFR2 gene, a receptor tyrosine kinase that is amplified and overexpressed in 5–10% of breast tumours [59]. The 16q *locus* contains the candidate genes *TNRC9* and *LOC643714*. The function of *TNRC9* genes is currently unknown; however, the presence of the HMG box motif suggests that it possibly acts as a transcription factor [60]. MAP3K1, located at the 5q *locus*, is a gene involved in signal transduction and has not been previously reported to be involved with cancer. LSP1 is located at 11p *locus* and is an F-actin bundling cytoskeletal protein expressed in hematopoietic and endothelial cells. Other evidence of association pointed to a SNP around the H19 gene, a maternally imprinted gene that encodes an untranslated mRNA closely involved in regulation of IGF2. The fifth *locus* is an interval of 110 kb lacking known genes and located in the genomic region 8q24. Despite the absence of genes in the segment of 110 kb, the region 8q24 contains *loci* associated with prostate and colorectal cancers. The second stage of this study identified 1792 SNPs with *P*-value < 0.05, while the estimated by chance would be 1343. These observations have indicated that many additional common susceptibility alleles might be identifiable by this approach, but the detection of further susceptibility *loci* is associated with the increased coverage and use of larger number of cases and controls [58].

In the following years, nine articles using GWAS to identify genetic factors linked with breast cancer were published [61–69]. These works have not only increased the number of new markers associated with the illness, but also validated the genetic factors that were previously identified. Furthermore, the cancer genetic markers of susceptibility (CGEMS) group detected the association of FGFR2 in a second genome scan, genotyping 528,173 SNPs in 1145 cases of invasive breast cancer among postmenopausal white women and 1142 controls they detected a set of four SNPs in intron 2 of FGFR2 [62]. All the variants are related with FGFR2 expression in normal breast tissue, and interesting two of them are likely related to biological mechanism for interrupting active transcription factor-binding sites [70]. The deCODE group later on, using approximately 1000 unselected breast cancer cases and illumina 317k panel, found two additional *loci* at 2q and 5p [61, 63]. A further *locus* on 6q was identified by Gold et al. [64] studying 249 familial Ashkenazi Jewish breast cancer cases. This region contains two potential candidate genes, ECHDC1 and RNF146. The CGEMS group again added two novel *loci* with genome-wide significance: (i) one SNP, on the genomic region 1p11.2 neighbouring NOTCH2 and FCGR1B, is predominantly associated with estrogen receptor-positive breast cancer; (ii) the second SNP is located on chromosome 14q24.1, localizes to RAD51L1, a prior candidate pathway for breast cancer susceptibility [67]. Additional *loci* associated with the breast cancer were found with a more refined analysis of the first GWAS. Accordingly, Ahmed et al. [66] tested over 800 promising associations in the two stages involving 37,012 cases and 40,069 controls from 33 studies in the CGEMS and BCAC, finding strong evidence for additional susceptibility *loci* on 3p24 and 17q23.2; the causative genes include SLC4A7 and NEK10 on 3p and COX11 on 17q. Finally, Zheng et al. [65] conducted a GWAS among Chinese women and studied 607,728 SNPs in 1505 cases and 1522 controls; this analysis revealed 29 promising SNPs. The SNP at 6q25.1, located upstream of the estrogen receptor 1 gene (ESR1), exhibited consistent association with breast cancer across all the three stages performed, providing strong evidence of a susceptibility *locus* for breast cancer.

In 2010, a group conducted a new GWAS in which 582,886 SNPs were genotyped in 3659 cases with a family history of the disease and 4897 controls. They identified five new susceptibility *loci* on the chromosomes 9, 10 and 11, and found three SNPs in the 6q25.1, 8q24 and 11p15 regions with a higher correlation risk to develop cancer than the ones reported previously [69]. In the same year, other group, based on the fact that the germline BRCA1 mutations predispose to breast cancer, aimed to identify genetic modifiers of this risk in 1193 individuals with BRCA1 mutations who were diagnosed with invasive breast cancer under the age 40. This group was contrasted with 1190 BRCA1 carriers without breast cancer diagnosis over age 35. The first stage of this study had led to the identification of 96 SNPs; after the further stages of analysis, five SNPs on 19p13 were highly associated with breast cancer risk and also associated with triple-negative breast cancer in a separate study of 2301 triple-negative cases and 3949 controls [68].

Three studies were published in 2011 revealing new *loci* associated with the breast cancer. Haiman et al. [71] searching for common risk alleles for ER-negative breast cancer, combined GWAS data from women of African ancestry (1004 ER-negative cases and 2745 controls) and European ancestry (1718 ER-negative cases and 3670 controls). This study was further replicated with an additional 2292 ER-negative cases and 16,901 controls of European ancestry. Their conclusion pinpointed a common risk variant for ER-negative breast cancer at the TERT-CLPT1L *locus* on chromosome 5p15 in multiple populations. Furthermore, the same variant was also significantly associated with the triple-negative breast cancer, particularly in younger women (<50 years old). Cai et al. [72] published a four-stage GWAS including 17,153 cases and 16,943 controls among East-Asian women, after analysing 684,457 SNPs. The final result revealed one SNP at 10q21.2 (ZNF365) strongly implicated as a genetic risk variant for breast cancer among East-Asian women. Fletcher et al. [73] compared 296,114 tagging SNPs in 1694 cases of breast cancer and 2365 controls, with validation in three independent series totalling 11,880 cases and 12,487 controls, identifying a novel *locus* risk for breast cancer at 9q31.2 (the nearest genes around the SNP found are KLF4, RAD23B and ACTL7A), as well two variants mapping to 6q25.1, a *locus* previously reported. Although approximately 25 common genetic susceptibility *loci* have been identified to be independently associated with breast cancer risk, the genetic risk variants reported only explain a small fraction of the heritability of breast cancer.

Long et al. [74] aimed to discover novel genetic susceptibility *loci* for breast cancer, therefore they conducted a four-stage GWAS in 19,091 cases and 20,606 controls of East-Asian descent (Chinese, Korean and Japanese women were included). It was analysed 690,947 SNPs, from this group the final stage showed an SNP in chromosome 6q25.1, near to TGF-β activated kinase (TAB2), with consistent association with breast cancer risk across all four stages, reaching a *P*-value of 3.8×10^{-12} when the analysis was done with all samples combined. In addition, they identified two possible susceptibility SNPs, one located in the intron 5 of the ESR1 gene and the other at 11q24.3, with consistent association in each of the four stages. Kim et al. [75] conducted a GWAS to evaluate previously identified *loci* in Korean woman and to identify additional novel breast cancer susceptibility variants. Accordingly, they conducted a three-stage GWAS that included 6322 cases and 5897 controls. The results revealed one SNP in the epidermal growth factor receptor (ERB4) gene, located at chromosome 2q34, and showed that seven breast cancer susceptibility *loci* that were previously identified in European and/or Chinese population could be directly replicated in Korean women. Another GWAS study was conducted in Japanese patients with hormone receptor-positive, invasive breast cancer receiving adjuvant tamoxifen therapy. This study detected significant associations with recurrence-free survival of15 SNPs on nine chromosomal *loci* 1p31, 1q41, 5q33, 7p11, 10q22, 12q13, 13q22, 18q12 and 19p13. Among them, the one in the C10orf11 gene in 10q22 was significantly associated with recurrence-free survival in breast cancer patients treated with tamoxifen [76]. Besides these articles, two more were published in the same year. Ghoussaini et al. [77] reported a follow up of 72 promising associations from two independent GWAS using approximately 70,000 cases and 68,000 controls from 41 case-control studies and nine breast cancer GWAS. Through this study, three new breast cancer risk *loci* on 12p11 (PTHLH gene), 12q24 and 21q21 (NRIP1 gene) were identified. An interesting fact was that two SNPs were associated only with ER-positive disease, whereas the SNP on 12p11 was associated with similar relative risks for both ER-negative and ER-positive breast cancer. Because the GWAS of breast cancer separated by immunohistochemical have revealed *loci* contributing to the susceptibility of ER-negative subtypes. Siddiq et al. [78] conducted a large meta-analysis of ER-negative disease, comprising 4754 ER-negative cases and 31,663 controls from three GWAS, to identify additional genetic variants for ER-negative breast cancer. They performed an *in silico* replication with 86 SNPs using a P-value $\leq 10^{-5}$ in an additional population of 11,209 cases of breast cancer, where 946 were with ER-negative disease, and 16,057 controls of Japanese, Latino and European ancestry. As result two novel *loci* were identified, one at 6q14 and other at 20q11. At the *locus* 6q14 the SNP was associated with breast cancer and both ER-positive and ER-negative disease. In contrast, the SNP at 20q11 was associated with ER-negative breast cancer, but showed weaker association with overall breast cancer and no association with ER-positive disease. This work also confirmed three known *loci* associated with both ER-negative and ER-positive breast cancer. These findings highlight the relevance of large-scale collaborative studies to identify novel breast cancer risk *loci*.

In order to obtain a more comprehensive knowledge on the genetic factors controlling breast cancer development, the project collaborative oncological gene-environment study (COGS) was created through collaboration among four consortia [56]. The project consisted of a meta-analysis of nine GWAS, involving 10,052 breast cancer cases and 12,575 controls of European ancestry. 29,807 SNPs were selected for further genotyping. The selected SNPs were genotyped in 41 studies in BCAC, using 45,290 cases and 41,880 controls in European ancestry population. Another important point of the study was the custom Illumina iSelect genotyping array (iCOGS) utilized that comprises more than 200,000 SNPs. The combined efforts identified SNPs at 41 new breast cancer susceptibility *loci* at genome-wide significance ($P < 5 \times 10^{-8}$). Two other studies were published in 2013. One aimed to identify further cancer risk-modifying *loci* using multi-stage GWAS of 11,705 BRCA1 carriers (5920 diagnosed with breast cancer and 1839 diagnosed with ovarian cancer); further replication was done with an additional sample of 2646 BRCA1 carriers. Looking specifically at breast cancer factors they identified a novel risk modifier *locus* at 1q32 for BRCA1 carriers [79]. The other study was focused on identification of susceptibility *loci* specific to ER-negative disease, using a meta-analysis of 3 GWAS with 4193 ER-negative breast cancer cases and 35,194 controls with a series of 40 follow-up studies and also used the iCOGS to genotype. Their conclusion reported SNPs at four *loci*, 1q32.1 (MDM4 and LGR6), 2p24.1 and 16q12.2 associated with ER-negative but not ER-positive breast cancer. Once again providing further evidence for distinct etiological pathways associated with invasive ER-positive and ER-negative breast cancer [80].

GWAS have also been proven to be a powerful strategy to identify genetic factors associated with adverse reactions caused by drugs. The first GWAS for chemotherapy-induced alopecia was conducted in Japanese breast cancer patients, and identified SNPs significantly associated with drug-induced grade 2 alopecia. For instance, the rs3820706 (calcium channel voltage-dependent subunit beta) on 2q23 and its nearby SNP rs16830728 could be associated with significant molecular alterations in genes such as ion channel-related genes and genes related to the β-catenin signalling pathway [81].

The lack of concordance among some studies for breast cancer led a group to study 41 common non-synonymous SNP (nsSNP) for which evidence of association with breast cancer risk had been previously reported. This work combined 38 studies of white European women (46,450 cases and 42,600 controls), and showed strong association for one previously reported, 7q21; one novel susceptibility *locus*, 3p21 and the third *locus* is located in an established breast cancer susceptibility region, 3p24 [82]. Another study with 22,780 cases and 24,181 controls provided additional insights into the genetics and biology of breast cancer in East Asian women. It was identified that three genetic *loci* located at 1q32.1, 5q14.3 and 15q26.1 were recently associated with breast cancer risk [83]. Purrington et al. [84], interested on identify *loci* that influence triple-negative breast cancer risk, conducted a two-stage GWAS of triple-negative breast cancer with 1529 cases and 3399 controls in the first stage and 2148 cases and 1309 controls in the second. Variants at 19p13.1 and PTHLH *loci* showed significant association in both stages. Moreover, 25 SNPs already known as breast cancer susceptibility were associated with risk of triple-negative breast cancer ($P < 0.05$).

One particular article published in 2014 called attention for running a meta-analysis of GWAS of three mammographic density phenotype: dense area, non-dense and percent density in up to 7916 women in stage 1 and 10,379 women in the second stage. The results showed *loci* that reached genome-wide significance for all three phenotypes, for dense area (AREG, ESR1, ZNF365, LSP1, IGF1, TMEM184B and SGSM3), non-dense area (8p11.23) and percent density (PRDM6, 8p11.23 and TMEM184B). Interestingly, some regions are known as breast cancer susceptibility *loci* and the others regions were found, after a large meta-analysis, to be associated with breast cancer ($P < 0.05$). Based on the ability to identify known as well as putative novel breast cancer *loci* by studying mammographic density phenotypes, the authors demonstrated the power of using quantitative intermediate phenotypes to discover new disease *loci* [85].

In 2015, there were more than 90 established breast cancer risk *loci*, with 57 new ones, revealed through GWAS during 2013 and 2014. Nevertheless, new studies were published identifying new susceptibility *loci*. A group performed a meta-analysis restricted to women of European ancestry. They worked with 11 GWAS comprising of 15,748 breast cancer cases and 18,084 controls, and 46,785 cases and 42,892 controls from 41 studies genotyped on iCOGS, and used imputation to estimate genotypes for more than 11 million SNPs, identifying 15 novel *loci* associated with breast cancer at $P < 5x10^{-8}$ [85]. Palomba et al. [86], also following the assumption that analyses in genetically-homogeneous population could represent an additional approach to detect low penetrance alleles, conducted a GWAS study comparing 1431 Sardinian patients with non-familial, BRCA1/2-mutation-negative breast cancer to 2171 healthy Sardinian blood donors, where 2,067,645 SNPs were analysed. The study concludes the role of TOX3 and FGRF2 as breast cancer susceptibility genes in BRCA1/2-wild-type breast cancer patients from Sardinian population.

In 2016, three GWAS were three GWAS were published describing novel genetic susceptibility *loci*. It was a study including 14,224 cases and 14,829 controls of East Asian women, where two SNPs in two *loci* were found to be associated with breast cancer risk at the genome-wide significance level, one at 1p22.3 and other at 21q22.12 [87]. The identification of four previously unidentified *loci* including the ones at 13q22 (KLF5), 2p23.2 (WDR43) and 2q33 (PPIL3) with genome-wide significant association with ER-negative breast cancer, performing a meta-analysis of 11 GWAS consisting of 4939 ER-negative cases and 14,352 controls, combined with 7333 ER-negative cases and 42,468 controls and 15,252 BRCA1 mutation carriers genotyped on the iCOGS array [88]. GWAS also can be useful to identify SNPs associated with response to anthracycline-based neoadjuvant chemotherapy in breast cancer patients. A group identified two SNPs that were significantly associated with pathologic complete response after neoadjuvant chemotherapy. After the validation using 401 patients who received anthracycline-based neoadjuvant regimens the authors found that only one SNP, located in the WT1 gene, was associated with the pathologic complete response after anthracycline-based neoadjuvant therapy, suggesting that WT1 may be a potential target of anthracycline-based neoadjuvant therapy for breast cancer [89].

4. Conclusion

GWAS have been successful in identifying many genetic variants that are significantly associated with human diseases. However, a gap has emerged between the ability to detect these associations and the ability to meaningfully interpret their biological significance [90]. Currently, the challenges facing GWAS include the translation of associated *loci* into suitable biological hypotheses, missing heritability [91], and the understanding of how multiple modestly associated *loci* within genes interact to influence a phenotype [92]. Thus, the new trend for susceptibility *loci* identification has moved forward to describe precisely the functional weffects and target genes. The post-GWAS include detailed genetic and epidemiological dissection, bioinformatics prediction of functionality and *in vitro* and *in vivo* experimental verification of the molecular mechanisms for the causal variants and their target genes [93, 94]. Although identification of common risk variants is an emerging field, it will create a routine screening method for earlier diagnosis and direct breast cancer treatment strategies.

Abbreviations

GWAS	Genome-wide association studies
BRCA 1	Breast cancer 1 gene
BRCA 2	Breast cancer 2 gene
SNP	Single-nucleotide polymorphisms
HER 2+	Human epidermal growth factor receptor 2 positive
HR	Progesterone receptor
LOD	Logarithm of odds
LD	Linkage disequilibrium
TP53	Tumour protein p53
PALB2	Partner and localizer of BRCA2
PTEN	Phosphatase and tensin homolog
CHEK2	Checkpoint kinase 2
ATM	Serine/threonine kinase
NF1	Nuclear factor 1
NBN	Nibrin
CDH1	Cadherin-1
STK11	Serine/threonine kinase 11
FGFR2	Fibroblast growth factor receptor 2
TNRC9	Trinucleotide-repeat-containing 9
LSP1	Lymphocyte-specific protein 1
IGF2	Insulin-like growth factor 2
CGEMS	Cancer genetic markers of susceptibility
RNF146	RING finger protein 146
RAD51L1	DNA repair protein RAD51 homolog 2
NOTCH2	Neurogenic *locus* notch homolog protein 2
FCGR1B	Cluster of differentiation 64
BCAC	Breast Cancer Association Consortium
SLC4A7	Solute carrier family 4, sodium bicarbonate cotransporter, member 7
NEK10	NIMA-related kinase 10
COX11	Cytochrome C oxidase copper chaperone

ER	Estrogen receptor
KLF4	Kruppel-like factor 4
RAD23B	UV excision repair protein RAD23 homolog B
ACTL7A	Actin-like protein 7A
ESR1	Estrogen receptor 1
ERB4	Epidermal growth factor receptor
PTHLH	Parathyroid hormone-related protein
NRIP1	Nuclear receptor-interacting protein 1
COGS	Collaborative oncological gene-environment study
LGR6	Leucine-rich repeat-containing G-protein coupled receptor 6
AREG	Amphiregulin
ZNF365	Zinc finger protein 365
IGF1	Insulin-like growth factor 1
TMEM184B	Transmembrane protein 184B
SGSM3	Small G protein signaling modulator 3
KLF5	Krueppel-like factor 5
WDR43	WD repeat domain 43
PPIL3	Peptidyl-prolyl cis-trans isomerase-like 3
WT1	Wilms tumour protein

Author details

Paulo C.M. Lyra-Junior[1], Nayara G. Tessarollo, Isabella S. Guimarães[1], Taciane B. Henriques[1], Diandra Z. dos Santos[1], Marcele L.M. de Souza[1], Hugo M. Victor Marques[2], Laura F.R.L. de Oliveira[2], Krislayne V. Siqueira[2], Ian V. Silva[3], Leticia B.A. Rangel[1]* and Alan T. Branco[2]

*Address all correspondence to: lbarangel@yahoo.com

1 Laboratory of Cellular and Molecular Biology of Human Cancer, Department of Pharmaceutical Sciences and Biotechnology Program, Federal University of Espirito Santo State, Vitória, Brazil

2 Laboratory of Cellular and Molecular Biology of Human Cancer, Department of Pharmaceutical Sciences, Vitória, Brazil

3 Department of Morphology, Health Sciences Center, Federal University of Espirito Santo State, Vitória, Brazil

References

[1] Monteiro ANA, Freedman ML. Lessons from postgenome-wide association studies: functional analysis of cancer predisposition loci. Journal International Medicine. 2013; **274**: 414–424. DOI: 10.1111/joim.12085

[2] Venter JC, et al. The sequence of the human genome. Science. 2001; **291**: 1304–1351. DOI:10.1126/science.1058040

[3] Lander ES, et al. Initial sequencing and analysis of the human genome. Nature. 2001; **409**: 860–921. DOI: 10.1038/35057062

[4] Altshuler D, et al. Haplotype map of the human genome. Nature. 2005; **437**: 1299–1320. DOI: 10.1038/nature04226

[5] Ferlay J, et al. Cancer incidence and mortality worldwide: sources, methods and major patterns in GLOBOCAN 2012. International Journal Cancer. 2015; **136**: 359–386. DOI: 10.1002/ijc.29210. Epub 2014 Oct 9.

[6] American Cancer Society. Cancer Facts & Figures 2016. Atlanta: American Cancer Society; 2016.

[7] Perou CM, et al. Molecular portraits of human breast tumours. Nature. 2000; **406**: 747–752. DOI: 10.1038/35021093

[8] Sorlie T, et al. Gene expression patterns of breast carcinomas distinguish tumor subclasses with clinical implications. Proceedings of the National Academy of Sciences of the United States of America. 2001; **98**: 10869–10874. DOI: 10.1073/pnas.191367098

[9] Rakha EA, Chan S. Metastatic triple-negative breast cancer. Clinical Oncology. 2011; **23**: 587–600. DOI: 10.1016/j.clon.2011.03.013

[10] Collaborative Group on Hormonal Factors in Breast Cancer. Familial breast cancer: collaborative reanalysis of individual data from 52 epidemiological studies including 58,209 women with breast cancer and 101,986 women without the disease. The Lancet. 2001**;** **358**: 1389–1399. DOI: 10.1016/S0140-6736(01)06524-2

[11] Pharoah PD, et al. Polygenic susceptibility to breast cancer and implications for prevention. Nature Genetics. 2002; **31**: 33–36. DOI: 10.1038/ng853

[12] Miki Y, et al. A strong candidate for the breast and ovarian-cancer susceptibility gene BRCA1. Science. 1994; **266**: 66–71. DOI: 10.1126/science.7545954

[13] Friedman LS, et al. Confirmation of BRCA1 by analysis of germline mutations linked to breast and ovarian cancer in ten families. Nature Genetics. 1994; **8**: 399–404. DOI: 10.1038/ng1294-399.

[14] Wooster R, et al. Identification of the breast cancer susceptibility gene BRCA2. Nature. 1995; **378**: 789–792. DOI: 10.1038/378789a0

[15] Gudmundsdottir K, Ashworth A. The roles of BRCA1 and BRCA2 and associated proteins in the maintenance of genomic stability. Oncogene. 2006; **25**: 5864–5874. DOI: 10.1038/sj.onc.1209874

[16] Lakhani SR, et al. Prediction of BRCA1 status in patients with breast cancer using estrogen receptor and basal phenotype. Clinical Cancer Research. 2005; **11**: 5175–5180. DOI: 10.1158/1078-0432

[17] Foulkes WD, Shuen AY. In brief: BRCA1 and BRCA2. The Journal of pathology. 2013; **230**: 347–349. DOI: 10.1002/path.4205

[18] King M.C, Marks J.H, Mandell J.B. Breast and ovarian cancer risks due to inherited mutations in BRCA1 and BRCA2. Science. 2003; **302**: 643–646. DOI: 10.1126/science.1088759

[19] Chen S, Parmigiani G. Meta-analysis of BRCA1 and BRCA2 penetrance. Journal of Clinical Oncology. 2007; **25**: 1329–1333. DOI: 10.1200/JCO.2006.09.1066

[20] Mavaddat N, et al. Cancer risks for BRCA1 and BRCA2 mutation carriers: Results from prospective analysis of EMBRACE. Journal of the National Cancer Institute. 2013; **105**: 812–822. DOI: 10.1093/jnci/djt095

[21] Gabai-Kapara E, et al. Population-based screening for breast and ovarian cancer risk due to BRCA1 and BRCA2. Proceedings of the National Academy of Sciences of the United States of America. 2014; **111**: 14205–14210. DOI: 10.1073/pnas.1415979111

[22] Brekelmans CT, et al. Survival and prognostic factors in BRCA1-associated breast cancer. Annals of Oncology. 2006; **17**: 391–400. DOI: 10.1093/annonc/mdj095

[23] Graeser MK, et al. Contralateral breast cancer risk in BRCA1 and BRCA2 mutation carriers. Journal of Clinical Oncology. 2009; **27**: 5887–5892. DOI:10.1200/JCO.2008.19.9430

[24] Van Der Kolk DM, et al. Penetrance of breast cancer, ovarian cancer and contralateral breast cancer in BRCA1 and BRCA2 families: high cancer incidence at older age. Breast Cancer Research and Treatment. 2010; **124**: 643–651. DOI: 10.1007/s10549-010-0805-3

[25] Bernstein JL, et al. Contralateral breast cancer after radiotherapy among BRCA1 and BRCA2 mutation carriers: A WECARE study report. European Journal of Cancer. 2013; **49**: 2979–2985. DOI: 10.1016/j.ejca.2013.04.028

[26] Evans DG, et al. Contralateral mastectomy improves survival in women with BRCA1/2-associated breast cancer. Breast Cancer Research and Treatment. 2013; **140**: 135–142.DOI: 10.1007/s10549-013-2583-1

[27] Van den Broek AJ, et al. Impact of age at primary breast cancer on contralateral breast cancer risk in BRCA1/2 mutation carriers. Journal of Clinical Oncology. 2015; **34**: 409–418. DOI: 10.1200/JCO.2015.62.3942

[28] Giardiello FM, et al. Very high risk of cancer in familial Peutz-Jehgers syndrome. Gastroenterology. 2000; **119**: 1447–1453. DOI: 10.1053/gast.2000.20228

[29] Antoniou A, et al. Average risks of breast and ovarian cancer associated with BRCA1 or BRCA2 mutations detected in case series unselected for family history: a combined analysis of 22 studies. The American Society of Human Genetics. 2003; **72**: 1117–1130. DOI: 10.1086/375033

[30] The CHEK2 Breast Cancer Case-Control Consortium. CHEK2*1100delC and susceptibility to breast cancer: A collaborative analysis involving 10,860 breast cancer cases and 9,065 controls from ten studies. The American Society of Human Genetics. 2004; **74**: 1175–1182. DOI: 10.1086/421251

[31] Thompson D, et al. Cancer risks and mortality in heterozygous ATM mutation carriers. Journal of the National Cancer Institute. 2005; **97:** 813–822. DOI: 10.1093/jnci/dji141

[32] Rahman N, et al. PALB2, which encodes a BRCA2-interacting protein, is a breast cancer susceptibility gene. Nature Genetics. 2006; **39**: 165–167. DOI: 10.1038/ng1959

[33] Robson M. CHEK2, breast cancer, and the understanding of clinical utility. Clinical Genetics. 2010; **78**: 8–10. DOI: 10.1111/j.1399-0004.2010.01444.x

[34] Meindl A, et al. Germline mutations in breast and ovarian cancer pedigrees establish RAD51C as a human cancer susceptibility gene. Nature Genetics. 2010; **42**: 410–414. DOI: 10.1038/ng.569

[35] Manolio TA. Genomewide association studies and assessment of the risk of disease. The New England Journal of Medicine. 2010; **363**: 166–176. DOI: 10.1056/NEJMra0905980

[36] García-Closas M, Malats N, Silverman D, et al. NAT2 slow acetylation, GSTM1 null genotype, and risk of bladder cancer: results from the Spanish Bladder Cancer Study and meta-analyses. The Lancet. 2005; **366**: 649–59. DOI: 10.1016/S0140-6736(05)67137-1

[37] Cox A, et al. A common coding variant in CASP8 is associated with breast cancer risk. Nature Genetics. 2007; **39**: 352–358. DOI: 10.1038/ng1981

[38] Easton DF, Eeles RA. Genome-wide association studies in cancer. Human Molecular Genetics. 2008; **17**: R109–R115. DOI: 10.1093/hmg/ddn287

[39] Bush WS, Moore JH. Chapter 11: Genome-Wide Association Studies. PLoS Computation Biology. 2012; **8**: e1002822. DOI:10.1371/journal.pcbi.1002822

[40] Haines JL, et al. Complement factor H variant increases the risk of age-related macular degeneration. Science. 2005; **308**: 419–421. DOI: 10.1126/science.1110359

[41] Edwards AO, et al. Complement factor H polymorphism and age-related macular degeneration. Science. 2005; **308**: 421–424. DOI: 10.1126/science.1110189

[42] Klein RJ, Zeiss C, Chew EY, et al. Complement factor H polymorphism in age-related macular degeneration. Science. 2005; **308**: 385–389. DOI: 10.1126/science.1109557

[43] The Wellcome Trust Case Control Consortium. Genome-wide association study of 14,000 cases of seven common diseases and 3,000 shared controls. Nature. 2007; **447**: 661–678. DOI: 10.1038/nature05911

[44] Welter D, et al. The NHGRI GWAS catalog, a curated resource of SNP-trait associations. Nucleic Acids Research. 2014; **42**: 1001–1006. DOI: 10.1093/nar/gkt1229

[45] Li Y, et al. Genotype imputation. Annual Review Genomics Human Genetics. 2009; **10**: 387–406. DOI: 10.1146/annurev.genom.9.081307.164242

[46] Kichaev G, Pasaniuc B. Leveraging functional-annotation data in transethnic fine-mapping studies. American Journal Human Genetics. 2015; **97**: 260–271. DOI: 10.1016/j.ajhg.2015.06.007

[47] Freedman ML, Monteiro AN, Gayther SA et al. Principles for the post-GWAS functional characterization of cancer risk loci. Nature Genetics. 2011; **43**: 513–8. DOI:10.1038/ng.840.

[48] Blattler A, et al. Global loss of DNA methylation uncovers intronic enhancers in genes showing expression changes. Genome Biology. 2014; **15**: 469. DOI: 10.1186/s 13059-014-0469-0

[49] Howie BN, Donnelly P, Marchini JA. Flexible and accurate genotype imputation method for the next generation of genome-wide association studies. PLoS Genetics. 2009; **5**: e1000529. DOI: 10.1371/journal.pgen.1000529

[50] Li Y, et al. Mach: using sequence and genotype data to estimate haplotypes and unobserved genotypes. Genetic Epidemiology. 2010; **34**: 816–834. DOI: 10.1002/gepi.20533

[51] Browning SR, Browning BL. Rapid and accurate haplotype phasing and missing-data inference for whole-genome association studies by use of localized haplotype clustering. American Journal of Human Genetics. 2007; **81**: 1084–1097. DOI: 10.1086/521987

[52] Genomes Project C, et al. A global reference for human genetic variation. Nature. 2015; **526**: 68–74. DOI: 10.1038/nature15393

[53] 1000 Genomes Project Consortium, et al. An integrated map of genetic variation from 1092 human genomes. Nature. 2012; **491**: 56–65. DOI: .1038/nature11632

[54] Trynka G, Hunt KA, Bockett NA et al. Dense genotyping identifies and localizes multiple common and rare variant association signals in celiac disease. Nature Genetics. 2011; **43**: 1193–201. DOI: 10.1038/ng.998

[55] Voight BF, et al. The metabochip, a custom genotyping array for genetic studies of metabolic, cardiovascular, and anthropometric traits. PLoS Genetics. 2012; **8**: e1002793. DOI: 10.1371/journal.pgen.1002793

[56] Michailidou K, et al. Large-scale genotyping identifies 41 new loci associated with breast cancer risk. Nature Genetics. 2013; **45**: 353–361. DOI: 10.1038/ng.2563

[57] Available from: http://epi.grants.cancer/gov/oncoarray/ [Accessed: 2016-07-14].

[58] Easton DF, et al. Genome-wide association study identifies novel breast cancer susceptibility loci. Nature. 2007; **447**; 1087–1093. DOI: 10.1038/nature05887.

[59] Adnane J, et al. BEK and FLG, two receptors to members of the FGF family, are amplified in subsets of human breast cancers. Oncogene. 1991; **6**: 659–663.

[60] Brantjes H, et al. All Tcf HMG box transcription factors interact with Groucho-related co-repressors. Nucleic Acids Research. 2001; **29**: 1410–1419. DOI: 10.1093/nar/29.7.1410

[61] Stacey SN, et al. Common variants on chromosomes 2q35 and 16q12 confer susceptibility to estrogen receptor-positive breast cancer. Nature Genetics. 2007; **39**: 865–869. DOI: 10.1038/ng2064

[62] Hunter DJ, et al. A genome-wide association study identifies alleles in FGFR2 associated with risk of sporadic postmenopausal breast cancer. Nature Genetics. 2007; **39**: 870–874. DOI: 10.1038/ng2075

[63] Stacey SN, et al. Common variants on chromosome 5p12 confer susceptibility to estrogen receptor-positive breast cancer. Nature Genetics. 2008; **40**; 703–706. DOI: 10.1038/ng.131

[64] Gold B, et al. Genome-wide association study provides evidence for a breast cancer risk locus at 6q22.33. Proceedings of the National Academy of Sciences of the United States of America. 2008; **105**: 4340–4345. DOI: 10.1073/pnas.0800441105

[65] Zheng W, et al. Genome-wide association study identifies a new breast cancer susceptibility locus at 6q25.1. Nature Genetics. 2009; **41**: 324–328. DOI: 10.1038/ng.318

[66] Ahmed S, et al. Newly discovered breast cancer susceptibility loci on 3p24 and 17q23.2. Nature Genetics. 2009; **41**: 585–590. DOI: 10.1038/ng.354

[67] Thomas G, et al. A multistage genome-wide association study in breast cancer identifies two new risk alleles at 1p11.2 and 14q24.1 (RAD51L1). Nature Genetics. 2009; **41**: 579–584. DOI: 10.1038/ng.353

[68] Antoniou AC, et al. A locus on 19p13 modifies risk of breast cancer in BRCA1 mutation carriers and is associated with hormone receptor-negative breast cancer in the general population. Nature Genetics. 2010; **42**: 885–892. DOI:10.1038/ng.669

[69] Turnbull C, et al. Genome-wide association study identifies five new breast cancer susceptibility loci. Nature Genetics. 2010; **42**: 504–507. DOI: 10.1038/ng.586

[70] Meyer KB, et al. Allele-specific up-regulation of FGFR2 increases susceptibility to breast cancer. PLoS Biology. 2008; **6**: e108. DOI: 10.1371/journal.pbio.0060108

[71] Haiman CA, et al. A common variant at the TERT-CLPTM1L locus is associated with estrogen receptor-negative breast cancer. Nature Genetics. 2011; **43**: 1210–1214. DOI: 10.1038/ng.985

[72] Cai Q, et al. Genome-wide association study identifies breast cancer risk variant at 10q21.2: results from the Asia Breast Cancer Consortium. Human Molecular Genetics. 2011; **20**: 4991–4999. DOI: 10.1093/hmg/ddr405

[73] Fletcher O, et al. Novel breast cancer susceptibility locus at 9q31.2: results of a genome-wide association study. Journal of the National Cancer Institute. 2011; **103**: 425–435. DOI: 10.1093/jnci/djq563

[74] Long J, et al. Genome-wide association study in East Asians identifies novel susceptibility loci for breast cancer. PLoS Genetics. 2012; **8**: e1002532. DOI: 10.1371/journal.pgen.1002532

[75] Kim HC, et al. A genome-wide association study identifies a breast cancer risk variant in ERBB4 at 2q34: results from the Seoul Breast Cancer Study. Breast Cancer Research. 2012; **14**: R56. DOI: 10.1186/bcr3158

[76] Kiyotani K, et al. A genome-wide association study identifies locus at 10q22 associated with clinical outcomes of adjuvant tamoxifen therapy for breast cancer patients in Japanese. Human Molecular Genetics. 2012; **21**: 1665–1672. DOI: 10.1093/hmg/ddr597

[77] Ghoussaini M, et al. Genome-wide association analysis identifies three new breast cancer susceptibility loci. Nature Genetics. 2012: **44**: 312–318. DOI: 10.1038/ng.1049

[78] Siddiq A, et al. A meta-analysis of genome-wide association studies of breast cancer identifies two novel susceptibility loci at 6q14 and 20q11. Human Molecular Genetics. 2012; **21**: 5373–5384. DOI: 10.1093/hmg/dds381

[79] Couch FJ, et al. Genome-wide association study in BRCA1 mutation carriers identifies novel loci associated with breast and ovarian cancer risk. PLoS Genetics. 2013; **9**: e1003212. DOI: 10.1371/journal.pgen.1003212

[80] Garcia-Closas M, et al. Genome-wide association studies identify four ER negative-specific breast cancer risk loci. Nature Genetics. 2013; **45**: 392–398. DOI: 10.1038/ng.2561

[81] Chung R, et al. Roles of Wnt/β-catenin signalling pathway in the bony repair of injured growth plate cartilage in young rats. Bone. 2013; **52**: 651–658. DOI: 10.1016/j.bone.2012.10.035

[82] Milne RL, et al. Common non-synonymous SNPs associated with breast cancer susceptibility: findings from the Breast Cancer Association Consortium. Human Molecular Genetics. 2014; **23**: 6096–6111. DOI: 10.1093/hmg/ddu311

[83] Cai Q, et al. Genome-wide association analysis in East Asians identifies breast cancer susceptibility loci at 1q32.1, 5q14.3 and 15q26.1. Nature Genetics. 2014; **46**: 886–890. DOI: 10.1038/ng.3041

[84] Purrington KS, et al. Genome-wide association study identifies 25 known breast cancer susceptibility loci as risk factors for triple-negative breast cancer. Carcinogenesis. 2014; **35**: 1012–1019 DOI: 10.1093/carcin/bgt404

[85] Michailidou K, et al. Genome-wide association analysis of more than 120,000 individuals identifies 15 new susceptibility loci for breast cancer. Nature Genetics. 2015; **47**: 373–380. DOI: 10.1038/ng.3242

[86] Palomba G, et al. Genome-wide association study of susceptibility loci for breast cancer in Sardinian population. BMC cancer. 2015; **15**: 383. DOI: 10.1186/s12885-015-1392-9

[87] Han MR, et al. Genome-wide association study in East Asians identifies two novel breast cancer susceptibility loci. Human Molecular Genetics. 2016; **0**: 1–11. DOI: 10.1093/hmg/ddw164

[88] Couch FJ, et al. Identification of four novel susceptibility loci for oestrogen receptor negative breast cancer. Nature Communication. 2016; **7**: 11375. DOI: 10.1038/ncomms11375

[89] Wu L, et al. A genome-wide association study identifies WT1 variant with better response to 5-fluorouracil, pirarubicin and cyclophosphamide neoadjuvant chemotherapy in breast cancer patients. Oncotarget. 2016; **7**: 5042–5052. DOI: 10.18632/oncotarget.5837

[90] Qian DC, et al. Identification of shared and unique susceptibility pathways among cancers of the lung, breast, and prostate from genome-wide association studies and tissue-specific protein interactions. Human Molecular Genetics. 2015; **24**: 7406–7420. DOI: 10.1093/hmg/ddv440

[91] Cantor RM, Lange K, Sinsheimer JS. Prioritizing GWAS results: A review of statistical methods and recommendations for their application. American Journal of Human Genetics. 2010; **86**: 6–22. DOI: 10.1016/j.ajhg.2009.11.017

[92] Peng G, et al. Gene and pathway-based second-wave analysis of genome-wide association studies. European Journal of Human Genetics. 2010; **8**: 111–117. DOI: 10.1038/ejhg.2009.115

[93] Edwards SL, et al. Beyond GWASs: illuminating the dark road from association to function. American Journal of Human Genetics. 2013; **93**: 779–797. DOI: 10.1016/j.ajhg.2013.10.012

[94] Fachal L. Dunning AM. From candidate gene studies to GWAS and post-GWAS analyses in breast cancer. Current Opinion in Genetics & Development. 2015; **30**: 32–41. DOI: 10.1016/j.gde.2015.01.004

[95] Manolio TA, et al. Finding the missing heritability of complex diseases. Nature. 2009; **461**: 747–53. DOI: 10.1038/nature08494

2

Radon Exposure and Human Health: What Happens in Volcanic Environments?

Diana Linhares, Patrícia Garcia and Armindo Rodrigues

Abstract

Volcanic activity can cause hazardous effects to the environment and the health of the exposed persons such as an increased risk for the development of several cancers. In geothermal areas, volcanic gases such as radon are continuously vented from the main crater, from fumarolic fields or diffused through soil. The continued long-term exposure to radon can enhance the risk of lung cancer being considered the leading cause of lung cancer following tobacco smoking. The chronic exposure to volcanogenic radon requires the development of biomonitoring methods that will assist in the evaluation of the effects of exposure to this genotoxic element. The Human Biomonitoring with the use of exfoliated buccal cells is minimally invasive, and the endpoints of the buccal micronucleus cytome (BMCyt) assay are the biomarkers of effect most recently used to measure genetic damage for the exposure to genotoxic and cytotoxic xenobiotics. The BMCyt assay has been used in a number of occupational studies, and positive results were detected as a consequence of exposure to pesticides, metals, and industrial chemicals that are suspected to cause cancer. Regarding the chronic exposure to volcanic environments, many studies revealed a rise in the numbers of MN in buccal exfoliated cells, indicating an increased risk for cancer. This chapter aims to cover the main health hazards and biomonitoring methods for populations chronically exposed to volcanic environments, allowing an estimate of health risks and to implement risk management measures regarding the exposure to certain compounds.

Keywords: radon, volcanic environments, biomonitoring, BMCyt assay

1. Radon

1.1. Definition, physical and chemical properties

Radon was discovered by Fredrich Ernst Dorn in 1898. The name is derived from radium, as it was first detected as an emission from radium during radioactive decay. It is a naturally occurring radioactive gas of the noble gas family, is odorless and tasteless and, is produced by the decay of radium in the uranium decay chain. Radon is measured in terms of its activity (curies or becquerels), and these measurements provide information regarding how much a radioactive material decays every second (1 Ci = 37 billion Bq = 37 billion decays per second).

Radon also undergoes to radioactive decay, being divided in two parts (one part is called radiation, and the other part is called a daughter or progeny). In the air, the radioactive daughters (isotopes of polonium, bismuth, and lead) tend to attach to surfaces and to aerosol particles such as dust and cigarette smoke [1, 2, 3].

1.2. Sources in the environment

Radon is a radioactive compound, which rarely occurs naturally in the environment, being mostly derived from human activities; some of the potential sources of anthropogenic radiation include x-rays and other types of radiation used in medicine, radioactive waste generated by nuclear power stations and scientific research centers, and even electromagnetic radiation from television sets and microwave ovens.

On the other hand, radon isotopes are formed naturally through the radioactive decay of uranium or thorium, being present in rocks and soil. The decay products of ^{222}Rn, such as ^{218}Po and ^{214}Pb, can attach to particles in the air and be transported this way in the atmosphere being deposited on land or water by settling or by rain [4]. The human exposure to radon can occur by uranium mining activities (since uranium minerals emit radon gas), the occurrence of granitic bedrocks located underneath buildings [5], the use of building materials that contain variable uranium and radium concentrations, and exposure to volcanic activity.

1.3. Volcanic environments

During and after eruptions, volcanoes release hazardous gases such as sulfur dioxide (SO_2), sulfuric acid (H_2SO_4), hydrogen sulfide (H_2S), hydrogen chloride (HCl), hydrogen fluoride (HF), carbon dioxide (CO_2), and radon (Rn) [6]. These gases have both acute and chronic health effects: carbon dioxide and sulfur gases are the main gases responsible for acute mortality due to their asphyxiating and/or toxic properties; radon, due to its radioactivity, has important chronic effects, and thus, even at low doses, a long-term exposure may also pose a significant health risk.

According to Gasparini and Mantovani [7], the radon release, in volcanic systems, occurs mainly due to (a) the radon presence in rocks, minerals, pore fluids, and groundwater; (b) the release of magma fluids ascent to the surface, heating the nesting rocks; and (c) the increase in temperature that causes removal of the radon present in interstitial fluids and even into groundwater. Radon is considered a useful tracer of volcanic activity due to the ability to be transported from depth (by carrier gases such as CO_2) without being chemically altered [8]. However, volcanic environments are complex, and the nature of the driving force can change during gas ascent, depending on the physical-geological conditions in the environment that the gas encounters. Variations in temperature, pressure, mechanical stresses, chemical reactions, and mineral precipitation can change the gas-bearing properties of geological formations [9].

In a study developed in all regions of the Former Yugoslav Republic of Macedonia, it was shown that indoor radon concentration measurements in dwellings were significantly different between seasons, being the highest values observed in the winter and autumn [10]. Also, in the Vulsini Volcanic district in Northern Latium (Central Italy), Cinelli et al. [11] performed a series of soil gas radon measurements to estimate the radon radiation risk; the authors observed that soil gas radon concentration ranged between 7 and 176 kBq/m^3, revealing a large degree of variability particularly related to the different lithologies of the studied sites.

Considering that, in volcanically active environments, radon can be continuously vented from the volcano main crater, from fumarolic fields, or diffusely emitted through soil [12]; these environments present continuous health risks to the populations living in their vicinity, as it happens in the volcanic islands of the Azores archipelago.

The Azores archipelago is located in the North Atlantic Ocean, in the triple junction of the North American, African, and Eurasian plates [13], and is formed by nine islands of volcanic origin that represent the emerged part of the Azores Plateau. As a result of the Azores archipelago location on an active plate boundary, the islands are subjected to frequent seismic and volcanic activity, including eruptions and degassing processes. The São Miguel Island, located in the eastern group of the archipelago, has one of the most active and dangerous volcanoes of the archipelago, the Furnas volcano. Its activity is marked by the presence of fumarolic fields [14] and extensive soil diffuse degassing areas [15, 16] that surge the radon concentration increase [17]. In 2014, Silva et al. [18] surveyed the indoor radon concentration in some buildings from the villages of Furnas and Ribeira Quente (located in degassing areas in the vicinity of Furnas volcano); the annual radon concentration ranges between 23 and 6403 Bq/m^3. The level of indoor radon exceeds the limit defined by the regional legislation (150 Bq/m^3) (D.L.R No. 16/2009/A Art. 51) in 33% of the Furnas village buildings and in 21% of the ones of Ribeira Quente. Further up, Silva et al. [19] applied a series of regression models demonstrating that barometric pressure, soil water content, soil temperature, soil CO_2 flux, air temperature, relative air humidity, and wind speed are the statistical meaningful variables explaining between 15.8 and 73.6% of ^{222}Rn variations in Furnas volcano vicinity.

2. Human exposure to radon

Human exposure to natural ionizing radiation is largely due to radon. It is estimated that the worldwide radon contribution constitutes as much as 50% of the overall radiation dose, reaching values of about 1.15 mSv/year per capita [20].

Although the atmospheric concentration of radon is usually low, this gas tends to accumulate within confined environments with reduced or no air exchange, such as buildings, dwellings, tunnels, caves, and mines. During the radon decay process, alpha, beta, and gamma radioactive particles are released and can be inhaled and deposited on the bronchial epithelium of exposed individuals; considering that the alpha particle can disrupt the DNA structure within cells of the lining epithelia, and especially lung cells, exposure to this irradiation can contribute to an increased risk of lung cancer [17].

The effects of radon exposure in human health have been known since the sixteenth century, although radon was only discovered at the turn of the twentieth century. Still, it was only in the 1940s that a causal link between lung cancer in miners and radon exposure was established [21]. Taking in consideration that the studies on underground miners consistently demonstrated an increased risk of lung cancer caused by radon and its progeny, International Agency for Research on Cancer (IARC) classified radon as a human carcinogen in 1988 [22]. Later on in the 1970s, indoor radon accumulation in domestic buildings was first observed being considered to play a role in the epidemiology of lung cancer [23]. Considering that the awareness of the potential for hazardous exposure, due to accumulation of radon in indoor environments, has increased during the times, several programs were established to carefully monitor and control radon concentration in closed spaces, such as households located in areas where geogenic radon is highly likely to occur.

3. Biomonitoring

Traditionally, the term biomonitoring can be simply defined as a way to provide information about exposures to chemicals in living organisms. Exposure is commonly assessed by a spectrum of questionnaire data and ecological, environmental, or biological measurements. Biological measures of exposure allow the assessment of internal dose, by measuring the parent chemical or its metabolite or reaction product in the human blood, urine, milk, saliva, and adipose or other tissues [24]. Nowadays, and ever since Wild [25] proposed an environmental complement to the genome in determining risk of disease, termed the exposome (totality of exposures throughout the lifespan), researchers started to include in biomonitoring studies the cumulative measure of exposures to both chemical and nonchemical agents, such as diet, stress, and socio-behavioral factors. The exposomic approaches go a step beyond traditional biomonitoring, aiming to capture all exposures that potentially affect health and disease.

3.1. Human biomonitoring

When individuals or populations are exposed to a chemical, it may be absorbed and distributed among the bodily tissues, metabolized, and/or excreted (i.e., absorption, distribution, metabolism, and excretion (ADME)). For the assessment of the human exposure to a given xenobiotic, biologic measurements of the chemical can be made after the absorption step or during each of the subsequent steps of ADME [26]. This is called human biomonitoring (HBM), which is an approach for assessing human exposures to natural and synthetic compounds from the environment, occupation, and lifestyle; this scientifically developed methodology allows an evaluation of factors, such as cumulative exposure or genetic susceptibility, to a certain chemical compound allowing the extrapolation for adverse risks and health effects, such as cancer.

The data obtained in HBM studies integrate exposure from all routes (oral, inhalation, dermal, transplacental) and allow (1) establishing population reference ranges, (2) identifying unusual exposures for subpopulations, (3) evaluating temporal variability and trends within a population, (4) validating questions designed to estimate individual exposure, and (5) examining associations with health outcomes in epidemiologic studies. Therefore, HBM has tremendous utility, providing an efficient and cost-effective means of measuring human exposure to chemical substances, handing unequivocal evidence that both exposure and uptake have been taken place [27, 28].

3.2. Biomarkers

Biomarkers are commonly used as "agents" to measure the concentrations of chemical substances, their metabolites, or reaction products in human tissues or specimens, representing an integrative measurement of exposure to a given agent (i.e., the internal dose), that result from complex pathways of human exposure and also incorporate toxicokinetic information and individual characteristics such as a genetically based susceptibility [29].

In 1993, the WHO [30] provided three classifications of biomarkers—exposure, effect, and susceptibility—but with the rise of genomics and other advances in molecular biology, the biomarker classification has suffered some changes through time. In 2001, the Biomarker working group defined five classifications: (1) antecedent biomarkers, to identify the risk of developing an illness; (2) screening biomarkers, to screen for subclinical disease; (3) diagnostic biomarkers, to recognize overt disease; (4) staging biomarkers, to categorize disease severity; and (5) prognostic biomarkers, to predict future disease course. In this paradigm, biomarkers are viewed on a continuum between markers of exposure and markers of effect, with markers of susceptibility spanning the continuum.

The markers of effect are applied in the comparison of case and control, target and nontarget tissues, or dose and time to response, where a correlation between the biomarker and biological effect can be demonstrated; the markers of susceptibility are defined as the genetic factors that influence the body's sensitivity to a chemical but can also include biological factors, such as age, nutritional status, and lifestyle.

The continuous progress in molecular and analytical methods to measure biomarkers for linking exposure with health outcomes and new approaches in exposome research will enable a more comprehensive and integrated analysis across the biomarker continuum [31].

3.3. Micronucleus

Micronucleus (MN) is defined by Schmid [32] as a microscopically visible, round, or oval cytoplasmic chromatin mass next to the nucleus that is formed from acentric chromosomes, chromatid fragments, whole chromosomes, or chromatids. Micronucleus formation results from two basic phenomena in mitotic cells, which are chromosome breakage and the dysfunction of the mitotic apparatus.

This aberration is induced by genotoxic stress caused by a clastogen or an aneugen xenobiotic; the clastogen involves the induction of either chromosome fragments that lag behind the separating chromosomes or a chromatin bridge between chromosomes at the anaphase of mitosis; the aneugen causes a daughter cell to have an abnormal number of chromosomes by disrupting the whole chromosomes bound to the mitotic spindle at anaphase; by disrupting the spindle checkpoint, the chromatin is separated from the newly forming nucleus and forms an independent nucleus-like structure, the micronucleus [33].

Since this chromosomal aberration is a frequent and significant response to exposure to mutagenic agents, it has been extensively used to identify potential genotoxic exposures and also chromosomal instability [34].

3.4. Buccal micronucleus cytome (BMCyt) assay

The continuous chromosomal damage in fully differentiated cells (as in the buccal epithelial cells) implies that damage occurred in the basal cell layer during earlier nuclear divisions. Considering that buccal epithelial cells are in direct contact with inhaled and ingested substances and/or elements and more than 90% of all human cancers are of epithelial origin, it can be argued that buccal epithelial cells represent a preferred target site for early genotoxic events induced by carcinogenic agents [35]. Therefore, the MN assay using exfoliated buccal cells can be considered the most suitable biomonitoring approach for the detection of increased cancer risk in humans, when the exposure to genotoxic agents occurs via inhalation or ingestion.

The buccal micronucleus cytome (BMCyt) assay is a useful and minimally invasive method that allows screening for both genomic damage and cytotoxicity events [36]. This technique is minimally invasive [37] and is frequently used in biomonitoring studies of occupational and environmental exposure to carcinogenic substances [38–40].

This assay involves the collection of exfoliated buccal epithelial cells from inside the cheeks by scraping the oral mucosa, smearing onto glass slides, and staining by the Feulgen method; this methodology allows the examination of cells to determine the frequency of MN and other genomic damage markers such as karyorrhexis (nuclear disintegration associated with the loss of nuclear membrane integrity), karyolysis (nuclei completely depleted of DNA and therefore appear as Feulgen-negative ghost-like), and pyknosis (small shrunken, intensively stained nucleus); these anomalies are associated with both cytotoxicity (necrosis and keratinization) and genotoxicity (apoptosis) being considered as effective biomarkers for populations exposed to mutagenic and carcinogenic agents [41].

Factors such as the minimal invasiveness of cell collection, high reliability, and low cost of BMCyt have contributed to the worldwide success for epidemiological studies enabling the early detection of carcinogenic effects in the cell exposed to various carcinogenic agents [42].

4. Case studies

It has been demonstrated that exposure to radon can induce lung tumors and other cancers in experimental animals [43]. Also, a radon dose-related carcinogenicity has been shown through epidemiologic studies of miners and case-control studies in the general population [44–47].

In Europe, Darby et al. [48] in a collaborative study that included 13 case-control studies in 9 European countries, each of which registered over 150 people with lung cancer and 150 or more controls and which included data about radon levels over 15 years, found that the risk of lung cancer (after stratification for study, age, gender, region of residence, and smoking) increased by 8% per 100 Bq/m^3 increase in radon concentration. In the United States, Krewski et al. [49] evaluated the risk associated with prolonged residential radon exposure, combining data from seven large-scale case-control studies (4081 cases and 5281 controls), and these authors also found that the risk of lung cancer due to exposure to residential radon was increased by 10% per 100 Bq/m^3.

For the biomonitoring of the human populations, the application of easy and noninvasive techniques is necessary; for the last 10–15 years, there has been an increase in the use of cytogenetic monitoring techniques, such as the buccal micronucleus cytome (BMCyt) over the use of MN in lymphocytes. Nevertheless, there are only a few studies, developed in the Azores, that apply this assay for the risk assessment of the chronic exposure to radon of volcanic origin.

Considering the geologic context of the archipelago, some studies have been developed to biomonitor the health effects of the chronic exposure the compounds released by the volcanic activity. In the study of Amaral et al. [50], it was observed that the population living in the vicinity (inside the crater) of Furnas volcano presented higher rates of cancer of the lip, oral cavity, and pharynx, in both sexes, and of female breast cancer. The relative risk analysis revealed a higher risk for lip, oral cavity, pharynx, and breast cancer in this population compared to a population inhabiting an island without historical records of volcanic activity. According to these authors, these higher cancer rates could be partially explained by the chronic exposure to environmental factors resulting from volcanic activity. More recently, Rodrigues et al. [51] in a study carried with inhabitants of Furnas volcano demonstrated that the chronic exposure to a volcanically active environment results in genotoxic and cytotoxic effects in human oral epithelial cells; this research group used the buccal micronucleus assay and observed that the frequencies of micronucleus and other nuclear anomalies were significantly higher in the Furnas inhabitants when compared to the inhabitants of an area without volcanic activity. Also, the inhabitants of Furnas village presented a 2.4-fold higher risk of having a higher frequency of micronucleated cells.

More recently, Linhares et al. [52] took a step forward in this investigation and evaluated the DNA damage in the buccal epithelial cells of individuals chronically exposed to indoor radon in Ribeira Quente inhabitants, a village within 7 km (in the south flank) of the Furnas volcano. The authors shown that indoor radon concentration correlated positively with the frequency of micronucleated cells and that the exposure to indoor radon is a risk factor for the occurrence of micronucleated cells in the inhabitants of the hydrothermal area.

The results obtained in these studies demonstrate a significant association between chronic exposure to indoor and the occurrence of DNA damage evidencing the usefulness of biological surveillance to assess mutations involved in pre-carcinogenesis, reinforcing the need for further studies with human populations. Likewise, these studies set the basis for the use of the BMCyt assay in volcanic areas worldwide to assess the effects of the chronic exposure to genotoxic substances and/or elements.

5. Risk management

It has been reported that more than 60% of the ionizing radiation a person receives every year can be caused by natural sources of radiation and more than 50% of this radiation can be due to radon and the products of its disintegration. Hence, maintaining radon safety is a critical challenge, and this has been actively discussed throughout the last few decades [53]. To assure a public health risk assessment, factors such as the source, the pathway, and the receptor must be considered.

The indoor radon concentration is associated with factors such as the building structure (such as construction material, pavement, ventilation, and the presence of basements or air boxes), as well as the ventilation measures taken. These factors are particularly relevant in households built on volcanic hydrothermal areas, where soil diffuse degassing can be very intense. As for the consequences of human exposure to indoor radon, these will depend of factors such as the concentration of radon indoors, the duration of exposure, the general health status of the individual, and the synergistic effect with smoking.

In order to manage the risk, primary strategies such as education and prevention activities must be established to prevent/diminish the entrance of radon into the buildings [54]. However, this may not be easily achieved, since the indoor radon varies considerably by region and locality and is greatly affected by the household structure as well as soil and atmospheric conditions. Consequently, often the development of secondary strategies to remediate the effects of indoor radon is required, such as taking measures in the construction of the household by selecting an adequate foundation type, location, building materials used, entry points for soil gas, and building ventilation systems.

At an individual level, it is necessary to ensure an adequate past medical history or family medical history, since individuals who have chronic respiratory diseases such as asthma, emphysema, and fibrosis may be more susceptible to the respiratory effects of radon and radon progeny. Due to the reduced expiration efficiency and the increased residual air volume of these individuals, radon and its progeny would be resident in the lungs for longer periods of time, increasing the risk of damage to the lung tissue.

The above-discussed epidemiologic studies clearly evidence the carcinogenicity of radon in volcanically active environments. However, radon control efforts appear to be held up, and the cost-effectiveness of current strategies and interventions is questionable; therefore, the continuous biomonitoring of the populations exposed to radon in volcanic areas is necessary to further implement risk management measures.

Author details

Diana Linhares[1,2*], Patrícia Garcia[1,3] and Armindo Rodrigues[1,2]

*Address all correspondence to: diana.ps.linhares@uac.pt

1 Faculty of Sciences and Technology, University of the Azores, Ponta Delgada, Portugal

2 IVAR, Institute of Volcanology and Risks Assessment, University of the Azores, Ponta Delgada, Portugal

3 cE3c, Centre for Ecology, Evolution and Environmental Changes, and Azorean Biodiversity Group, University of the Azores, Ponta Delgada, Portugal

References

[1] Edling C (1985) Radon daughter exposure and lung cancer. British Journal of Industrial Medicine, **42**:721-722

[2] Biermann AH, and Sawyer SR (1995) Attachment of radon progeny to cigarette-smoke aerosols. Lawrence Livermore Natl. Lab., CA (United States). Technical Report UCRL-CR-120647

[3] Ojo TJ, and Ajayi IR (2014) A review on environmental radon and its potential health risk on humans. Journal of Environmental Science, Toxicolology and Food Technology, **8**, 1-8

[4] Agency for Toxic Substances and Disease Registry (ATSDR) (2012) Public Health Statement for Radon. Atlanta, GA: U.S. Department of Health and Human Services, Public Health Service

[5] Denton GRW and Namazi S (2013) Indoor Radon Levels and Lung Cancer Incidence on Guam. Procedia Environmental Sciences, **18**:157-166

[6] Durand M, Florkowski C, George P, Walmsley T, Weinstein P, Cole J (2004) Elevated trace element output in urine following acute volcanic gas exposure. Journal of Volcanology and Geothermal Research, **134**:139-48

[7] Gasparini P and Mantovani MSM (1978) Radon anomalies and volcanic eruptions. Journal of Volcanology and Geothermal Research, **3**, 325-341

[8] Barbosa SM, Donner RV, Steinitz G (2015) Radon applications in geosciences–Progress & Perspectives. The European Physical Journal Special Topics, **224**:597-603

[9] Padilla GD, Hernández P, Padrón E, Barrancos J, Pérez NM, Melián G et al. (2013) Soil gas radon emissions and volcanic activity at El Hierro (Canary Islands): The 2011-2012 submarine eruption. Geochemistry, Geophysics, Geosystems, **14**:432-447

[10] Stojanovska Z, Januseski J, Bossew P, Zunic ZS, Tollefsen T, Ristova M (2011) Seasonal indoor radon concentration in FYR of Macedonia. Radiation Measurements, **46**:602-610

[11] Cinelli G, Tositti L, Capaccioni B, Brattich E, Mostacci D (2015) Soil gas radon assessment and development of a radon risk map in Bolsena, Central Italy. Environmental Geochemistry and Health, **37**(2):305-319

[12] Hansell A, Horwell C, Oppenheimer C (2006) The health hazards of volcanoes and geothermal areas. Occupational and Environmental Medicine, **63**:149-156

[13] Searle R (1980) Tectonic pattern of the Azores spreading centre and triple junction. Earth and Planetary Science Letters, **51**:415-434

[14] Ferreira T, Gaspar JL, Viveiros F, Marcos M, Faria C, Sousa F (2005) Monitoring of fumarole discharge and CO2 soil degassing in the Azores: contribution to volcanic surveillance and public health risk assessment. Annals of Geophysics, **48**:4-5

[15] Viveiros F, Cardelllini C, Ferreira T, Caliro S, Chiodini G, Silva C (2010) Soil CO2 emissions at Furnas Volcano, São Miguel Island, Azores archipelago: Volcano monitoring perspectives, geomorphologic studies, and land use planning application. Journal of Geophysical Research, **115**, B12208, 1-17

[16] Viveiros F, Cardellini C, Ferreira T, Silva C (2012) Contribution of CO2 emited to the atmosphere by diffuse degassing from volcanoes: The Furnas Volcano case study. International Journal of Global Warming, **4**(3-4): 287-304

[17] Appleton JD (2013) Radon in air and water. In: Essentials of medical geology. O. Selinus et al. (Eds), Dordrecht, Netherlands, pp. 239-277. Springer Netherlands

[18] Silva C, Ferreira T, Viveiros F, Allard P (2014) Indoor radon (222Rn) monitoring in some buildings at Furnas and Ribeira Quente villages (Furnas Volcano, Azores): public health risk assessment. Comunicações Geológicas, **101**, Especial II, 927-931

[19] Silva C, Ferreira T, Viveiros F, Allard P (2015) Soil radon (222Rn) monitoring at Furnas Volcano (São Miguel, Azores): applications and challenges. The European Physical Journal Special Topics, **224**(4): 659-686

[20] UNSCEAR (United Nations Scientific Committee on the effects of Atomic Radiation). (2008). Sources and effects of ionizing radiation. Report to General Assembly, Annex B, United Nations, New York

[21] Hueper WC (1942) Occupational Tumors and Allied Diseases. Springfield, Ill. Charles C Thomas

[22] International Agency for Research on Cancer Monographs on the Evaluation of Carcinogenic Risks to Humans (IARC) (1988) Man-Made Mineral Fibres and Radon. Lyon, France: IARC Press; **43**:33-171

[23] Axelson, O (1984) Room for a role for radon in lung cancer causation? Medical Hypotheses, **13**(1):51-61

[24] Needham LL, Barr DB, Calafat AM (2005) Characterizing children's exposures: beyond NHANES. Neurotoxicology, **26**:547-553

[25] Wild CP (2005) Complementing the genome with an "exposome": the outstanding challenge of environmental exposure measurement in molecular epidemiology. Cancer Epidemiology, Biomarkers and Prevention, **14**:1847-1850

[26] LaKind JS, Sobus JR, Goodman M, Barr DB, Furst P, Albertini RJ, et al. (2014) A proposal for assessing study quality: biomonitoring, environmental epidemiology, and short-lived chemicals (BEES-C) instrument. Environment International, **73**:195-207

[27] Sexton K, Needham L, Pirkle J (2004) Human Biomonitoring of Environmental Chemicals. American Scientist, **92**, 38

[28] Angerer J, Ewers U, Wilhelm M (2007) Human biomonitoring: state of the art. International Journal of Hygiene and Environmental Health, **210**(3-4): 201-228

[29] Ladeira C and Viegas S (2016) Human Biomonitoring – An overview on biomarkers and their application in Occupational and Environmental Health. Biomonitoring, **3**:15-24

[30] World Health Organization (WHO). 1993. Biomarkers - Biomarkers and risk assessment: Concepts and principles, Environmental Health, Criteria No.155(93), Geneva

[31] Dennis KK, Marder ME, Balshaw DM, Cui Y, Lynes MA, Patti GJ, et al. (2017) Biomonitoring in the era of the exposome. Environmental Health Perspectives, **125**(4), 502-510

[32] Schmid W (1975) The micronucleus test. Mutation Research, **31**(1):9-15

[33] Utani K, Kohno Y, Okamoto A, Shimizu N (2010) Emergence of Micronuclei and Their Effects on the Fate of Cells under Replication Stress. PLoS ONE, **5**(4): e10089. https://doi.org/10.1371/journal.pone.0010089

[34] Tolbert PE, Shy CM, Allen JW (1992) Micronuclei and other anomalies in buccal smears: method development. Mutation Research, **271**:69-77

[35] Holland N, Bolognesi C, Volders MK, Bonassi S, Zeiger E, Knasmueller S (2008) The micronucleus assay in human buccal cells as a tool for Biomonitoring DNA damage: The HUMN project perspective on current status and knowledge gaps. Mutation research, **659**:93-08

[36] Thomas P, Holland N, Bolognesi C, Kirsch-Volders M, Bonassi E, Zeiger S, et al. (2009) Buccal micronucleus cytome assay. Nature Protocols, **4**:825-837

[37] Bolognesi C, Knasmueller S, Nersesyan P, Thomas P, Fenech M (2013) The HUMNxl scoring criteria for different cell types and nuclear anomalies in the Buccal Micronucleus Cytome Assay: an update and expanded photogallery. Mutation Research-Reviews in Mutation Research, **753**(2):100-13

[38] Çelik A, Yildirim S, Ekinci SY, Taşdelen B (2013) Bio-monitoring for the genotoxic assessment in road construction workers as determined by the buccal micronucleus cytome assay. Ecotoxicology and Environment Safety, **92**:265-270

[39] Hallare AV, Gervasio MK, Gervasio PL, Acacio-Claro PJ (2009) Monitoring genotoxicity among gasoline station attendants and traffic enforcers in the City of Manila using the micronucleus assay with exfoliated epithelial cells. Environmental Monitoring and Assessment, **156**:331-341

[40] Garcia PV, Linhares D, Amaral AFS, Rodrigues AS (2012) Exposure of thermoelectric power-plant workers to volatile organic compounds from fuel oil: Genotoxic and cytotoxic effects in buccal epithelial cells. Mutation Research, **747**:197-201

[41] Fenech M (2007Cytokinesis-block micronucleus cytome assay. Nature Protocols, **2**: 1084-1104

[42] Bonassi S, Ugolini D, Kirsch-Volders M, Strömberg U, Vermeulen R, et al. (2005) Human population studies with cytogenetic biomarkers: review of the literature and future prospectives. Environmental and Molecular Mutagenesis, **45**:258-270

[43] Monchaux G, Morlier J, Morin M, Chameaud J, Lafuma J, Masse R (1994) Carcinogenic and Cocarcinogenic Effects of Radon and Radon Daughters in Rats. Environmental Health Perspectives, **102**(1):64-73

[44] Schoenberg JB, Klotz JB, Wilcox HB, Nicholls GP, Gil-del-Real MT, Stemhagen A, et al. (1990) Case–control study of residential radon and lung cancer among New Jersey women. Cancer Research, **50**(20):6520-6524

[45] Lubin JH, Boice Jr JD, Edling C, Hornung RW, Howe GR, Kunz E, Kusiak RA, Morrison HI, Radford EP, Samet JM et al. (1995) Lung cancer in radon-exposed miners and estimation of risk from indoor exposure. Journal of the National Cancer Institute, **87**(11):817-27

[46] Duport P (2002) Is the radon risk overestimated? Neglected doses in the estimation of the risk of lung cancer in uranium underground miners. Radiation Protection Dosimetry, **98**(3):329-338

[47] Wichmann HE, Rosario AS, Heid IM, Kreuzer M, Heinrich J, Kreienbrock L (2005) Increased lung cancer risk due to residential radon in a pooled and extended analysis of studies in Germany. Health Physics, **88**(1):71-79

[48] Darby S, Hill D, Auvinen A, Barros-Dios JM, Baysson H, Bochicchio F, et al. (2005) Radon in homes and risk of lung cancer: collaborative analysis of individual data from 13 European case-control studies. British Medical Journal, **330**(7485): 223-226

[49] Krewski D, Lubin JH, Zielinski JM, Alavanja M, Catalan VS, William Field R, et al. (2006) A combined analysis of North American case-control studies of residential radon and lung cancer. Journal of Toxicology and Environmental Health, Part A, **69**(7-8), 533-597

[50] Amaral A, Rodrigues V, Oliveira J, Pinto C, Carneiro V, Sanbento R, et al. (2006) Chronic exposure to volcanic environments and cancer incidence in the Azores, Portugal. Science of the Total Environment, **367**:123-128

[51] Rodrigues A, Arruda M, Garcia P (2012) Evidence of DNA damage in humans inhabiting a volcanically active environment: A useful tool for biomonitoring. Environment International, **49**:51-56

[52] Linhares D, Garcia P, Silva C, Barrosos J, Kazachkova N, Pereira R, Lima M, Camarinho R, Ferreira T, Rodrigues A (2016) DNA damage in oral epithelial cells of individuals chronically exposed to indoor radon (222Rn) in a hydrothermal area. Environmental Geochemistry and Health. DOI: 10.1007/s10653-016-9893-2

[53] Bissett RJ and McLaughlin JR (2010) Radon. Chronic Diseases in Canada, **29**:38-50

[54] Larsson LS (2014) Risk-Reduction Strategies to Expand Radon Care Planning with Vulnerable Groups. Public Health Nursing (Boston, Mass.), **31**(6), 526-536

3

Cancer Causing Chemicals

Maher Soliman

Abstract

Carcinogens are substances that induce cancer by damaging the genome or through disruption of cellular metabolic processes. Some compounds interact directly with DNA, while others are activated to reactive molecules that can bind with DNA by covalent adducts causing mutations in genes crucial to biological processes. Cigarette smoke is by far the most important and notorious carcinogen. Cigarette smoke contains many carcinogenic substances including polycyclic aromatic hydrocarbons (PAHs), which are known to cause cancer. Nitrites, which are present in many foods, are converted into nitrous acid in the stomach and may then react with amines in food to produce nitrosamines, which are carcinogenic. Aflatoxins produced by Aspergillus flavus are promoter for hepatic cancer. Several cytotoxic drugs are carcinogens especially alkylating agents that interact with DNA. Individuals exposed to certain pesticides may be at risk to the development of certain cancers. Inorganic arsenic exposure has been suggested to be associated with the development of several cancers. Sufficient evidence indicated an association between dioxins and various cancers including soft tissue sarcoma, lymphoma and leukemia. Asbestos has been found to be significantly associated with lung cancer and mesothelioma.

Keywords: aflatoxins, cancer, carcinogens, carcinogenesis, chemicals, smoking

1. Introduction

Worldwide, cancer is a leading cause of mortality [1]. According to GLOBOCAN estimates, about 14.1 million new cancer cases and 8.2 million deaths occurred in 2012 worldwide [1]. The incidence and mortality rates of cancer differ between countries. However, over the last decades, the burden of cancer has shifted to less developed countries due to later stage of diagnosis and unavailability of treatment. Currently about 57% of cancer cases and 65% of cancer deaths occurs in less developed countries [1, 2]. The cancer profile also varies between countries. The incidence rates of prostate, colorectal, female breast and lung cancer are several times higher in more developed countries compared with less developed countries. Liver, stomach, and cervical cancers are more frequent in less developed countries; these cancers are predominantly attributable to infection. However, lung cancer remains the leading cause of cancer death globally [1].

The burden of cancer is rising because of the aging of the population, and increasing exposure to established carcinogenic chemicals, viruses and radiations, as well as adoption of unhealthy lifestyle behaviors such as smoking, alcohol intake, overweight, and limited physical activity. Moreover, the success of screening programs and earlier detection of cancer have contributed to the rise of cancer problem [1, 2].

Carcinogens are substances which induce cancer, by damaging the genome or through disruption of cellular metabolic processes. Carcinogens have usually an insidious toxic effect rather than an acute toxic effect. Carcinogens could be either from synthetic chemicals or natural substances. Carcinogens can be classified as genotoxic or nongenotoxic agents according to mechanism of carcinogenesis. Genotoxins bind directly to DNA causing irreversible damage to the genome like polycyclic aromatic hydrocarbons (PAHs). Nongenotoxins do not directly affect DNA but could promote growth, like hormones and some organic compounds. Procarcinogens are not carcinogenic themselves, but turn into carcinogenic substances in the body, e.g. nitrates taken in the diet change into nitrosamines which is carcinogenic. Co-carcinogens are substances that promote the activity of other carcinogens in causing cancer but they are not carcinogenic on their own [3].

Chemical carcinogenesis was first described in 1775 by an eminent English physician and surgeon, Percivall Pott who observed the occurrence of cancer of the scrotum in a number of his patients who were chimney sweepers when they were young [3, 4]. Accordingly, Pott suggested that the occupation of these men as young boys and their exposure to large amounts of soot could be the causative agent of the cancer. One hundred years later, the high incidence of skin cancer among certain German workers was recognized to be associated to their exposure to coal tar, the chief constituent of the chimney sweeps' soot [5].

Only after 140 years of Dr. Pott's report of the association of epidermal cancer of the scrotum with the exposure to soot from the combustion of coal, the first experimental laboratory animal study on carcinogenesis was reported. In 1915, Yamagawa and Ichikawa first published a comprehensive paper describing the production of a malignant epidermal neoplasm by repeatedly applying crude coal tar to the ears of rabbits for a number of months [6]. Afterwards, several studies tried to define and isolate the causative carcinogenic substance from the crude tar. In 1930s, the first carcinogenic chemical compound, dibenz[a,h]anthracene was produced, followed by several polycyclic aromatic hydrocarbons (PAHs) were isolated from active crude tar fractions.

Since 1971, The International Agency for Research on Cancer (IARC) has evaluated more than 1000 agents, and has classified them into five groups as follows [7]:

- Group 1: Carcinogenic to humans (120 agents).
- Group 2A: Probably carcinogenic to humans (81 agents)

- Group 2B: Possibly carcinogenic to humans (299 agents)
- Group 3: Not classifiable as to its carcinogenicity to humans (502 agents)
- Group 4: Probably not carcinogenic to humans (1 agent)

2. Mechanisms of action of carcinogens

Carcinogenesis could be classified into four phases; initiation, promotion, progression and metastasis. Carcinogenic chemicals can initiate and/or promote this process by affecting the expression and activity of certain genes responsible for cell growth, differentiation, DNA repair, cell-cycle control, and apoptosis. Some compounds interact directly with DNA, while others are activated to reactive molecules that can bind with DNA by covalent adducts causing mutations in genes crucial to biological processes. Polycyclic aromatic hydrocarbons (PAHs) are known to cause cancer by forming covalent adducts with DNA, resulting in altered cell growth and repair [3].

Chemical carcinogens can target certain genes termed proto-oncogenes and tumor suppressor genes, which when become mutated, allow cells to grow without control like in breast, colon and lung cancers. Two well studied proto-oncogenes are MYC and RAS, which are responsible for regulation of the cell cycle and apoptosis. MYC function is involved in protein-protein interactions with various cellular factors such as in Burkitt's Lymphoma. RAS function as GTP-binding protein; important in signal transduction cascade such as in Pancreatic, Colorectal, Bladder Breast, Kidney, & Lung Neoplasms; Leukemia; Melanoma [8, 9]. Mutations in these genes can cause dysregulated cell division. The mutant proteins maintain their normal functions but are no longer under control of orders that regulate these processes. The products of RAS gene are essential components of kinase signaling pathways that regulate cell growth and differentiation. Mutations in RAS can be caused by organochlorine pesticide and exposure to arsenic [3].

One of the most well recognized tumor suppressor genes is p53 also known as TP53 or tumor protein (EC:2.7.1.37) is a gene that codes for a protein that regulates the cell cycle and hence functions as a tumor suppression. Under suboptimal conditions such as DNA damage, tumor suppressor genes produce products that inhibit cell division for growth. Mutations in p53 have been discovered in breast cancer and bronchial cancer exposed to organophosphorus pesticides and PAHs [10].

3. Some chemical carcinogens

3.1. Cigarette smoking

Cigarette smoking is the most important carcinogen. Cigarettes are the predominant type of tobacco product consumed in the world. Worldwide, more than 1 million cancer deaths are attributed to cigarette smoking annually. Cigarette smoking is the major cause of lung cancer.

Polycyclic aromatic hydrocarbons and the tobacco-specific nitrosamine 4-(methylnitrosamino)-1-(3-pyridyl)-1-butanone are likely to play major roles lung cancer induction [11].

Cigarette smoking is a major risk factor for cancers of oral cavity, oropharynx hypopharynx and Larynx, and the risk is greatly increased by alcohol consumption. Most cases of esophageal cancer, sinonasal and nasopharyngeal cancer, liver cancer, pancreatic cancer, stomach cancer, cervical squamous cell carcinoma, transitional cell carcinomas of the bladder, ureter, and renal pelvis and myeloid leukemia in adults are linked to cigarette smoking [12].

Laboratory studies clearly demonstrate that inhalation of cigarette smoke and topical application of cigarette smoke condensate (CSC) cause cancer in experimental animals. Studies identified the carcinogenic polycyclic aromatic hydrocarbons (PAHs) in cigarette smoke and showed that CSC has both carcinogenic and cocarcinogenic (tumor-promoting activity) effect. Tumors are not induced by the PAHs alone, using doses equivalent to their concentrations in CSC. However, carcinogenesis appears to depend on the composite interaction of the tumor initiators such as PAHs and tumor promoters [12].

Cigarette smoke contains more than 60 carcinogenic compounds that have been evaluated for carcinogenicity in laboratory animals, and 15 of them are considered as carcinogenic to humans. PAHs are a group of compounds produced from tobacco smoking. PAHs have a direct local carcinogenic effect. Benzo[a]pyrene, one of PAHs, has powerful carcinogenic activity to humans. Heterocyclic compounds are also combustion products and include nitrogen-containing analogues of PAHs such as furan, which is carcinogenic to liver [12].

N-nitrosamines are a large group of potent carcinogens. N-nitrosamines in cigarette smoke can induce lung tumors, tumors of the pancreas, nasal cavity, and liver and esophageal tumors. Aromatic amines such as 2-naphthylamine and 4-aminobiphenyl, which is the first identified carcinogens resulting from dye industry exposures, causes bladder cancer. Aldehydes such as formaldehyde and acetaldehyde are commonly present in our daily life from smoking. Other carcinogens present in cigarette smoke are vinyl chloride, and ethylene oxide [12, 13].

Cigarette smoke also contains oxidants such as nitric oxide and free radicals that are involved in oxidative damage produced by cigarette smoke. Cigarette smoke contains diverse carcinogens. PAH, N-nitrosamines, aromatic amines, 1,3-butadiene, benzene, aldehydes, and ethylene oxide are among the most important carcinogenic compounds present in cigarette smoke [12].

3.2. Polycyclic aromatic hydrocarbons

Polycyclic aromatic hydrocarbons (PAHs) are a group of organic compounds composed of two or more fused aromatic (benzene) rings containing only carbon and hydrogen atoms. PAHs containing two and three rings are present in vapor phase in atmosphere as they have low molecular weight. However, PAHs with five rings or more are largely bound to particles and considered the most hazardous to humans. PAHs with intermediate molecular weight (four rings) are allocated between vapor and particulate phases. More than 11 carcinogenic PAHs were detected in the air of industrial countries. The most widely-spread PAHs compound is benzo[a]pyrene which is used as a marker for total exposure to carcinogenic PAHs.

Polycyclic hydrocarbons differ in their carcinogenicity; some have weak carcinogenic effect like, the compound dibenzo[a,c]anthracene, while others have potent carcinogenicity like 3-methylcholanthrene and 7,12-dimethylbenzo[a]anthracene [14].

PAHs are released into the environment form the combustion of carbon containing materials at high temperature. Indoor air contamination by PAHs occurs from indoor emission sources such as smoking, cooking, domestic heating with fuel stoves and open fireplaces, as well as from intrusion of outdoor air [14].

PAHs emissions from motor vehicle, power generation plants, waste incinerators and open burning are considered the main component of outdoor sources in industrialized countries. In developing countries, cooking and heating with solid fuels such as wood, agricultural residues or coal remains the main contributing source of indoor PAHs air pollution [14].

Individual exposure to PAHs occurs via inhalation of air, consumption of food and water, and dermal contact with soil and dust. Indoor air would be the major source contributing to the PAHs exposure through inhalation, as people spent 80–93% of their time indoors [14].

PAHs are easily absorbed from the gastrointestinal tract of human, as they are highly lipid soluble. Then they are rapidly distributed in a various tissues with a tendency for localization in fatty tissues. PAHs metabolized via the cytochrome P450s and epoxide hydrolase enzymes [14].

The carcinogenic potential of PAHs has been well established for decades, and evidence to date has resulted in many of these compounds being labeled as reasonably carcinogenic. Lung tumors have been detected in animals exposed to PAHs. In vitro studies showed that c-myc expression, adduct formation, and cell-cycle progression are altered in lung epithelial cells exposed to PAHs [15].

The mechanisms of carcinogenesis of PAHs have been extensively investigated. PAHs might cause DNA adducts. Recent studies indicate that PAHs can alter cell signaling cascades that control cell communication, growth, and immune functions. PAHs have been shown to act through nuclear receptors [15].

3.3. Nitrosamines

Nitrosamines are a class of approximately 300 compounds and about 90% of them have been found to be carcinogenic. For example dimethylnitrosamine causes liver cancer, whereas some of the tobacco specific nitrosamines cause lung cancer. Nitrates and nitrites occur naturally in fruit and vegetables, which are considered as an important part of a healthy diet in most countries. Nitrates and nitrites are often used as food additives in processed meats such as ham, bacon, sausages and hot dogs to prevent toxin production by Clostridium Botulinum (the microorganism responsible for botulism), and preserve meat products recognizable appearance and flavor as well [13].

Nitrosamines are produced by chemical reactions of nitrates or its reduced form nitrites with amines in the meat during its processing, storage, and cooking. N-nitrosodimethylamine

(NDMA) is one of the most frequently occurring nitrosamines in our dietary foods. NDMA is a potent carcinogen, associated with increased risk of malignant tumors of liver, lung, and stomach [13].

Nitrates (NO_3) and nitrites (NO_2) are inorganic compounds, composed of a single nitrogen atom (N) and a number of oxygen atoms (O). It is believed that nitrates themselves are relatively inert, and activated by nitrate reductase enzyme from bacteria in the mouth into to nitrites. Then nitrites are converted to nitrous acid by the acidic juices in stomach, which further reacts with amines to form nitrosamines. The carcinogenesis of nitrosamines could be through gene mutation and DNA adductions. A high consumption of processed meats was correlated to an increased gastric cancer risk, and many people consider nitrates/nitrites as the main reason for that [13].

3.4. Aflatoxins

Aflatoxin is a potent human carcinogen. It is a naturally occurring toxic metabolite produced by certain fungi (Aspergillus flavis). Aflatoxins are an interesting example of DNA damaging agents from a natural source. Among the aflatoxins of natural origin, aflatoxin B1 is the most potent hepatocarcinogen and considered to be the most toxic. Aflatoxins are regularly found in improperly stored staple commodities such as cassava, corn, cotton seed, millet, peanuts, rice, sesame seeds, and wheat [16].

Aflatoxins may be metabolized in the liver to a reactive epoxide intermediate or hydroxylated to become the less harmful aflatoxin M_1. Aflatoxins are commonly ingested through contaminated food. Animals fed contaminated food can pass aflatoxin transformation products into eggs, milk products, and meat. However the most toxic type of aflatoxin B_1, can permeate through the skin. It has been suggested that aflatoxins induce p53 gene mutations in hepatocytes [16].

3.5. Drugs and chemotherapy

Many drugs have carcinogenic potential such as intercalating antibiotics or nitroimidazole derivatives like metronidazole. The mechanism of action of nitroimidazoles is through reduction of the nitro group in predominantly anaerobic environments leads to formation of reactive intermediate products and hence destruction of DNA strands. Antimicrobial agents can be directly toxic, can interact with other drugs to increase their toxicity, or can alter microbial flora to cause infection by organisms that are normally saprophytic [17].

The majority of cytostatic agents (like: melphalan, nitrosourea, etoposide) are potentially carcinogenic. Certain tumors have been triggered by chemotherapy. Furthermore, some cytostatic agents have an immunosuppressive effect which renders the organism unable to eliminate mutated cells efficiently.

Owing to increased survival rates after chemotherapy, some patients develop years after primary therapy secondary malignancy. Most of secondary malignancies appear in the first 10 years after chemotherapy, especially after alkylating agents or nitrosourea derivatives. Of the alkylating agents, ALKERAN (melphalan), also known as L-phenylalanine mustard, phenylalanine mustard, LPAM, or L-sarcolysin, is a phenylalanine derivative of nitrogen mustard.

According to previous studies, alkylating agents such as cyclophosphamide, melphalan or procarbazine have the strongest leukemogenic potential [18].

3.6. Pesticides

Pesticides are a group of biologically active natural and synthetic chemicals, which are used to kill unwanted harmful insects, fungi, rodents and plants. All pesticides contain biologically active compounds that are purposely designed to interfere with normal biologic processes in target organisms. Therefore, individuals exposed to certain pesticides may be at risk to the development of certain cancers. Exposure to these pesticides could be through occupational exposures, the ingestion of contaminated food and water, by absorption through the skin, or by inhalation during application [19].

Currently, evidence supports that pesticides containing arsenic and ethylene oxide have the potential to cause cancer in humans. Pesticides may cause cancers by affecting cellular proliferation, apoptosis, and cell communication and inducing oxidative stress through non-genotoxic mechanisms. For example, 1,1,1-Trichloro-2,2-bis(*p*-chlorophenyl)-ethane (DDT) is one of the most well-known organochlorine carcinogenic pesticides. DDT tumorigenesis has been shown to be caused by tissue damage through oxidative mechanisms, alter cell signaling pathways (MAPK) that regulate growth, or activate the oncogene erb-B2 [20].

Though DDT was banned in the United State in the early 1970s, it is still used in other countries, and high levels of DDT has been detected in air, water, soil, plants, animals, and human tissues. The organochlorine pesticide 1,1,1-trichloro-2,2-bis (p-chlorophenyl)-ethane (DDT), is a well-known and widely dispersed "environmental estrogen" (World Health Organization Criteria no. 9; Geneva, Switzerland (1979)".

3.7. Arsenic

Inorganic arsenic has been suggested to be a human carcinogen since 1977. Arsenic is emitted into the atmosphere mainly from anthropogenic sources and a small amount from natural sources. Individuals may be exposed to arsenic compounds through contaminated food and drinking water or air emissions from industrial facilities that manufacture pesticides, glass, and cigarette tobacco [21].

Evidence suggests that there is a strong association between arsenic exposure and the development of skin, lung, bladder, kidney, liver, and colon cancers. The mechanism by which arsenic causes cancer is not well understood. It has been proposed that Arsenic does not interact with DNA, but indirectly causes chromosome aberrations, genomic instability, and aberrant DNA methylation in promoter regions of genes [22].

3.8. Dioxins

Dioxins are a group of structurally related compounds produced from industrial and combustion activities such as bleaching of paper, the manufacture of some pesticides, waste incineration, and fuels burning. They could be released from natural sources such as volcanic eruptions and forest fires. Dioxins are found in air, soil, water and food sources. Sufficient evidence from human epidemiologic and mechanistic studies showed an association between dioxins and various cancers including soft tissue sarcoma, lymphoma, leukemia, and Hodgkin disease. TCDD is the well-studied dioxin, which is known to be human carcinogen [23].

The mechanism responsible for dioxin-mediated carcinogenesis is via activation of the aryl hydrocarbon (Ah) receptor resulting in a wide spectrum of biologic responses, including altered metabolism, growth, and differentiation. It has been suggested that Dioxin alters multiple integrated cell signaling pathways, namely, the MAPK-ERK pathway through activation of tumor necrosis factor-alpha (TNF-a) and epidermal growth factor (EGF). Others suggested mutations in the proto-oncogene H-ras [24].

3.9. Asbestos

Asbestos is a group of six naturally occurring fibrous silicate minerals, namely: chrysotile, actinolite, amosite, anthophyllite, crocidolite, and tremolite. Chrysotile constitutes about 90% of the commercially used asbestos worldwide. Asbestos is released into the environment from natural and man-made sources and has been detected in air, soil, drinking water, food, and medicines. Asbestos toxicity occurs after a long latent period of about 15–40 year after initial fiber exposure. Occupational exposure to any type of asbestos increases the risk of lung cancer and mesothelioma [25].

More than 50 countries have banned the mining and/or use of all types of asbestos. However, past and current occupational asbestos exposures, and non-occupational domestic asbestos exposure originating from existing buildings that contain enormous amounts of the fibers and neighborhood exposures in communities living near asbestos mining, remains a global health challenge [26].

The carcinogenesis of asbestos is not fully understood. However, asbestos is a genotoxic agent that can induce direct DNA damage, gene transcription, and protein expression important in modulating cell proliferation, cell death, and inflammation [25].

Author details

Maher Soliman

Address all correspondence to: maher.soliman@daad-alumni.de

Oncology Department, Faculty of Medicine, Alexandria University, Alexandria, Egypt

References

[1] Torre LA, Bray F, Siegel RL, Ferlay J, Lortet-Tieulent J, Jemal A. Global cancer statistics, 2012. CA: A Cancer Journal for Clinicians. 2015;**65**(2):87-108

[2] Bray F, Moller B. Predicting the future burden of cancer. Nature Reviews. Cancer. 2006; **6**:63-74

[3] Pitot CH, Loeb DD. Fundamentals of Oncology. 4th ed. New York: Marcel Dekker; 2002. 41p

[4] Pott P. The Chirurgical Works of Percivall Pott, Vol. 5, Chirurgical Observations Relative to the Cataract, the Polypus of the Nose, the Cancer of the Scrotum, the Different Kinds of Ruptures, and the Mortification of the Toes and Feet. London: L. Hawes, W. Clarke and R. Collins; 1775

[5] Miller EC. Some current perspectives on chemical carcinogenesis in humans and experimental animals: Presidential address. Cancer Research. 1978;**38**:1479-1496

[6] Yamagawa K, Ichikawa K. Experimentelle Studie über die Pathogenese der Epithelialgeschwülste. Mitteilungen of Medical Faculty of Imperial University of Tokyo. 1915;**15**: 295-344

[7] "IARC Monographs". Monographs.iarc.fr. Retrieved 2017-10-5

[8] Gibbs WW. Untangling the roots of cancer. Scientific American. 2003;**289**(1):56-65

[9] Kling J. Put the blame on methylation. The Scientist. 2003;**16**(12):27-28

[10] Barrett JC, Shelby MD. Mechanisms of human carcinogens. Progress in Clinical and Biological Research. 1992;**374**:415-434

[11] Hecht SS. Tobacco smoke carcinogens and lung cancer. Journal of the National Cancer Institute. 1999;**91**:1194-1210

[12] Hecht SS. Etiology of cancer: Tobacco. In: TV DV, Lawrence ST, Rosenberg SA, editors. Devita, Hellman & Rosenberg's Cancer: Principles & Practice of Oncology. 8th ed. Philadelphia: Lippincott Williams & Wilkins; 2008. p. 148-165

[13] Oliver CP, Gloria MBA, Barbour JF, Scanlan RA. Nitrate, nitrite and volatile nitrosamines in whey-containing food products. Journal of Agricultural and Food Chemistry. 1995;**43**:967-969

[14] Air Quality Guidelines for Europe. 2nd ed. Copenhagen: WHO Regional Office for Europe; 2000 Polycyclic Aromatic Hydrocarbons. (WHO Regional Publications, European Series, No. 91)

[15] Menzie CA, Potocki BB, Santodonato J. Exposure to carcinogenic PAHs in the environment. Environmental Science and Technology. 1992;**26**:1278-1284

[16] McPherson M. Mycotoxin testing with aran gas: Aflatoxin B1 mycotoxin destruction using allotropic oxygen O4, O5, and O6. The Journal of Microbiology. 2015;**2**(6):00068

[17] Neu HC, Gootz TD. Medical Microbiology. 4th ed. University of Texas Medical Branch; Galveston; 1996. ISBN-10: 0-9631172-1-1

[18] Jones RB, Frank R, Mass T. Safe handling of chemotherapeutic agents: A report from the Mount Sinai Medical Center. CA: A Cancer Journal for Clinicians. 1983;**33**:258-263

[19] Alavanja MC, Samanic C, Dosemeci M, et al. Use of agricultural pesticides and prostate cancer risk in the agricultural health study cohort. American Journal of Epidemiology. 2003;**157**:800-814

[20] Bounias M. Etiological factors and mechanism involved in relationships between pesticide exposure and cancer. Journal of Environmental Biology. 2003;**24**:1-8

[21] Guo HR, Wang NS, Hu H, Monson RR. Cell type specificity of lung cancer associated with arsenic ingestion. Cancer Epidemiology, Biomarkers & Prevention. 2004;**13**:638-643

[22] Shi H, Shi X, Liu KJ. Oxidative mechanism of arsenic toxicity and carcinogenesis. Molecular and Cellular Biochemistry. 2004;**255**:67-78

[23] Bertazzi PA, Zocchetti C, Guercilena S, et al. Dioxin exposure and cancer risk: A 15-year mortality study after the "Seveso accident." Epidemiology. 1997;**8**:646-652

[24] Cole P, Trichopoulos D, Pastides H, Starr T, Mandel JS. Dioxin and cancer: A critical review. Regulatory Toxicology and Pharmacology. 2003;**38**:378-388

[25] MacDonald L. The health hazards of asbestos removal. JAMA. 1992;**267**:52-53

[26] Mossman BT, Bignon J, Corn M, Seaton A, Gee JB. Asbestos: Scientific developments and implications for public policy. Science. 1990;**247**:294-301

4

Early Metastasis in Colorectal Cancer Poses an Option for New Diagnostic and Treatment Strategies

Hassan Adwan, Dina Elharouni, Danira Habashy, Nadine Banna, Rania Georges, Asim Pervaiz and Martin R. Berger

Abstract

Metastasis is the spread of tumor cells from a primary site to a secondary site within the host's body. It is initiated by the detachment of the tumor cells from the primary tumor followed by invasion into the surrounding tissue. Thereafter the cells migrate across the endothelium and into the blood vessels (intravasation). During the intravasation the cells have to survive the sheer forces and the immune response. Upon arrival to the target organ, the cells leave the circulation and cross the endothelium to reach the host organ. Once there, the tumor cells are greeted with the organ's local immune cells and with a hostile or inappropriate environment, where they finally have to form proliferating colonies. Metastasis is therefore far from being a straight-forward or efficient process with less than 0.1% of disseminating tumor cells (around 1 × 109 cells per day for a 1 cm size tumor) succeeding in colonizing distal organs. The identification of the involved marker during the early metastasis process will be essential for establishment of new diagnostics tools, as well as development of novel treatment strategies.

Keywords: colorectal cancer, early metastasis, migration, invasion, homing

1. Introduction

Cancer metastasis is the major cause of cancer morbidity and mortality, and accounts for about 90% of cancer deaths [1]. Metastasis is a complex process requiring several processes, which involves the spread of cancer cells from the primary tumor to surrounding tissues and to distant organs. Cancer cells require the capacity to invade the surrounding tissues, then migrate and survive in the circulation, colonize the foreign organ and eventually resume growth, to gain metastatic capability [2], Metastasis alone is an inefficient process because the tumor cells have to acquire some necessary abilities to regenerate a tumor at a distant site [3, 4]. Over the past few years, the main determinants of metastatic competence in CRC have begun to be characterized. In fact, the acquirement of a stem-like phenotype by cancer cells is very important for the tumor cells to regenerate in a foreign organ, in the absence of mutations associated with the metastatic process in CRC. These metastatic stem cells adopt multiple phenotypes and behaviors and critically depend on their interaction with the microenvironment to migrate, survive in the circulation and flourish in a foreign organ. The metastatic cascade consists of four essential steps. The first of which is the detachment of the tumor cells from the primary tumor. There after the separated cells undergo local invasion into the surrounding tissue, e.g. into the mesenchyma, followed by migration of the tumor cells across the endothelium and into the vessels in a process known as intravasation where disseminating tumor cells have to survive the circulatory system's sheer forces and swarming immune cells. Upon arrival to the target or appropriate organ, tumor cells have to leave the circulation and cross once again the endothelium to reach the host organ. Once there, the disseminated tumor cells are greeted with the organ's local immune cells as well as with a hostile or inappropriate environment where they finally have to form proliferating colonies. Metastasis is therefore far from being a straight-forward or efficient process with less than 0.1% of disseminating tumor cells (around 1×10^9 cells per day for a 1 cm size tumor) succeeding in colonizing distal organs. The cells have to face multiple ordeals, such as the immune system, at each step of the process thus making metastasis a process possible mostly out of the sheer number of disseminating cells entering the bloodstream [5]. Multi-biochemical events and other parameters affect the metastatic cascade such as extracellular matrix structure, growth factors, chemokines, matrix metalloproteinases. Hence, the biochemical markers along with the tumor microenvironment may serve as a crucial target for the inhibition and prevention of metastasis [5].

2. Metastasis in colorectal cancer

2.1. Cancer cell detachment

Cancer cell detachment is a process usually occurring from the extracellular matrix (ECM). Cell detachment involves both mechanical forces and protease-mediated cleavage, but also decreased expression of adhesion molecules and changes in glycosylation of cell membrane glycoproteins and proteoglycans. Mechanical forces are generated by actomyosin-driven contraction. The cytosolic dissociation of cell–substrate adhesions can also be performed by the calpain cysteine proteases, by phosphorylation/dephosphorylation of cytosolic adapter proteins and by posttranslational modification of integrins or adapter proteins.

Extracellular dissociation of cell-substrate adhesions can be achieved by proteolytic cleavage of matrix constituents that are mediated by matrix proteases. Moreover, the detachment could occur by the shedding of matrix receptors such as integrins [6]. Anoikis is a form of programmed cell death that occurs when anchorage-dependent cells detach from their ECM [7]. When cells are detached from the ECM, there is a loss of normal cell-matrix interactions, and subsequently anoikis can occur through the down-regulation of Bcl-xL (an anti-apoptotic component of the mitochondrial pathway) and the up-regulation of Fas ligand (FasL) (an activator of the death receptor pathway) [8].

However, during the metastatic detachment, the tumor cells resist and escape the anoikis process. This escape includes the alteration of enzyme systems in the signaling pathways that regulate anoikis, such as small GTPases and effectors, receptor tyrosine kinases and other kinases such as NF-κB, and EMT factors [6, 9].

Furthermore, there are multiple anoikis-independent mechanisms by which normal epithelial cells would die once detached from the ECM. Metastatic cancer cells must overcome these anoikis-dependent and anoikis-independent barriers in order to survive once they lose the attachment to the ECM [6].

2.2. Detachment in mCRC

Metastatic colorectal cancer (mCRC) is a long and complex process involving several mechanisms, and molecular pathways. CRC is currently considered the third most common neoplasm in the world according to the World Cancer Research Fund International, and the second most frequent malignancy causing death [10] mCRC is a multi-step biological process (**Figure 1**). This process starts with a series of mutations in colonic epithelial cells, continues with their detachment from the large intestine, dissemination through the blood and/or lymphatic circulation, attachment to the hepatic sinusoids and interactions with the sinusoidal cells, such as sinusoidal endothelial cells, Kupffer cells, stellate cells, and pit cells. The metastatic sequence terminates with colorectal cancer cell invasion, adaptation and colonization of the hepatic parenchyma. All these events are termed the colorectal cancer invasion-metastasis cascade, which includes multiple molecular pathways. The cellular and molecular pathways of the metastatic process in CRC have been extensively analyzed over the last decades. The metastatic process in CRC involves a series of steps such as:

1. Lysis of the extracellular matrix

Enzymes produced by cancer cells alter the extracellular matrix and thus enable cancer cells to leave the original site of the primary tumor.

Matrix metalloproteinases (MMPs) are crucial components of cells that can degrade a range of extracellular matrix proteins allowing cancer cells to detach and migrate. MMPs are a family of zinc-dependent endoproteinases with an enzymatic activity directed against main Extra Cellular Matrix (ECM) components.

The mechanism by which MMPs aid cancer cells to escape and degrade the ECM consists of two main steps. First, proteinase acts by removing any physical barriers to invasion by the degradation of ECM macromolecules such as collagens, laminins, and proteoglycans. Second,

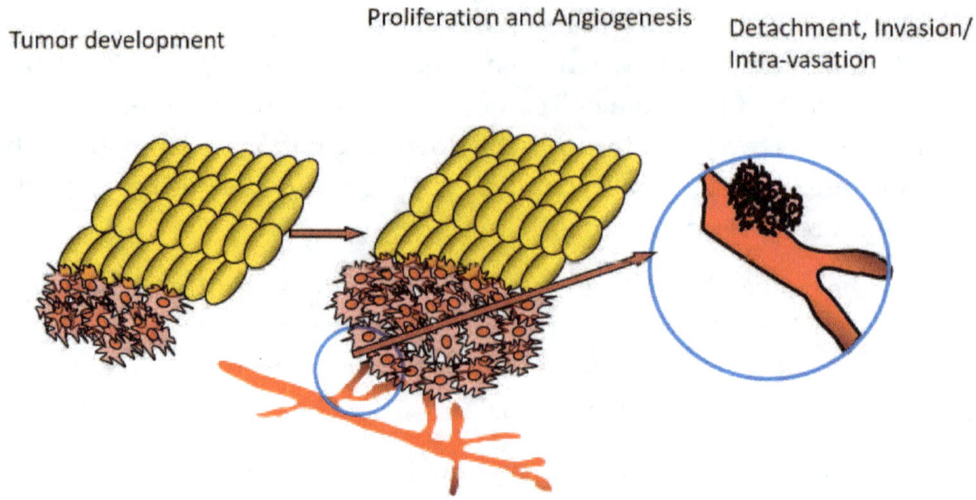

Figure 1. Illustration of the initial stages of the metastasis process. The tumor development is followed by tumor growth and angiogenesis. This stage is characterized by the down-regulation of cell attachment proteins such as the cadherins, as well as the tight junction proteins such as the claudins. In addition the expression of the matrix metalloproteinase is increased in this stage.

MMPs modulate cell adhesion. For cells to move through the ECM, they must be able to form new cell–matrix and cell–cell attachments and break existing ones. Overexpression of MMP-1, -2, -3, -7, -9, -13, and MT1-MMP has been demonstrated in human colorectal cancers (**Figure 1**). The degree of overexpression of some MMPs has been noted to be correlated with different stages of disease and/or prognosis [12].

2. Cellular adhesion

Cancer cells express adhesion molecules as cadherins, integrins, and carcinoembryonic antigen (CEA) that favor their adhesion to the extracellular matrix. These adhesion molecules have been under exclusive research regarding their roles concerning their regulation and expression in the process of early metastasis during detachment from the primary tumor.

A. Cadherins

Cell adhesion molecules (CAMs) regulate cell–cell and cell-matrix adhesion and are implicated in almost all stages of metastasis, therefore alterations in normal levels of CAMs such as E-cadherin will be significant in tumor progression. E-cadherin is the prototypical member of the type-1 classical cadherins and is found at adherens junctions (AJs), which are structures that mediate cell-cell interactions. E-cadherin is a single-pass transmembrane glycoprotein containing five extracellular repeats that mediate its Ca^{2+}-dependent homophilic interaction with opposing molecules on neighboring cells [11].

Studies exploring the expression of E-cadherin and α-catenin in tumor tissues have shown that loss of both molecules is linked to an increased invasiveness of tumor cells [12]. Evidence for this comes from in vitro and in vivo studies, which demonstrate that E-cadherin expression is inversely correlated with the motile and invasive behavior of tumor cells and also with metastasis in cancer patients [12]. Further studies have revealed that the relocalization of β-catenin to the nucleus correlates with the acquisition of the mesenchymal phenotype [13], and is associated with the loss of E-cadherin.

Loss of the E-cadherin molecule is thought to enable metastasis by disrupting intercellular contacts. This can occur due to somatic mutations, chromosomal deletions, proteolytic cleavage, and silencing of the *CDH1* promoter. Silencing can also occur either by DNA hypermethylation or through the action of transcription factors such as Slug, Snail, and Twist [14].

B. Integrins

Integrins are heterodimeric cell-surface glycoproteins that serve to mediate cell–ECM interactions, thereby linking cues from the extracellular environment to the actin cytoskeleton [15]. These membrane-spanning proteins consist of 2 subunits, termed a and b, of which there are at least 18 a-subunits and 8 b-subunits. The resulting multitude of possible combinations gives rise to more than 20 different integrins, which act to differentially control a range of biological processes through selective binding to extracellular substrates.

The crosstalk between epithelial cell-cell adhesion and cell- matrix adhesion signaling, and the dynamic interplay between the two, contribute to the plasticity within tumor cells that allows them to respond to external cues, which in turn drives effective migration and invasion. Below, we will review data on the key signaling intermediates that regulate this crosstalk, as well as discuss recent work that is in support of a physical interaction between integrin- and E-cadherin-mediated adhesions that governs the adhesive strength of E-cadherin.

C. EMT

Epithelial-mesenchymal transition (EMT) is a reversible morphogenetic biological process that involves the transition from stationary polarized epithelial cells to motile, multipolar or spindle-shaped mesenchymal cells. The EMT is described in detail in another part of this chapter.

2.3. Hypoxia

Hypoxia in cancer cell metastasis is a tumor oxygen deficiency termed as the environmental stressor (**Figure 2**). This condition is known to induce genes involved in the regulation of cell proliferation, extracellular matrix production, cell adhesion, and other hallmarks of tumorigenesis [16].

The mechanism behind the hypoxia induced metastasis is influenced by transcription factors like the hypoxia-inducible factor (HIF) family. This family consists of three members, HIF-1, -2, and -3, that regulate vital cellular processes such as glucose metabolism, angiogenesis, cell proliferation, and tissue remodeling [17].

Hypoxia is linked to tumor early metastasis by several known molecular mechanisms. The first mechanism is the HIF-1α binding to hypoxia-response elements within the c-met promoter activating transcription of this gene. Overexpression of the Met protein on the cell surface of tumor cells leads them to be more susceptible to hepatocyte growth factor stimulation. This causes extracellular matrix degradation, cell dissociation, and escape from hypoxic areas

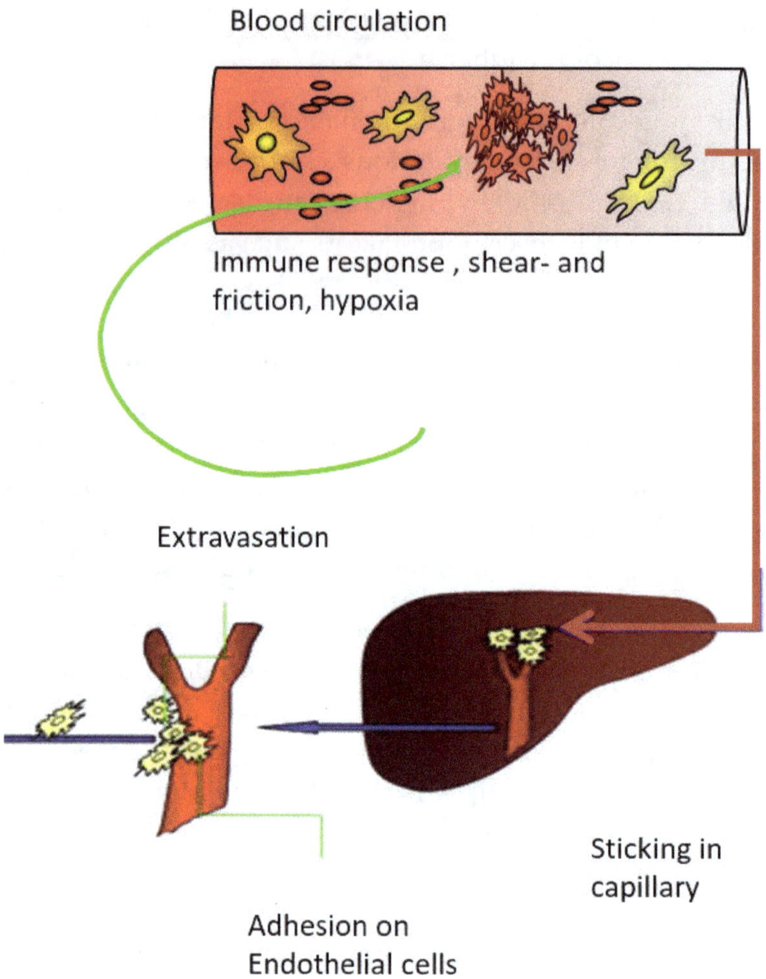

Figure 2. The post tumor cell intravasation stage poses the greatest obstacles for the tumor cells in the metastasis process. The immune response, shear and friction forces as well as hypoxia are responsible for considerable highest elimination of the tumor cells. The EMT is a special feature that defined the tumor cells in this time period.

to more oxygen-rich environments at a secondary [18]. Moreover, the HIF expression is necessary and sufficient to cause E-cadherin loss, a critical step in EMT [19].

While hypoxia has been strongly linked to tumor metastasis and poor clinical outcome of patients, it seems to actually have a dual role: insufficient oxygen limits tumor cell division while at the same time selecting for more malignant cells and inducing cell adaptations allowing for more invasive behavior. This is likely because low oxygen tension is able to increase cell invasiveness, cause cells to switch to anaerobic metabolism, increase genetic instability, and promote angiogenesis [20].

2.4. Invasion and endothelial transmigration

2.4.1. Mechanisms of invasion in CRC

The colonic epithelium in particular is composed of polarized cells with a characteristic apical membrane, forming a barrier with the components of the colon lumen, a basal membrane attached to the basement membrane and lateral membranes attaching to adjacent cells. In order to invade other tissues, tumor cells may move individually, as clusters or as collective sheets by changing their phenotype and morphological features either by epithelial to mesenchymal transition (EMT), collective to amoeboid transition (CAT) or mesenchymal to amoeboid transition (MAT). EMT is the process of transition of the tumor cells from an epithelial phenotype into a mesenchymal phenotype by losing E-cadherin and upregulating vimentin [21]. This mechanism of invasion has been observed in colorectal cancer (CRC), breast cancer, hepatocellular carcinoma, pancreatic cancer, prostate carcinoma and lung cancer cells. CAT involves individual tumor cells detaching from cell clusters and developing amoeboid migration such as in melanomas. MAT describes the transition of mesenchymal tumor cells to amoeboid cells as observed in fibrosarcomas, melanomas and breast cancer. Amoeboid cells decrease their interactions with the extra-cellular matrix (ECM), which allows them to move easily through intact ECM gaps without resorting to proteolysis or ECM degradation and thus independent of protease activity [22]. EMT is the mode of invasion most observed and described in CRC.

2.4.2. EMT

EMT was first described as a process in developmental biology in embryogenesis. It was observed that a similar mechanism was employed by invading tumor cells, which undergo several phenotypical changes to resemble mesenchymal cells. This process requires the loss of cell–cell interactions such as the loss of epithelial cadherin (E-cadherin), α-catenin, claudins [23], occludin and ZO-1, with transcription factors' activation increasing the expression of mesenchymal proteins such as neuronal cadherin (N-cadherin), fibronectin and vimentin, reorganization of the cytoskeleton and production of proteases and ECM degrading enzymes [24]. The entirety of these processes is linked together, starting with the loss of E-cadherin. It binds extracellularly with its adjacent cell's E-cadherin while it binds intracellularly to α- and β-catenin and p-120 catenin, which is responsible for signal transduction and connecting the junctions to the cytoskeleton. Factors that have been known to induce EMT include transforming growth factor β (TGF-β), which plays an essential role in the transition and progression by activating Smad, integrins, platelet derived growth factor (PDGF), hepatocyte growth factor (HGF), vascular endothelial growth factor (VEGF) and fibroblast growth factor (FGF). They induce the expression of EMT-related transcription repressors such as Snail, Slug, Twist and zinc finger E-box binding homeobox 1 (ZEB1). The downregulation of E-cadherin is generally accompanied by the upregulation of mesenchymal proteins, notably N-cadherin. This transition from E- to N-cadherin is called "cadherin shift" and is essential in EMT [25]. Upon loss of E-cadherin, the membrane-bound β-catenin is translocated to the nucleus where it regulates several genes' transcription, notably cyclin D1 and c-myc thus contributing to the progression of malignancy. In turn, N-cadherin expression mediated the formation of Rho-induced stress fibers forming lamellipodia (major actin projection leading the cell forward) by Ras-related C3 botulinum toxin substrate 1 (Rac1) protein activation and filopodia (thin actin projections from the leading edge of the cell) by cell division control protein 42 homolog (Cdc42) activation. Therefore, invading tumor cells undergoing EMT are able to detach themselves from clusters of epithelial cells; they lose their epithelial phenotype and are capable of moving individually similar to a mesenchymal cell.

Furthermore, EMT is known to preserve stem cell properties, evade apoptosis and the immune response as well as confer resistance to radiotherapy and chemotherapy, which was described in CRC. As of late, various microRNAs (miRs) have been shown to regulate EMT such as miR-9, which interacts with E-cadherin thus facilitating cell detachment and motility and increases VEGF levels leading to neoangiogenesis. Interestingly, epithelial cell differentiation may be driven by the miR-200 family including miR-200a, miR-200b, miR-200c, miR-429 and miR-141. Zinc Finger E-Box Binding Homeobox 1 and 2 (ZEB1 and ZEB2) transcription factors repress the miR-200 family at transcription, while this miR family itself inhibits ZEB1 and ZEB2 (EMT inducers) at a post-transcriptional level. Furthermore, ZEB induces EMT and stem cell characteristics by upregulating Sox2, Klf4 and Bmi1, which are ordinarily inhibited by the miR-200 family. This process has been conjectured to occur in CRC [26].

2.4.3. *Collective cell invasion*

Epithelial cancers such as breast and colorectal cancers witness the occurrence of collective cell or bulk invasion. The cells maintain their intercellular junctions, adherence and desmosomes, and thus stay attached together during movement [27]. However, there is a front to back polarity where tip or leader cells at the front of migration are phenotypically different than following cells. The asymmetry in actomyosin filaments affecting the tip cells are mediated by Rho GTPases and myosin II. Tip cells therefore become more similar to a mesenchymal cell as opposed to the following cells which maintain an epithelial phenotype with intact intercellular contacts. Cell movement occurs due to coordination in the polar CRC cells' cytoskeleton generating traction [28]. In order for movement to be possible, ECM and BM remodeling is required [29]. Stromal-cell derived factor (SDF1/CXCL12), FGF and TGF-β family are factors known to provoke collective cell migration. A two-dimensional invasion by a monolayer of cells, three-dimensional invasion or detachment of a cell cluster from the primary tumor are, among others, all different possible types of collective cell invasion (**Figure 2**).

In order to pull cells at the front and push those at the back, it is crucial to generate traction force. This is done by integrins present in the tip cells such as β1 and β3 integrins expressed therein, which attach to constituents of the ECM such as fibronectin by focal adhesion complexes [27]. Leading cells also express $\alpha 2\beta 1$ integrins, which bind to collagen and $\alpha v\beta 3$ integrins, which attach to fibrin. Following cells also form lamellipodia underneath the cells at the front whose $\alpha 6\beta 1$ integrins attach to the BM formed by the invading leading cells paving the way. Integrin binding to the ECM causes cytoskeletal changes such as activation of contractin, talin, paxilin and vinculin, which are cytoskeletal adaptor proteins. This induces actin reorganization, which is important for the formation of filopodia. Pseudopodia are regulated by Rac while filopodia are regulated by Cdc42. On the other hand, Rho is mainly involved in individual rather than collective cell invasion [30].

ECM degradation and remodeling is crucial for paving the way for migrating cells and is highly dependent on ECM density, gap size, orientation and dimensions as well as on the migrating cell [22]. Leading cells produce membrane type 1 matrix metalloproteinase; MMP14 (MT1-MMP), which degrades the initial outlet for movement through the ECM, which is then widened by the following cells. The latter continue ECM degradation followed by the production and deposition of laminin, perlecan, nidogen 1 and collagen type IV [31].

2.4.4. *Mesenchymal cell invasion after EMT*

In carcinomas, mesenchymal cells mainly originate from clusters of epithelial cells, which have undergone EMT. They generally invade as single cells [27]. Mesenchymal cell migration is a five-step process starting with pseudopodia formation at the front of the cell, which initiates focal contact with the ECM. Then focal proteolysis is followed by the contraction of the actomyosin filaments to pull the cell forward, which is finally followed by detachment of the trailing end from the ECM in order for the cell to be pulled forward [32]. The mesenchymal cell is partially polarized due to reorganization of the cytoskeletal F-actin resulting in a front able to bind tightly to the ECM and a trailing end or a tail that contracts refraction fibers in order to move [33].

TGF-β and nuclear accumulation of Smad2 were found to be the primary culprit in the detachment and de-differentiation of single tumor cells from moving epithelial clusters. On the other hand, it was found that Smad2 was retained in the cytoplasm in collectively invading cells and non-moving cells. Interfering with TGF-β type II receptor hindered intravasation or hematogenous metastasis for individual mesenchymal cells but tumor cell clusters moving by collective invasion were still observed in the lymphatic system [30]. Therefore, this study showed that TGF-β is crucial for individual cell movement via activation of the EGF receptor, fibrinogen/angiopoietin-related protein (FARP), E3 ubiquitin-protein ligase (Nedd4), Myosin phosphatase Rho-interacting protein (M-RIP), Smad4 and RhoC. However, it is necessary that TGF-β is downregulated thereafter to allow for tumor cell adhesion and subsequent colony formation at distal sites [12].

2.4.5. *Role of TME*

EMT is promoted by TGF-β, HGF, FGF, endothelial growth factor (EGF) and insulin-like growth factor (IGF). Along with interleukin (IL)-1α, these factors act on the tip cells and activate collective cell invasion. TGF-β in particular plays a major role in invasion by inducing EMT, and myofibroblast formation, as well as by producing autocrine mitogens and targeting CD8+ T cells to evade the immune response [34].

MMPs are upregulated in most cancers and are related to enhanced tumor growth, angiogenesis, invasiveness and metastasis. They are secreted from tumor cells, leading cells from collective invading cells, myofibroblasts and immune cells. They are central in the degradation of ECM proteins, the cleavage of cellular adhesion molecules like E-cadherin and the activation of cytokines and growth factors [35].

Immune cells from the TME were found to play tumor-promoting functions as demonstrated the observation that chronic inflammation often leads to the development of cancer, as for chronic Hepatitis C infection which causes hepatocellular carcinoma by its sustained and persistent inflammation. NF-κB is secreted by tumor cells and tumor-associated immune cells. It induces expression of the inflammatory cytokines IL-1, IL-6, TNF and RANKL, which stimulate invasion and metastasis. Tumor cells can actively regulate the tumor microenvironment (TME) to shield themselves from the immune system as part of the cancer immunoediting process. They do so by secreting and expressing a variety of immunosuppressive molecules that downregulate or inhibit the immune system, such as TGF-β, thus converting macrophages from an antitumor state to a pro-tumor state. Macrophages in the protumorigenic state help the growth and propagation of tumor cells by inducing ECM cleavage, tissue remodeling, angiogenesis, chemoresistance, and tumor-associated macrophage recruitment. Mutations in cancer cells may also result in the exposure of different epitopes on the surface of the cells, thus equally modulating the immune system [36].

The most relevant tumor-related cells in the TME are tumor-associated macrophages (TAMs) and cancer associated fibroblasts (CAFs) or myofibroblasts, both of which aid in tumor progression. TAMs stimulate metastasis while myofibroblasts re-organize the ECM to facilitate metastasis and epithelial tumor cell migration.

2.4.6. TAMS

TAMs or macrophages infiltrating the tumor bed are found to stimulate angiogenesis as well as tumor development and progression. Macrophages represent the largest percentage of the immune cell population present in the TME. Ideally as a part of the immune system, the macrophages should eradicate tumor cells and halt progression when activated correctly. However, macrophages were found to be mostly pro-tumoral in the TME. Their presence in the TME was significantly related to poor prognosis in several types of cancer such as breast, ovarian cancers, and lymphomas [37]. These two opposing states, pro and anti-tumoral, can be classified as M1 and M2. M1 or classically activated macrophages are generally anti-tumorigenic, expressing pro-inflammatory cytokines such as TNF-α, IL-6, IL-12, and inducible NO synthase (iNOS). However, M2 or alternatively activated macrophages have increased expression of anti-inflammatory cytokines such as IL-10 and IL-1 decoy receptor, which inhibits T effector cells. This classification is however simplified. It has been shown that within each polarization, macrophage activation states are heterogeneous calling forth further subdivisions, each initiated by different regulators and having different functions. In the liver, additional phenotypes for macrophages have been identified such as the one associated with hepatocarcinoma. These TAMs exhibit mainly the M2 phenotype and promote angiogenesis by increased expression of VEGF, they also facilitate matrix remodeling to accommodate angiogenesis by producing matrix metalloproteases [38].

Tumor cells secrete colony stimulating factor 1 (CSF1), also known as macrophage colony-stimulating factor (M-CSF), which recruits CSF1 receptor-expressing macrophages to the TME [39]. TAMs secrete enzymes that help degrade the ECM as well as various growth factors such as EGF, which promotes EMT and invasiveness. They also express Chemokine (C-C motif) ligand 18 (CCL18), which stimulates the clustering of integrin in tumor cells thus providing an anchor to the ECM and facilitating invasion and tumor cell motility. Furthermore, TAMs secrete MMP, produce cysteine cathepsins and serine proteases, which contribute to the re-organization of the ECM to facilitate metastasis. For instance, collective cell invasion is promoted by MMP2 and MMP9 secretion from immature myeloid cells at the leading edge of the invading cluster in CRC.

2.4.7. CAFs

CAFs play an important role in the TME by secreting various cytokines such as IL-8, or growth factors such as VEGF, or MMPs or chemokines such as chemokine (C-X-C motif) ligand 12

(CXCL12) which drive tumor growth, neoangiogenesis and local invasion [34]. They were found to communicate with tumor cells via the CXCL12/CXCR4 axis, which promotes tumor migration. More importantly, CAFs rearrange the ECM forming channel-like structures through which cancer cells may grow and invade the surrounding tissue without having to undergo EMT, thus maintaining their characteristic epithelial features. In a study, CAFs were incubated with supernatants from CRC cells, which led to marked activation of the TGF-β pathway [40]. As seen previously, TGF-β is a known pro-tumoral factor inducing metastasis, which is also secreted from CAFs upon interaction with the TME. The secreted TGF-β in turn stimulates CAFs for further TGF-β secretion in an autocrine loop.

CAFs are also the primary source of ECM and connective tissue formation, such as collagens I, III, IV, V, and XII, and proteoglycans [41]. CAFs treated with TGF-β in vitro showed an overexpression of collagen type I, fibronectin, urokinase type plasminogen activator (u-PA), MMPs such as MMP-2 and MMP-9, and tissue inhibitors of metalloproteinases (TIMPs) [40]. On the genetic level, tenascin-C and laminin-B1 were also upregulated when compared with normal colon fibroblasts [41]. CAFs produce more MMPs when compared to CRC cells, thus making it the major player in ECM remodeling. Interestingly, collagen type IV, which is the main constituent of the basement membrane, is degraded by MMP-2 and MMP-9, which thus facilitate mesenchymal invasion [40].

Co-culturing of spheroid CRC cells and CAFs in a collagen invasion experiment showed that the spheroidal CRC cells in contact with CAFs had irregular edges with both individual cell and collective cell invasion of the matrix as opposed to the smooth-edged control CRC spheroids [42]. In another collagen invasion experiment, CRC cells treated with CAFs supernatants were found to have a five-fold increase in matrix invasion as opposed to control CRC cells [43]. Treated cells were also found to have a more elongated shape compared to the control CRC cells. CAFs were indeed shown to over-produce FGF-1, which activates FGFR-3, a receptor tyrosine kinase, leading to local invasion and cellular migration [44]. The pro-invasion morphological changes induced in CRC cells upon contact with CAFs supernatant confirm the multi-functional role they play in metastasis [45]. A recent study showed that CAFs were able to induce metastasis at a very early stage in tumor development, even when the tumor was of microscopic size, in a small number of cancer cells which remained associated with CAFs upon entering the circulation, potentially forming micrometastatic niches in distal organs which are only visible upon progression [46]. These mechanisms that induce tumor cell invasion and migration may be an interesting target for novel therapies in order to inhibit metastasis.

2.4.8. Role of the ECM

The ECM in particular may be defined as the collection of molecules surrounding the cells in a certain tissue, generally structural proteins such as collagens and elastins, enzymes such as metalloproteinases, polysaccharides, glycoproteins, water, signaling molecules and ECM bound growth factors. The ECM is vital for maintaining tissue homeostasis, proper scaffolding and structure. It is characteristic and unique for each type of tissue. It is a dynamic pool of molecules constantly edited by the surrounding cells in order to cater for their needs. Furthermore, ECM is an important motor for tissue growth, healing and cellular differentiation as demonstrated by studies in the developmental biology field. ECM is not only altered by the type of cells present in the tissue but also by their state such as inflammation, injury, etc. Tumor beds in general share characteristic abnormalities in their ECM such as disorganized and disrupted ECM with extensive and uncontrolled neoangiogenesis. These changes in the ECM may drive the progression and invasiveness of tumors.

The colonic epithelium in particular is composed of polarized cells with a characteristic apical membrane, forming a barrier with the components of the colon lumen, a basal membrane attached to the basement membrane and lateral membranes attaching to adjacent cells. The basement membrane (BM) is a distinct structure of the ECM composed mainly of collagen type IV rich in disulfide bridges conferring the BM its rigidity, and of laminin, fibronectin and proteoglycans. Collagen type I replaces collagen type IV from the BM in the stromal ECM, which does not form disulfide bonds, making it less stiff than the BM [47].

Generally, tumors share common features with the ECM of unhealed wounds such as increased stiffness and epithelial contractility. They are characterized by dense growth in connective and fibrous tissues known as *desmoplasia* following injury or BM degradation [48]. Degradation of the BM is currently considered a marker for CRC and carcinoma progression in general. It has been associated with higher metastasis rates and worse prognosis as well as reduced patient survival [49]. Local tumor invasion is driven by two main consecutive mechanisms: enzymatic breakdown of the BM and migration of the malignant epithelial cells through the cleared ECM. A decrease in lateral cell–cell adhesion molecules like E-cadherin [50] is expected to allow for malignant cell detachment and migration. However, it has been shown that CRC may migrate as collective sheets [51]. Along with the enzymatic cleavage of the BM by MMPs, metastatic clones undergo cytoskeletal changes and form cell protrusions such as pseudopodes in order to migrate across the BM towards the mesenchyma, thus initiating tissue invasion [52]. BM degradation actively contributes to the progression of CRC since the ECM initially binds and presents growth factors and other modulators to surrounding cells. Disruption of the BM then releases these signaling molecules lodged within it such as angiogenic factors, growth factors and chemokines [53] thus advancing tumor growth, metastasis, neoangiogenesis and modulation of the immune system to a pro-tumoral state.

Laminin, a glycoprotein abundant in the BM, binds to integrin in epithelial cells, controls cell adhesion to the ECM, interacts with cell-surface receptors and adheres to other laminins thus giving the BM its strength [54]. Laminin-332 is ubiquitous and unique to the epithelium and was thus hypothesized to play a role in carcinoma development. Indeed laminin-332 cleavage products were found to activate the endothelial growth factor receptor (EGFR) pathway known to drive tumor proliferation, loss of cellular adhesion to the ECM and boosting migration [57]. It is a heterotrimeric structure composed of $\alpha3$, a $\beta3$ and $\gamma2$ chains. The $\alpha3$ chain, specifically its large globular domain 3 (LG3 domain) interacts with $\alpha3\beta1$ integrin thus enhancing cellular migration, adhesion and spreading on the ECM. Laminin-332 also interacts and binds to $\alpha6\beta4$ and $\alpha6\beta1$ integrins regulating actin-cytoskeletal protrusion, cellular migration and tissue invasion [55]. Degradation of the $\alpha3$ chain resulting in cleaved LG3 and 4 domains were shown to be over-expressed in carcinomas which activate phosphoinositide 3-kinase (PI3K) and matrix metalloproteinases precipitating tumor growth and invasiveness. This was reversed in vivo with the use of antibodies against this domain of the $\alpha3$ chain [56]. In colon and breast cancer, $\gamma2$ chain cleavage by membrane type-1 MMP was found to stimulate cellular migration [57]. The migration-inducing effects of laminin-332 cleavage products contrast with that of intact laminin-332 itself, which promote epithelial cell adherence to the BM. These opposing effects are hypothesized to alternate under the effects of MMPs cleaving the laminin, thus maintaining tissue homeostasis. In CRC, MMPs are secreted by the tumor cells and surrounding inflammatory cells causing a shift in laminin activity to its cleaved form's migration and invasion inducing effects. All of these cleavage products expose a repeat of an EGF-like domain in the short arm of laminin-332 and become ligands to cell-surface EGFR, thus activating its proliferative and anti-apoptotic pathway [58].

In addition the non-collagenous proteins bone sialoprotein II and osteopontin have been found to be involved in the regulation of the ECM proteins MMP-7 and 9. The inverse regulation of Hoxc8, Runx2 implicates that these genes may be regulated in a feed-back loop manner [59, 60].

The formed dense collagen reorganized by the overexpressed LOX and the various metalloproteinases has a different orientation in CRC compared to normal healthy tissue. The collagen fibers become radially disposed at the interface between the epithelium and the stroma at an angle of 50°C as opposed to 10°C in the healthy colon. This structural change helps tumor cells migrate along the steeply aligned collagen fibers, thus aiding in local invasion of adenocarcinoma cells beyond the epithelium to the mesenchyma transformation [61]. High grade dysplasia was found to hoard changes in the ECM, harboring a denser and ordered collagenous fibers deposition, which reinforces the importance of ECM changes in malignancy, tumor progression and local invasion [62].

2.5. Intravasation

2.5.1. Mechanism

Intravasation is the process of invasion of the tumor cells into the blood or lymphatic vessels. In order for tumor cells to make contact with endothelial cells, complex interactions are needed with proteins lipids and carbohydrates. Carcinoma cells release various mediators and growth factors such as VEGF or vascular endothelial growth factor to promote the process of forming new blood vessels, also known as angiogenesis. The newly formed blood vessels have a leakier endothelial membrane than normal blood vessels, which may aid the process of intravasation and metastasis [63]. The lymphatic vessels are known to be formed of a mono-layer of endothelial cells without intercellular tight junctions. They also lack a basement membrane and smooth muscle cells to cover the endothelial cell layer unlike blood vessels making them an easy target for invasion [64]. Tumor cells are known to release VEGF-A, which is a potent activator of vascular endothelial receptor 1 (VEGF-R1) and R2, known to induce angiogenesis as well as the release of VEGF-C and –D, which activate VEGF-R3 known to induce lymphangiogenesis oriented towards the tumor cells. In turn, lymphatic vessels are thought to secrete chemokines such as CCL21, which might attract invading tumor cells [64].

It remains a topic for debate as to whether tumor cells migrate actively towards the blood and lymph vessels or whether it is a passive migratory process. The fact that the newly formed tumor blood vessels are immature, lacking organization and intercellular junctions may support the claim that tumor cells simply grow through the fragile endothelium, forming clumps in the lumen due to intravascular proliferation [65]. However, strong evidence exists to support active migration, such as the change in tumor cell expression of growth factors and their receptors influenced by TME components such as TAMs and CAFs. Transient TGF-β activation of TGF-β type 2 receptor/Smad4 induced EMT and stimulated their invasion of blood vessels whereas prolonged TGF-β activation hindered the process [30]. In the lymphatic vessels, on the other hand, invading cells were found to be organized solely in non-EMT clusters and independent of TGF beta signaling [66]. It is therefore safe to assume that both active and passive mechanisms occur in the intravasation process of tumor cells, requiring both EMT and non-EMT cells for hematogenous intravasation (**Figure 2**).

2.5.2. Survival of tumor cell against circulating immune cells and sheering forces

In order for metastasis to be successful, disseminated tumor cells have to survive the immune system as well as the shearing forces of the circulation. It was shown that disseminating tumor cells are shielded by adherent platelets which protect the cancer cells from shearing forces and natural killer cells, as well as aid in extravasation [67]. Disseminating tumor cells were found to express membrane-bound tissue factor, which is activated by coagulation factors such as VIIa and X. Proteinase activated receptor 2 (PAR2) is activated by the Tf-VIIa complex causing immunomodulation, angiogenesis and evasion of apoptosis in the tumor cells [68]. Elevated platelet count and concentration was found to be correlated in a clinical setting with lower survival in colorectal, breast and lung cancers while treatment with anticoagulants lowered metastasis in cancer patients [69].

2.6. Extravasation

2.6.1. Mechanism

Once circulating tumor cells (CTCs) have found their way into the lumen of the blood vessels, they will extravasate and attempt to invade foreign tissues. Knowledge of CTC extravasation is modeled after leukocyte migration across the endothelium into target inflammatory tissue [35]. The extravasation process maybe both, active or passive. Organ specificity or tissue tropism of certain carcinomas may be due to a number of factors. The vascular structure may be more favorable in certain organs such as in the bone marrow, which has a single layer of endothelial cells thus facilitating the movement of red blood cells in and out of the bone marrow. This route constitutes an easy target for CTC extravasation, making the bone marrow a preferred destination for metastasis of various carcinomas such as breast, gastric and prostate cancers [70].

In the case of CRC, the organization and arrangement of the circulation is the major determinant of CRC metastasis. CRC is known to have a strong tropism for metastasis to the liver although the cells themselves may be poorly adapted to the liver environment. However, the portal circulation, draining directly from the mesentery into the liver, transports millions of tumor cells over from the colon to the liver microvasculature, making liver metastasis possible although otherwise it would have been highly unlikely. In these cases, extravasation and homing into a certain tissue is passive and dependent of the organization of the circulation as well as its structure [5]. However, active processes are also at work where CTCs bind to specific features in the organ of interest such as TIMP1, which drives CRC metastasis to the liver by stimulating the HGF pathway [71]. We may thus conclude that extravasation at a certain site or homing of CTCs is dependent on mechanical and organizational features of the circulation as well as on specific interactions between the tumor cells and the endothelium in question (**Figure 3**).

2.6.2. Passive extravasation

Passive extravasation entails no active migration involving molecular interactions between CTCs and endothelial cells. The endothelium often sheds endothelial cells from its wall creating an opening through which CTCs enter into the parenchyma of the invaded tissue. The CTCs may also proliferate inside of the lumen which causes an increase in size and ends with the rupture of the vascular wall, giving full access to the target organ [72]. Furthermore CTCs are known to associate with platelets for protection within the circulation, therefore damage in the blood vessel wall, exposing fibrinogen on endothelial cells, attracts platelets and tumor cells alike. Fibrin clots can further damage the blood vessels, which attract even more platelets in CTC to the site of injury. Furthermore tumor cells may also migrate into other tissues following the migration pattern of white blood cells within the circulation.

2.6.3. Active extravasation

Countless studies have shown that homing and extravasation might be more than simply a mechanical response to a faulty environment. TAMs were shown to secrete TNF-α, VEGF and TGF-β into the circulation to distal tissues where they activate tissue macrophage production of S100A8, which is a chemoattractant for CTCs [46]. CTC attachment to the endothelium is allowed by endothelial cell P- and E-selectins binding to tumor cells as well as tumor glycan patterns and adhesion molecule interactions such as integrin and CD44 interactions [73]. Overexpression of mucin carbohydrate is correlated with increased metastasis in CRC. Constituents of the ECM such as laminin and fibronectin may increase the arrest of

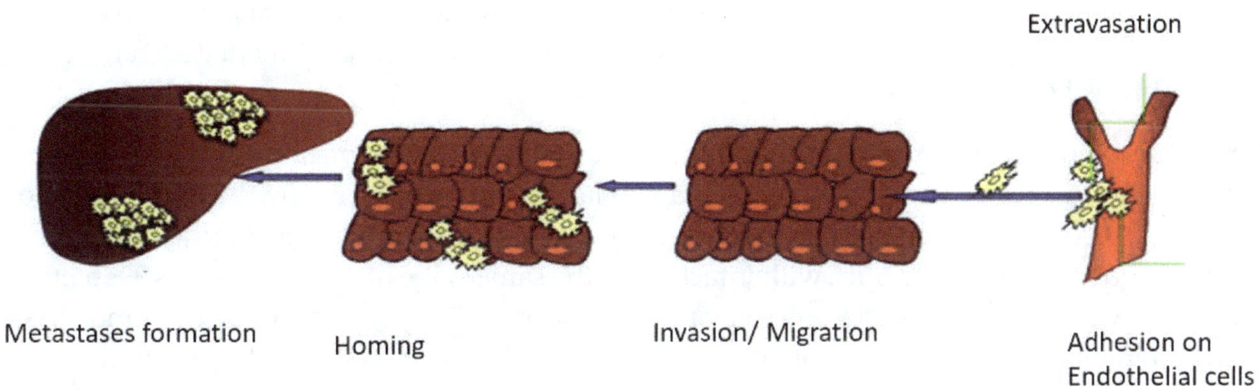

Figure 3. The tiny fraction of the disseminated tumor cells that were able to survive the previous steps must undergo extravasation, migration and homing into the distant organ with different histological nature. Adaption of the new environment demands further physiologic elasticity from the cells.

tumor cells at a certain site in the vasculature. However, when this interaction is counteracted by targeting peptides against fibronectin and laminin, it was found that it reduces the formation of metastasis. Circulating tumor cells may also increase vascular permeability and cause retraction of endothelial cells to expose the ECM for attachment by secreting VEGF which activates SRC (**Figure 3**).

2.6.4. Chemokines and colorectal cancer

Multiple interactions between tumor and stromal cells often contribute to the tumor progression. These interactions are mediated by a variety of growth factors, enzymes and chemokines. In this regard, chemokines play their role in three possible routes, which are enhanced proliferation by auto-or paracrine manner (a), modulating the immune response (b) or favoring the angiogenesis (c). Effects of chemokines in CRC are quite vital in terms of tumor growth and its metastasis. Many of the clinical studies have indicated the expressional changes of chemokines in CRC development and progression. CXC-chemokines are more important in this regard, as these chemokines have been shown to modulate the anti-tumor immune response, behavior of the epithelial cells and cross talk with the stroma. Chemokines are of vital importance in CRC metastasis, where chemotactic signals from different organs facilitate the directional migration of CRC cells, which lead to the metastatic state of the disease. In this context, several studies have highlighted the high expression of chemokine receptors (e.g. CXCR4, CXCR3, CCR6, CCR1 and CCRL2, CCR7 and CCR5) which favor the metastasis of CRC to lymph nodes and liver [47, 74, 75, 23].

2.7. Homing

For the immune response in host tissues, a focus is made on Kupffer cells in CRC liver metastasis. In the case of CRC metastasis to the liver, Kupffer cells (KC), which are the resident liver macrophages, have been reported to directly kill cancer cells through the secretion of cytotoxic molecules such as TNF-α, reactive oxygen species and enhancing the antitumor response of other immune cells such as T effector cells. They have also been reported to have a protumorigenic effect by producing signaling molecules such as cytokines and chemokines, which promote angiogenesis, ECM remodeling and cleavage and recruitment of TAMs. KC are the only characterized macrophages that exhibit dectin-2 receptor mediated cancer cell phagocytosis [76].

In a mouse model of colorectal cancer liver metastasis, KC were chemically depleted by gadolinium chloride before tumor induction and at a later stage of tumor growth, after liver colonization. Absence of KC at the early stage of liver metastasis and invasion led to an increase in tumor burden compared to mice with intact KC at the same stage of liver metastasis. Depletion of KC however in the later stages of liver colonization (18 days) decreased the tumor load with an increase in the number of activated cytotoxic T-cells (CD3+ T cells) and infiltrating cells expressing iNOS with a decrease in the number of VEGF-expressing infiltrating cells, as opposed to non-depleted animals. These results point towards a bimodal role of KC in liver metastasis and tumors, with an antitumor effect in early stages of metastasis, before tumor establishment in the liver, and a protumorigenic effect at later stages of liver colonization and metastasis. Deeper understanding of the precise contribution of KC in CRC liver metastasis may be beneficial for timing immunomodulatory therapies [77]. It was also observed that the occurrence of CRC liver metastasis is rare in patients with cirrhotic livers. Upon closer investigation, it was found that a rat colon cancer cell line (RCN-9) pretreated with conditioned media of KC from cirrhotic rat livers and then inoculated into rat liver showed a reduced incidence of hepatic colonization. In vitro, RCN-9 cells were found to be sensitized to TIL-FasR-mediated killing after treatment with cirrhotic KC media by upregulation of FasR on RCN-9 cells [78]. This further confirms the versatility and importance of the role KC may play in tumor progression.

3. Antimetastatic treatment for CRC

3.1. Targeted therapies for metastatic detachment

To effectively eliminate metastatic cancer cells, it is suggested that both anoikis-dependent and anoikis-independent pathways should be targeted. Fortunately, many of the signaling pathways are already the targets of current FDA-approved therapeutic drugs such as bevacizumab (Avastin) against VEGF, ramucirumab (Cyramza) against VEGF receptor, cetuximab (Erbitux) and panitumumab (Vectibix) against EGF receptor [6].

However, there are significant molecular differences between tumors, which can affect both prognosis and response to treatment. Personalized medicine aims to tailor treatment according to the characteristics of the individual patient and is now a clinical reality as testing for *KRAS* mutations to guide treatment with the anti-EGFR monoclonal antibodies cetuximab and panitumumab is now part of routine clinical practice. However, not all patients who are *KRAS* wild type respond to anti-EGFR therapy and a validated biomarker for antiangiogenic therapy is still lacking. Therefore, other molecular biomarkers are needed to assist with predicting response to both existing drugs as well as to drugs currently under investigation [79].

3.1.1. Role of personalized medicine in metastatic detachment

Advances in the treatment of metastatic colorectal cancer have led to an improvement in survival from 12 months with fluorouracil monotherapy to approximately 2 years. However, there are significant molecular differences between tumors which can affect both prognosis and response to treatment. Personalized medicine aims to tailor treatment according to the characteristics of the individual patient, specifically for early metastatic prognosis and biomarker precision application to personalized treatments. In metastatic colorectal cancer an improved understanding of the underlying pathology and molecular biology has successfully merged with advances in diagnostic techniques and local/systemic therapies as well as improvements in the functioning of multidisciplinary teams, to enable tailored treatment regimens and optimized outcomes. Indeed, as a result of these advancements, median survival for patients with mCRC is now in the range of 20–24 months, having approximately tripled in the last 20 years.

3.1.2. Anti-epidermal growth factor receptor therapies in mCRC personalized treatment

The first true use of personalized medicine in mCRC was the clinical testing of *KRAS* mutations (which occur in approximately 45–50% of patients with CRC) [80]. Subsequently the anti-EGFR treatment is given only to patients who are *KRAS* wild type. However, not all patients who are *KRAS* wild type respond to anti-EGFR therapy and therefore there has been substantial research into other potential predictive biomarkers for future precision application [81].

3.1.3. BRAF mutation in personalized therapy of mCRC

After KRAS mutations, BRAF V600E mutations currently have the strongest evidence to support their use as a predictive biomarker for EGFR-targeted mAb activity. Overall, BRAFV600E activating mutations occur in approximately 10–15% of CRC tumors and are generally mutually exclusive to KRAS mutations [82]. Most but not all of the available evidence links BRAF V600E mutations with resistance to EGFR-targeted mAb therapy [83], however, the impact of tumor BRAF status on efficacy of these treatments has not yet definitively been addressed due to the relatively small number of patients with BRAF mutations.

3.1.4. The PI3K pathway in mCRC personalized therapy

The main alterations in the PI3K pathway in CRC are mutations in PIK3CA and loss of PTEN protein expression. These molecular alterations may coexist with KRAS and BRAF mutations and this makes it more challenging to ascertain their clinical significance [84]. However, PTEN loss correlates with advanced and metastatic tumors and has been associated with worse survival outcomes in CRC.

Several studies revealed that PIK3CA mutations or PTEN loss are associated with a lack of response to anti-EGFR therapies and these alterations therefore appear to have a negative predictive role [85].

Moreover, the personalized strategy has yet developed to be exon specific. For example, mutations in exon 20 of PIK3CA have been associated with a low response rate to anti-EGFR therapy, whereas mutations in exon 9 do not appear to have this effect, which leads to taking research on mutation correlation with the metastatic therapy more specific [86].

Huge advances have already been made, which can be exemplified by recent progress in the management of mCRC, particularly the discovery and implementation of *KRAS* as a predictive biomarker. Indeed, the implementation of new technologies is leading to the accumulation of huge amounts of genomic and proteomic data and the identification and validation of predictive biomarkers for existing and new targeted therapies and will likely improve patient outcomes in the future.

True personalized medicine in mCRC currently remains an aspiration for the future rather than a clinical reality. However, it is likely that a molecular screening approach to treatment will become increasingly used in the future to fully characterize tumors and identify patients who are most likely to benefit from targeted treatments. This holds great promise for the improvement of patient outcomes but brings its own logistical and financial challenges as well as new complexities, such as how to overcome tumor heterogeneity, how to interpret a patient's molecular profile to select the most appropriate treatment and how to prevent rapid development of treatment resistance.

Author details

Hassan Adwan[1*], Dina Elharouni[1], Danira Habashy[1], Nadine Banna[1], Rania Georges[2], Asim Pervaiz[3] and Martin R. Berger[2]

*Address all correspondence to: hassan.adwan@guc.edu.eg

1 Department of Pharmacology and Toxicology, Faculty of Pharmacy and Biotechnology, The German University in Cairo, Cairo, New Cairo City, Egypt

2 Toxicology and Chemotherapy Unit, German Cancer Research Center, Heidelberg, Germany

3 Department of Allied Health Sciences, University of Health Sciences, Lahore, Pakistan

References

[1] Seyfried TN, Huysentruyt LC. On the origin of cancer metastasis. Critical Reviews in Oncogenesis. 2013;**18**(1-2):43-73

[2] Valastyan S, Weinberg RA. Tumor metastasis: Molecular insights and evolving paradigms. Cell. Oct 2011;**147**(2):275-292

[3] Massagué J, Obenauf AC. Metastatic colonization by circulating tumour cells. Nature. Jan 2016;**529**(7586):298-306

[4] Oskarsson T, Batlle E, Massagué J. Metastatic stem cells: Sources, niches, and vital pathways. Cell Stem Cell. Mar 2014;**14**(3):306-321

[5] Chaffer CL, Weinberg RA. A perspective on cancer cell metastasis. Science. Mar 2011; **331**(6024):1559-1564

[6] Buchheit CL, Weigel KJ, Schafer ZT. Cancer cell survival during detachment from the ECM: Multiple barriers to tumour progression. Nature Reviews. Cancer. Sep 2014; **14**(9):632-641

[7] Frisch SM, Screaton RA. Anoikis mechanisms. Current Opinion in Cell Biology. Oct 2001; **13**(5):555-562

[8] Sakamoto S, Kyprianou N. Targeting anoikis resistance in prostate cancer metastasis. Molecular Aspects of Medicine. Apr 2010;**31**(2):205-214

[9] Douma S, Van Laar T, Zevenhoven J, Meuwissen R, Van Garderen E, Peeper DS. Suppression of anoikis and induction of metastasis by the neurotrophic receptor TrkB. Nature. Aug 2004;**430**(7003):1034-1039

[10] Al-Ahwal MS, Shafik YH, Al-Ahwal HM. First national survival data for colorectal cancer among Saudis between 1994 and 2004: What's next? BMC Public Health. Jan 2013;**13**:73

[11] van Roy F, Berx G. The cell-cell adhesion molecule E-cadherin. Cellular and Molecular Life Sciences. Nov 2008;**65**(23):3756-3788

[12] Jiang WG. E-cadherin and its associated protein catenins, cancer invasion and metastasis. The British Journal of Surgery. Apr 1996;**83**(4):437-446

[13] Stockinger A, Eger A, Wolf J, Beug H, Foisner R. E-cadherin regulates cell growth by modulating proliferation-dependent beta-catenin transcriptional activity. The Journal of Cell Biology. Sep 2001;**154**(6):1185-1196

[14] Bolós V, Peinado H, Pérez-Moreno MA, Fraga MF, Esteller M, Cano A. The transcription factor slug represses E-cadherin expression and induces epithelial to mesenchymal transitions: A comparison with snail and E47 repressors. Journal of Cell Science. Feb 2003;**116**(Pt 3):499-511

[15] Hynes RO. Integrins: Bidirectional, allosteric signaling machines. Cell. Sep 2002;**110**(6): 673-687

[16] Chan DA, Giaccia AJ. Hypoxia, gene expression, and metastasis. Cancer Metastasis Reviews. Jun 2007;**26**(2):333-339

[17] Chan DA, Sutphin PD, Denko NC, Giaccia AJ. Role of prolyl hydroxylation in oncogenically stabilized hypoxia-inducible factor-1alpha. The Journal of Biological Chemistry. Oct 2002;**277**(42):40112-40117

[18] Pennacchietti S, Michieli P, Galluzzo M, Mazzone M, Giordano S, Comoglio PM. Hypoxia promotes invasive growth by transcriptional activation of the met protooncogene. Cancer Cell. Apr 2003;**3**(4):347-361

[19] Esteban MA et al. Regulation of E-cadherin expression by VHL and hypoxia-inducible factor. Cancer Research. Apr 2006;**66**(7):3567-3575

[20] Jun JC, Rathore A, Younas H, Gilkes D, Polotsky VY. Hypoxia-inducible factors and cancer. Current Sleep Medicine Reports. Mar 2017;**3**(1):1-10

[21] Kalluri R, Weinberg RA. The basics of epithelial-mesenchymal transition. The Journal of Clinical Investigation. Jun 2009;**119**(6):1420-1428

[22] Friedl P, Wolf K. Plasticity of cell migration: A multiscale tuning model. The Journal of Cell Biology. Jan 2010;**188**(1):11-19

[23] Akram IG, Georges R, Hielscher T, Adwan H, Berger MR. The chemokines CCR1 and CCRL2 have a role in colorectal cancer liver metastasis. Tumour Biology. Feb 2016; **37**(2):2461-2471

[24] Škovierová H, Okajčeková T, Strnádel J, Vidomanová E, Halašová E. Molecular regulation of epithelial-to-mesenchymal transition in tumorigenesis (review). International Journal of Molecular Medicine. Mar 2018;**41**(3):1187-1200

[25] Christofori G. New signals from the invasive front. Nature. May 2006;**441**(7092):444-450

[26] Wellner U et al. The EMT-activator ZEB1 promotes tumorigenicity by repressing stemness-inhibiting microRNAs. Nature Cell Biology. Dec 2009;**11**(12):1487-1495

[27] Friedl P, Hegerfeldt Y, Tusch M. Collective cell migration in morphogenesis and cancer. The International Journal of Developmental Biology. 2004;**48**(5-6):441-449

[28] Hegerfeldt Y, Tusch M, Bröcker E-B, Friedl P. Collective cell movement in primary melanoma explants: Plasticity of cell-cell interaction, beta1-integrin function, and migration strategies. Cancer Research. Apr 2002;**62**(7):2125-2130

[29] Wolf K et al. Multi-step pericellular proteolysis controls the transition from individual to collective cancer cell invasion. Nature Cell Biology. Aug 2007;**9**(8):893-904

[30] Giampieri S, Manning C, Hooper S, Jones L, Hill CS, Sahai E. Localized and reversible TGFbeta signalling switches breast cancer cells from cohesive to single cell motility. Nature Cell Biology. Nov 2009;**11**(11):1287-1296

[31] Artym VV, Zhang Y, Seillier-Moiseiwitsch F, Yamada KM, Mueller SC. Dynamic interactions of cortactin and membrane type 1 matrix metalloproteinase at invadopodia: Defining the stages of invadopodia formation and function. Cancer Research. Mar 2006; **66**(6):3034-3043

[32] Friedl P, Wolf K. Tumour-cell invasion and migration: Diversity and escape mechanisms. Nature Reviews. Cancer. May 2003;**3**(5):362-374

[33] Condeelis J, Segall JE. Intravital imaging of cell movement in tumours. Nature Reviews. Cancer. Dec 2003;**3**(12):921-930

[34] Massagué J. TGFbeta in cancer. Cell. Jul 2008;**134**(2):215-230

[35] Joyce JA, Pollard JW. Microenvironmental regulation of metastasis. Nature Reviews. Cancer. Apr 2009;**9**(4):239-252

[36] Wessler S, Krisch LM, Elmer DP, Aberger F. From inflammation to gastric cancer-The importance of Hedgehog/GLI signaling in *Helicobacter pylori*-induced chronic inflammatory and neoplastic diseases. Cell Communication and Signaling. Apr 2017;**15**(1):15

[37] Jarosz-Biej M et al. M1-like macrophages change tumor blood vessels and microenvironment in murine melanoma. PLoS One. 2018;**13**(1):e0191012

[38] Chanmee T, Ontong P, Konno K, Itano N. Tumor-associated macrophages as major players in the tumor microenvironment. Cancers (Basel). Aug 2014;**6**(3):1670-1690

[39] Goswami A et al. Binding and phosphorylation of par-4 by akt is essential for cancer cell survival. Molecular Cell. Oct 2005;**20**(1):33-44

[40] Hawinkels LJAC et al. Interaction with colon cancer cells hyperactivates TGF-β signaling in cancer-associated fibroblasts. Oncogene. Jan 2014;**33**(1):97-107

[41] Rupp C et al. IGFBP7, a novel tumor stroma marker, with growth-promoting effects in colon cancer through a paracrine tumor-stroma interaction. Oncogene. Feb 2015;**34**(7): 815-825

[42] De Boeck A et al. Differential secretome analysis of cancer-associated fibroblasts and bone marrow-derived precursors to identify microenvironmental regulators of colon cancer progression. Proteomics. Jan 2013;**13**(2):379-388

[43] Herrera M et al. Cancer-associated fibroblast and M2 macrophage markers together predict outcome in colorectal cancer patients. Cancer Science. Apr 2013;**104**(4):437-444

[44] Henriksson ML et al. Colorectal cancer cells activate adjacent fibroblasts resulting in FGF1/FGFR3 signaling and increased invasion. The American Journal of Pathology. Mar 2011;**178**(3):1387-1394

[45] Tommelein J, Verset L, Boterberg T, Demetter P, Bracke M, De Wever O. Cancer-associated fibroblasts connect metastasis-promoting communication in colorectal cancer. Frontiers in Oncology. 2015;**5**:63

[46] Liu C et al. A zebrafish model discovers a novel mechanism of stromal fibroblast-mediated cancer metastasis. Clinical Cancer Research. Aug 2017;**23**(16):4769-4779

[47] Müller A et al. Involvement of chemokine receptors in breast cancer metastasis. Nature. Mar 2001;**410**(6824):50-56

[48] Bissell MJ, Radisky D. Putting tumours in context. Nature Reviews. Cancer. Oct 2001; **1**(1):46-54

[49] Delektorskaya VV, Kushlinskii NE. Clinical significance of the content of biomolecular markers in invasive front of colon carcinomas. Bulletin of Experimental Biology and Medicine. Jan 2011;**150**(3):368-371

[50] Bracke ME, Van Roy FM, Mareel MM. The E-cadherin/catenin complex in invasion and metastasis. Current Topics in Microbiology and Immunology. 1996;**213**(Pt 1):123-161

[51] Friedl P, Bröcker EB. The biology of cell locomotion within three-dimensional extracellular matrix. Cellular and Molecular Life Sciences. Jan 2000;**57**(1):41-64

[52] Jia Z et al. Tumor cell pseudopodial protrusions. Localized signaling domains coordinating cytoskeleton remodeling, cell adhesion, glycolysis, RNA translocation, and protein translation. The Journal of Biological Chemistry. Aug 2005;**280**(34):30564-30573

[53] Tlsty TD, Coussens LM. Tumor stroma and regulation of cancer development. Annual Review of Pathology. 2006;**1**:119-150

[54] Aumailley M, Smyth N. The role of laminins in basement membrane function. Journal of Anatomy. Jul 1998;**193**(Pt 1):1-21

[55] Mercurio AM, Rabinovitz I, Shaw LM. The alpha 6 beta 4 integrin and epithelial cell migration. Current Opinion in Cell Biology. Oct 2001;**13**(5):541-545

[56] Tran M et al. Targeting a tumor-specific laminin domain critical for human carcinogenesis. Cancer Research. Apr 2008;**68**(8):2885-2894

[57] Gilles C et al. Contribution of MT1-MMP and of human laminin-5 gamma2 chain degradation to mammary epithelial cell migration. Journal of Cell Science. Aug 2001;**114**(Pt 16):2967-2976

[58] Guess CM, Quaranta V. Defining the role of laminin-332 in carcinoma. Matrix Biology. Oct 2009;**28**(8):445-455

[59] Georges R, Adwan H, Zhivkova M, Eyol E, Bergmann F, Berger MR. Regulation of osteopontin and related proteins in rat CC531 colorectal cancer cells. International Journal of Oncology. Aug 2010;**37**(2):249-256

[60] Uhlmann ME et al. Influence of osteopontin expression on the metastatic growth of CC531 rat colorectal carcinoma cells in rat liver. Cancer Gene Therapy. Nov 2011;**18**(11):795-805

[61] Adur J, Carvalho HF, Cesar CL, Casco VH. Nonlinear optical microscopy signal processing strategies in cancer. Cancer Informatics. 2014;**13**:67-76

[62] Birk JW et al. Second harmonic generation imaging distinguishes both high-grade dysplasia and cancer from normal colonic mucosa. Digestive Diseases and Sciences. Jul 2014;**59**(7):1529-1534

[63] Tong RT, Boucher Y, Kozin SV, Winkler F, Hicklin DJ, Jain RK. Vascular normalization by vascular endothelial growth factor receptor 2 blockade induces a pressure gradient across the vasculature and improves drug penetration in tumors. Cancer Research. Jun 2004;**64**(11):3731-3736

[64] Alitalo K, Tammela T, Petrova TV. Lymphangiogenesis in development and human disease. Nature. Dec 2005;**438**(7070):946-953

[65] Chung JY et al. Competitive enhancement of HGF-induced epithelial scattering by accessory growth factors. Experimental Cell Research. Feb 2011;**317**(3):307-318

[66] Tsuji T, Ibaragi S, Hu G. Epithelial-mesenchymal transition and cell cooperativity in metastasis. Cancer Research. Sep 2009;**69**(18):7135-7139

[67] Im JH et al. Coagulation facilitates tumor cell spreading in the pulmonary vasculature during early metastatic colony formation. Cancer Research. Dec 2004;**64**(23):8613-8619

[68] Schaffner F, Ruf W. Tissue factor and PAR2 signaling in the tumor microenvironment. Arteriosclerosis, Thrombosis, and Vascular Biology. Dec 2009;**29**(12):1999-2004

[69] Nash GF, Turner LF, Scully MF, Kakkar AK. Platelets and cancer. The Lancet Oncology. Jul 2002;**3**(7):425-430

[70] Alix-Panabières C, Riethdorf S, Pantel K. Circulating tumor cells and bone marrow micrometastasis. Clinical Cancer Research. Aug 2008;**14**(16):5013-5021

[71] Kopitz C et al. Tissue inhibitor of metalloproteinases-1 promotes liver metastasis by induction of hepatocyte growth factor signaling. Cancer Research. Sep 2007;**67**(18):8615-8623

[72] Sahai E. Illuminating the metastatic process. Nature Reviews. Cancer. Oct 2007;**7**(10): 737-749

[73] Gout S, Huot J. Role of cancer microenvironment in metastasis: Focus on colon cancer. Cancer Microenvironment. 2008;**1**(1):69-83

[74] Zabel BA, Lewén S, Berahovich RD, Jaén JC, Schall TJ. The novel chemokine receptor CXCR7 regulates trans-endothelial migration of cancer cells. Molecular Cancer. Jun 2011;**10**:73

[75] Pervaiz A, Ansari S, Berger MR, Adwan H. CCR5 blockage by maraviroc induces cytotoxic and apoptotic effects in colorectal cancer cells. Medical Oncology. May 2015;**32**(5):158

[76] Lee JH, Lee S-W. The roles of carcinoembryonic antigen in liver metastasis and therapeutic approaches. Gastroenterology Research and Practice. 2017;**2017**:7521987

[77] Wen SW, Ager EI, Christophi C. Bimodal role of Kupffer cells during colorectal cancer liver metastasis. Cancer Biology & Therapy. Jul 2013;**14**(7):606-613

[78] Song RX et al. Effect of long-term estrogen deprivation on apoptotic responses of breast cancer cells to 17beta-estradiol. Journal of the National Cancer Institute. Nov 2001;**93**(22):1714-1723

[79] Moorcraft SY, Smyth EC, Cunningham D. The role of personalized medicine in metastatic colorectal cancer: An evolving landscape. Therapeutic Advances in Gastroenterology. Sep 2013;**6**(5):381-395

[80] Yamauchi M et al. Assessment of colorectal cancer molecular features along bowel subsites challenges the conception of distinct dichotomy of proximal versus distal colorectum. Gut. Jun 2012;**61**(6):847-854

[81] Zhao B et al. Mechanisms of resistance to anti-EGFR therapy in colorectal cancer. Oncotarget. Jan 2017;**8**(3):3980-4000

[82] Pritchard CC, Grady WM. Colorectal cancer molecular biology moves into clinical practice. Gut. Jan 2011;**60**(1):116-129

[83] Mao C, Liao R-Y, Qiu L-X, Wang X-W, Ding H, Chen Q. BRAF V600E mutation and resistance to anti-EGFR monoclonal antibodies in patients with metastatic colorectal cancer: A meta-analysis. Molecular Biology Reports. Apr 2011;**38**(4):2219-2223

[84] Bardelli A, Siena S. Molecular mechanisms of resistance to cetuximab and panitumumab in colorectal cancer. Journal of Clinical Oncology. Mar 2010;**28**(7):1254-1261

[85] Di Fiore F, Sesboüé R, Michel P, Sabourin JC, Frebourg T. Molecular determinants of anti-EGFR sensitivity and resistance in metastatic colorectal cancer. British Journal of Cancer. Dec 2010;**103**(12):1765-1772

[86] De Roock W et al. Effects of KRAS, BRAF, NRAS, and PIK3CA mutations on the efficacy of cetuximab plus chemotherapy in chemotherapy-refractory metastatic colorectal cancer: A retrospective consortium analysis. The Lancet Oncology. Aug 2010;**11**(8):753-762

5

Epithelial-Mesenchymal Transition in Tumor Microenvironment Induced by Hypoxia

Görkem Eskiizmir and Erdoğan Özgür

Abstract

A tumor microenvironment contains various noncancerous cells including adipocytes, fibroblasts, immune and inflammatory cells, neuroendocrine cells, pericytes, vascular and lymphatic endothelial cells, and the extracellular matrix that surrounds cancerous cells. In the tumor microenvironment, cancer cells interact and cross talk with noncancerous cells and orchestrate different mechanisms of cancer such as tumorigenesis, angiogenesis, and metastasis. Moreover, the expansive nature of cancer cells and chaotic angiogenesis affect microcirculation as well as alter the oxygen concentration progressively. Hypoxia, a key player in the multistep process of cancer metastasis, is important in different regions of the tumor microenvironment. Hypoxia may transform cancer cells to become more aggressive and invasive by triggering overexpression of several hypoxia-related factors that activate epithelial-mesenchymal transition (EMT). Herein, the current knowledge of how hypoxia-driven EMT is presented in the tumor microenvironment of solid cancers is discussed.

Keywords: cancer, cancer metastasis, epithelial-mesenchymal transition, hypoxia, tumor microenvironment

1. Tumor microenvironment: current perspective

The tumor microenvironment contains a multinetwork of cells, soluble factors, extracellular matrix (ECM) components, and signaling molecules that surround and neighbor cancer cells. It mediates aberrant tissue function and modulates subsequent progression in solid cancers [1]. In this microenvironment, the main structures are the parenchyma, stroma, growth factors, lymphokines and cytokines, and inflammatory and matrix metalloproteinase enzymes

(**Figure 1**). While cancer cells are located in the parenchyma, noncancerous cells and ECM constitute the stroma. Currently, it is known that noncancerous cells have key roles in several mechanisms of carcinogenesis, tumor progression, and metastatic cascade [2]. Noncancerous cells behave differently in the tumor microenvironment than healthy tissue. However, it is still unclear how noncancerous cells and noncellular components of the tumor niche collaborate and assist cancer cells to acquire invasive and metastatic features.

It is known that chronic inflammation is an important factor in shaping the tumor microenvironment. The major inflammatory cells located in the tumor microenvironment are T lymphocytes, natural killer cells, and tumor-associated macrophages (TAMS). TAMs are important in ECM destruction/restructuring of the tumor microenvironment, tumor cell motility, and triggering angiogenesis. These cells have both tumor-progressive and tumor-suppressive effects.

In the tumor microenvironment, fibroblasts have various roles under inflammatory conditions. However, they attain new characters and called as "*carcinoma-associated fibroblasts*" after the beginning of the neoplastic process. They constitute 50–70% of the volume of many solid epithelial tumors, such as pancreas, stomach, and breast cancers [3]. In addition, they are particularly effective in carcinogenesis, tumor progression, and metastasis [4, 5]. Studies on carcinoma-associated fibroblasts demonstrated that during the chronic inflammation and wound healing, only activated fibroblasts promote tumor growth. There are hypotheses about the production of cancer-associated fibroblasts. Genetic changes in normal fibroblast or exposure to EMT may directly arise from mesenchymal stem cells [6].

Cancer stem cells (CSCs) are also tumor microenvironment-specific cells. CSCs have been intensively researched recently. Today, we know many cancer types consist CSCs in their microenvironment, which is associated with aggressive tumor biology and treatment resistance. Moreover, CSCs are responsible for immune modulation during the carcinogenesis [7].

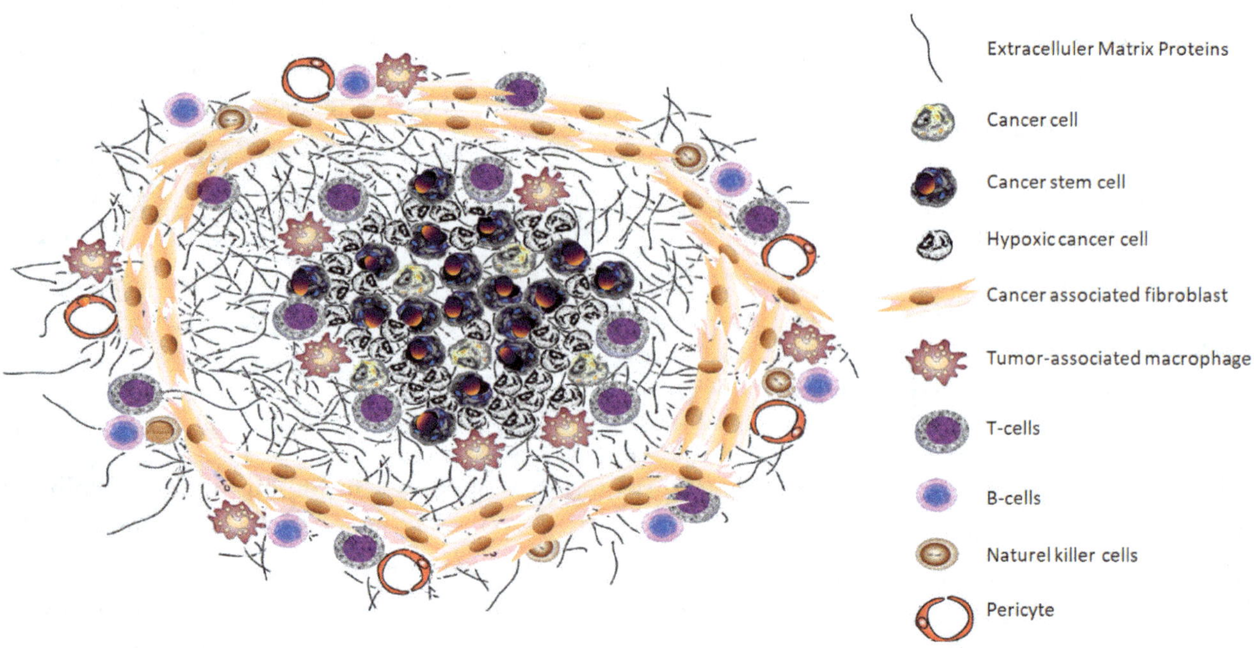

Figure 1. A schematic view of the tumor microenvironment.

In the tumor microenvironment, a unique network has been shown to be created by mainly carcinoma-associated fibroblasts and CSCs with the participant of other noncancerous cells. This network modulates and regulates different mechanisms of the neoplastic processes, such as carcinogenesis, tumor progression, angiogenesis, and metastasis.

Similar to healthy tissue, tumor tissue supplies oxygen and substances from blood and lymphatic vessels. Therefore, angiogenesis is a crucial step for tumor growth [8]. However, due to the rapid growth of tumor tissue, new blood vessel production is usually insufficient. This situation results with decrease of tissue oxygen levels termed as *hypoxia*. This new condition forces cells to acquire new and devastating behaviors such as resistance to environmental changes, invasiveness, and also metastatic phenotypes via different mechanisms. In this review, we aim to focus on the role of hypoxia and hypoxia-driven EMT in tumor microenvironment from the current perspective.

2. Hypoxia in tumor microenvironment

Hypoxia is a hallmark of tumor microenvironment. It emerges due to an inadequate blood source, which keeps proliferation cells viable. The cellular machinery uses several mechanisms in response to hypoxia. When a decrease in the level of oxygen develops, changes in numerous transcriptional regulators are altered.

2.1. Hypoxia: definition

Basically, hypoxia refers to the imbalance between the level of oxygen that the tissues require and that can be supplied. It is noteworthy that *normoxia* describes the "atmospheric" oxygen level which is approximately 20–21% (160 mmHg). However, every healthy tissue has lower and distinct oxygen levels; therefore, *physoxia* is a better terminology that defines the normal range of oxygen levels in different tissues [9]. The oxygen level of different tissues and cancers is presented in **Table 1** [10]. Therefore, hypoxic conditions often occur when the oxygen

Tissue/organ	Physoxia (% O_2)	Cancer	Hypoxia (% O_2)
Brain	4.6	Brain tumor	1.7
Breast	8.5	Breast cancer	1.5
Cervix	5.5	Cervix cancer	1.2
Kidney (cortex)	9.5	Renal cancer	1.3
Liver	4.0–7.3	Liver cancer	0.8
Lung	5.6	Lung cancer (nonsmall cancer)	2.2
Pancreas	7.5	Pancreas tumor	0.3
Rectal mucosa	3.9	Rectal cancer	1.8

Table 1. Physoxia and hypoxia of several tissues/organs and cancers.

tension (pO_2) decreases lower than 2.5 mmHg, even though tumor oxygen levels are dictated by the initial tissue and tumor microenvironment [11, 12]. Moreover, hypoxic regions are heterogeneously distributed particularly in the locally advanced tumors [13].

Cancer cells respond to hypoxia in two ways through apoptosis or resistance and survival, which is driven by the exposure time. If cancer cells are able to survive, they acquire new and unique features. Hypoxic conditions affect the gene transcription, which affords the ability of the cancer to survive through invasiveness, genetic instability, and metastasis. Furthermore, treatment (radiotherapy and/or chemotherapy) resistance may emerge [14]. A hypoxic response is mediated by hypoxia-inducible factors (HIFs), which control many facets of cancer cell viability [15].

2.2. Hypoxia-inducible factors

The HIFs orchestrate the responses to hypoxia in normal and cancer cells. Recently, three subtypes of HIFs have been introduced: HIF-1, -2, and -3. They are heterodimeric complexes and mainly act to mediate cellular processes including angiogenesis, cell proliferation, and tissue remodeling in response to hypoxia. HIFs are composed of basic helix-loop-helix-PER-ARNT-SIM (bHLH-PAS) proteins including an O_2-labile alpha subunit (HIF-1α, -2α, and -3α) and a stable beta subunit (HIF-β). They interact with hypoxia-responsive elements that contain a conserved RCGTG core sequence [16]. HIF-1α was the first introduced prototypic member of HIF family, and has been shown to regulate O_2-dependent transcriptional responses [17]. After a while from the discovery of HIF-1α, a new HIF protein, HIF-2α, was introduced by independent research groups [18–21]. Currently, it is known that HIF-1α is the first biomolecule that responds to acute hypoxia, and HIF-2α is the major regulator under chronic hypoxic conditions. This phenomenon has been referred as the "*hypoxic shift*" [22]. Holmquist-Mengelbier et al. demonstrated that HIF-1α is active for a short duration particularly under hypoxia or anoxia (O_2 level <0.1%). However, HIF-2α is active for a long duration under less severe hypoxia (O_2 level <5.0%) [23]. Furthermore, Pietras et al. reported that the activation of HIF-2α may cause aggressive and infiltrative histopathological features under normal oxygen levels, which is termed as "*pseudohypoxic phenotype*" [24–26]. Tian et al. reported a correlation between HIF-2α and vascular endothelial growth factor mRNA expression levels in the endothelium [21]. Therefore, HIF-2α overexpression may lead to an increase in chaotic vascularization in the tumor microenvironment. In 2002, HIF-3 was introduced by Makino et al. [27]. Although the functions of HIF-3 are not clear yet, Heikkila et al. indicated that HIF-3 might regulate the activity of other HIF complexes [28].

Hypoxic conditions occur heterogenically in almost all types of solid cancers, which lead to HIF protein overexpression. Under physiologic conditions, HIF-1α is constitutively expressed; however, it is degraded rapidly upon its hydroxylation by prolyl hydroxylases (PHDs) [29]. In contrast, the O_2-dependent PHD inhibition develops under hypoxia and HIF-1α protein expression is increased [30]. Under physiological conditions, HIF-1α regulates the expression of important genes that regulate numerous biological processes. In the tumor microenvironment, elevated HIF-α protein expression, which was induced by hypoxia or other oncogenic signals, promotes tumor growth, angiogenesis, and proliferation through the regulation of critical genes (**Figure 2**). Recent evidence has shown that HIF-1α/-2α can impact tumor development through critical oncoproteins and tumor-suppressor genes such as MYC, p53, and mTOR signaling pathway [31–35]. HIFs may also promote the immune-suppressive mechanisms that promote apoptotic resistance in the tumor microenvironment [36]. Therefore, HIF-1α overexpression due to pathological hypoxia is generally related to poor prognosis and tumor progression in solid cancer [37, 38]. Moreover, HIFs promote the progression of cancer through EMT induction. During the EMT, carcinoma cells undergo migration and invasion, leading to cancer progression and metastasis [39].

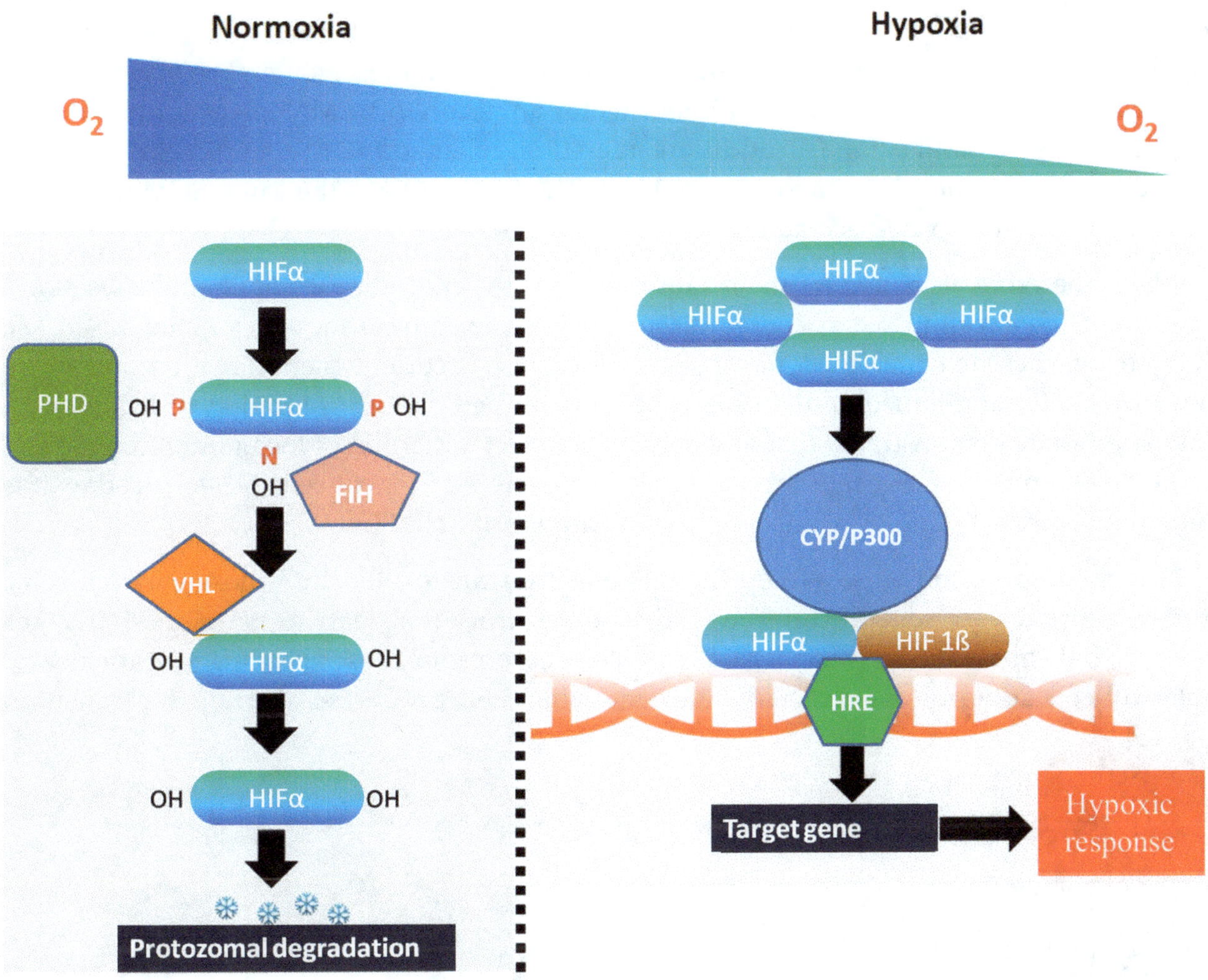

Figure 2. Regulation of HIF in normoxia and hypoxia. During normoxia, PHD enzymes and FIH take role in hydroxylation of HIF-α. Hydroxylation of HIF-α by PHDs creates a binding site for the Von Hippel-Lindau (VHL), HIF-α-VHL interaction leads to proteasomal degradation. Under hypoxic conditions, PHDs and FIH are inhibited due to lack of oxygen. Inhibition of PHDs and FIH lead to HIF-α stabilization and dimerization with its transcriptional partner HIF-1β. HIF-α-HIF-1β interaction leads to translocation to the nucleus and binding to consensus hypoxia-responsive elements (HRE) within the promoters or enhancers of HIF target genes.

3. EMT in cancer: an overview

3.1. Epithelial-mesenchymal transition: definition

Epithelial and mesenchymal cells have various functional characteristics. The epithelium is a thin layer which consists of the collection of cells with similar features that have been associated with one to another by cell-to-cell junctions such as tight junctions, adherens junctions, desmosomes, and gap junctions. Epithelium layer is polarized because apical side and the basal side have different properties that are referred as *apicobasal polarity*. Of note, cell-to-cell junctions consist of cadherins; however, cell-to-basal lamina or ECM junctions consist *laminin*. Moreover, actin is another cell-to-cell adhesion complex which has strong apicobasal polarity. All of these junctions provide immobility to the epithelium. On the other hand, mesenchymal cells do not have these features and only have focal points that adhere to their neighbor mesenchymal cells. Similar to epithelial cells, adhesions between mesenchymal cells can involve cadherin for cell-to-cell junctions and integrins for adhesion to ECM. However, they do not have junctions for basal lamina. In addition, interstitial collagen and fibronectin are important for the ECM adhesion of the mesenchymal cell. They do not have the same ECM molecules associated with the apical-basolateral surface (**Figure 3**).

In 1953, Abercrombie and Heaysman observed that the migration of epithelial cells slows down and they realign when contact each other by forming adhesive junctions [40, 41]. Conversely, mesenchymal cells, particularly fibroblasts, reorient their direction and move away by generating lamellipodia. This process is termed contact inhibition of locomotion. Thereafter, they demonstrated that any defect in contact inhibition of locomotion contributes to the development of invasive and aggressive characters of cancer cells [42–44]. Today, it is known that contact inhibition of locomotion is important in EMT.

EMT is a complex course where epithelial cells are transformed into mesenchymal cells. It is coordinated by several different influential factors that lead to behavioral changes in epithelial cells. Concisely, epithelial cells lose core properties including the apicobasal polarity, cell adhesion, and increase mesenchymal cell properties during the transition [45, 46].

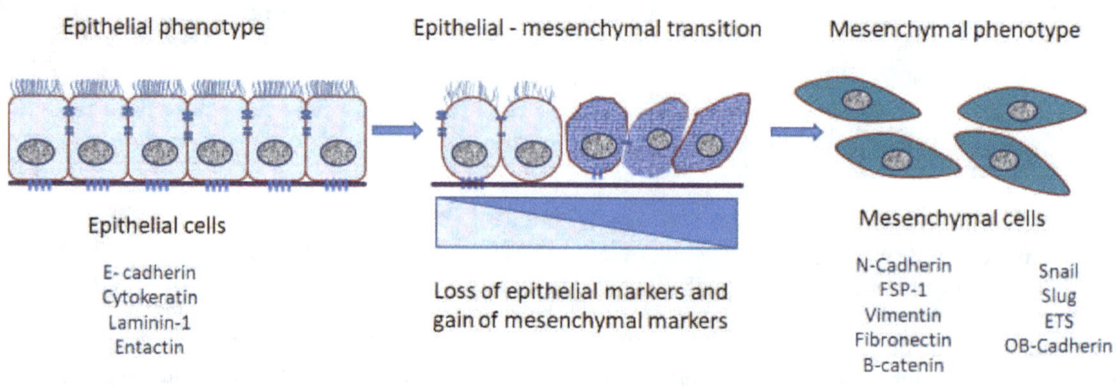

Figure 3. A schema for epithelial-mesenchymal transition. Loss of epithelial markers and gain of mesenchymal markers during the transition from epithelial phenotype to mesenchymal phenotype.

EMT is a naturally occurring transdifferentiation process and is critical during embryonic development and organogenesis. This phenomenon also occurs during wound healing, tissue regeneration, organ fibrosis, and carcinogenesis. In addition, a post-EMT behavior of a part of cells may include reverse transition, which is referred as the *mesenchymal-epithelial transition* [47].

The majority of tumors originate from epithelial tissues of lung, colon, breast, pancreas, prostate, bladder, ovary kidney, liver, and head and neck. Currently, EMT is important in cancer progression and metastasis. Epithelial cells may acquire several abilities such as motility, invasion, and malignant features via EMT [48]. Moreover, it is known that inflammation is the key inducer of EMT in cancer progression. Inflammation may trigger a number of signaling pathways involved in carcinogenesis. However, the specific signals that are induced during the pathologic EMT in epithelial cancers remain unclear [49].

3.2. EMT in physiology and diseases

The mechanisms under the induction and progression of EMT vary dramatically, even though motile cells with mesenchymal phenotype develop consequently. EMT is classified into three different subtypes: type-1, -2, and -3. Type-1 EMT (physiologic EMT) is related to implantation, embryogenesis, and organ development. It is impacted by remodeling and diversification of tissue during morphogenesis. Type-1 EMT is not related with inflammation, fibrosis, and systemic dissemination and generally occurs transiently. Type-2 EMT impacts tissue regeneration and fibrosis, and the process depends on continued inflammation in adults. It continues until the underlying injuries or infections are resolved/repaired. Type-2 EMT may produce mesenchymal cells that are activated. Most notably are the myofibroblasts that produce extreme levels of collagen-rich ECM. Type-3 EMT happens in the context of tumor growth/cancer progression and the tumors transform to a mesenchymal phenotype. The type-3 EMT induction is assisted by genomic changes by cancer cells. It may produce cells that have aggressive properties, which promote movement into the bloodstream in order to spread to other organs.

3.2.1. Type-1 EMT

Type-1 EMT is the exchange from epithelial cells to mesenchymal cells in the embryonic phase events such as implantation, embryogenesis, and organ development. After early embryogenic stages, fertilized egg implantation to the endometrium is associated with an EMT [50, 51]. This is the first step of type-1 EMT that is accompanied by embryonic morphogenesis. At the gastrulation stage, EMT continues with the generation of three germ layers and a primitive streak is made in the epiblast layer [52]. The formation of the primitive streak is the most important part of gastrulation. Primitive streak leads to three germ layers. Thereafter, all tissues are generated during organogenesis by cell migration and differentiation. The EMT coordinates almost every stage of this process [53].

At gastrulation level, the EMT is mainly orchestrated by Wnt signaling [54]. Of note, the TGF-β superfamily, including Nodal and Vg1, and FGF receptors are in close relation to Wnt signaling. Moreover, different signaling modalities through BMPs, c-Myb, and msh homeobox 1 (Msx-1) play roles in the regulation of type-1 EMT [55].

3.2.2. *Type-2 EMT*

Type-2 EMT is the transition of epithelial cells to mesenchymal cells, which occurs during wound healing and fibrosis due to inflammation. It is orchestrated by fibroblasts and inflammatory cells, which release multiple inflammatory molecules, signals, and ECM components such as collagens, laminins, elastin, tenascin, and other matrix molecules. A variety of studies demonstrated an association between EMT and progressive organ fibrosis such as kidney and lung disease [56, 57].

Inflammatory cells and fibroblasts produce proteins such as FSP1, S100 cytoskeletal proteins, α-SMA, and collagen I that develop during the development of organ fibrosis [57]. These proteins have been used as a biomarker for fibrosis of organs, which are undergoing an EMT associated with chronic inflammation. However, epithelial markers, including cytokeratin and E-cadherin, continue to be expressed until they gain a complete fibroblastic phenotype [58]. Rastaldi et al. evaluated the EMT in human renal biopsies of 133 patients with kidney fibrosis. The EMT was detected in the fibrotic kidney based on the staining for cytokeratin, vimentin, α-SMA, and zona occludens 1 (ZO-1) [59]. Kidney fibrosis has been associated with multiple inflammatory cells that induce EMT with various growth factors such as TGF-β, EGF, and FGF-2 [60]. As the role of TGF-β has been determined in kidney fibrosis, several researchers focused on the inhibition of TGF-β using BMP-7 [61]. Morrissey et al. demonstrated that BMP-7 provided the reversal of EMT and repaired tubular structural damage and repopulation of healthy tubular epithelial cells of mice with kidney fibrosis [62].

3.2.3. *Type-3 EMT*

Type-3 EMT is the transmission of epithelial cells to mesenchymal cells in cancer progression, also known as the "*oncogenic epithelial-mesenchymal transition.*" Due to its complexity, oncogenic EMT is more complex than physiologic EMT. The role of type-3 EMT has been demonstrated in different cancer cells. For example, breast and prostate cancer cells can be classified as epithelial predominated or mesenchymal predominated [63, 64]. Zajchowski et al. studied different molecules to predict invasiveness of breast cancer by using gene array method and showed that epithelial proteins are related to noninvasiveness, whereas mesenchymal proteins are related to invasiveness [65]. Currently, several *in vitro/in vivo* studies demonstrated that mesenchymal status leads to an invasive phenotype, motility, and metastasis in cancers.

In solid tumors, loss of E-cadherin [66], cadherin transformation [67], adhesion loss, changes in apicobasal polarity, and tissue architecture modifications have been demonstrated in EMT. In addition, vimentin, N-cadherin, fibronectin, that are the mesenchymal markers, are highly expressed during the EMT [48]. In carcinogenesis and tumor progression, the loss of E-cadherin and increase in the N-cadherin, which is referred as "*cadherin switch,*" are the most significant indicators of the EMT. Currently, it is known that cadherin switch breaks down cell-to-cell junctions and controls the contact inhibition of locomotion. Moreover, it may modulate signal transduction in metastatic cascade [68]. The association between tumor progression and cadherin switch has been demonstrated in prostate cancer, urothelial bladder carcinoma, and malignant melanoma [67, 69, 70].

In literature, there are evidences that support the idea of *"high levels of mesenchymal markers are often related to aggressive tumor behavior and poor prognosis."* In cervix cancers, the correlation between lymph node metastasis and vimentin positivity was also determined [71]. Nevertheless, this correlation has been reported in a small number of cancer types. Therefore, it is hard to mention that vimentin is a definitive predictor of aggressiveness for all cancer types. Ahmad et al. suggested another biomarker for metastatic breast cancer: *stromelysin-3*. Stromelysin-3 is a matrix metalloproteinase and marker for mesenchymal cells. Breast carcinoma cells that undergo EMT are able to express stromelysin-3, which may partly explain the increased metastatic propensity detected in these tumors [72].

Recently, the genetic and biochemical properties that underlie acquirement of cancer cell invasiveness and metastasis are the major areas of intensive research. Xue and colleagues demonstrated that cancer cells departing HER-2/neu expressed a GFP transgene that was facilitated by FSP-1. Moreover, the low rate of metastasis was detected in FSP-1 null mice [73]. This research provided important evidences for the mechanism of metastasis related to EMT. In addition, Yang et al. reported that tumor cells were able to behave like mesenchymal cells and express mesenchymal markers [74]. Besides the evidences about EMT in the metastatic process, some studies have also shown data on reverse EMT. They suggest that the reversibility of EMT is observed during embryonic development and also during the tumor growth at metastatic side. Tumor cells try to undergo not only growth but also cell differentiation to resemble the originating epithelium. Brabletz et al. demonstrated the similarity of epithelial nature between primary tumor side and metastatic tissue for colorectal cancers [75]. It indicates that the induction of an EMT is likely to be central and crucial for the metastatic cascade and implicates EMT during the colonization process.

3.3. Molecular mechanisms and pathways of EMT

In pathologic or physiologic events, the EMT is triggered and controlled by different signaling pathways. Several transcription factors have been described for the regulation of EMT. Tumor growth factor-β signaling appears to be one of the most important pathways. It generally acts as an epithelial cell proliferation suppressor. However, it may also positively affect the tumor progression and metastasis [76, 77]. TGF-β can induce the EMT via two signaling pathways. The first pathway involves Smad proteins that regulate the action of tumor growth factor-β by affecting ALK-5 receptors. Smad proteins mediate signaling pathway effects on motility of cells [61, 78]. Inhibitory Smad can induce autocrine production of TGF-β, thereby, reinforcing epithelial-mesenchymal transition [79]. Recently, β-catenin and LEF found to be relevant with Smad in PDGF-induced EMT [80]. Currently, it is known that TGF-β/Smad/LEF/PDGF axis has important effects on EMT during cancer progression. The second mechanism for TGF-β-induced EMT is MAPK-dependent pathway [81].

Several studies have demonstrated the association between reduced cancer cell E-cadherin levels and activation of EMT [82, 83]. Eger et al. showed that the cFos oncogene induction in mouse mammary epithelial cells induced the EMT by decreasing E-cadherin [84]. The movement of β-catenin from the cytoplasm to nucleus causes acquisition of mesenchymal phenotype by affecting E-cadherin expression. Nuclear buildup of β-catenin has been shown to reduce E-cadherin expression and acquisition of invasive phenotype [85]. Scarpa et al. described the E-cadherin loss as an activation and contact-dependent cell polarity process via Rac signaling [86]. Currently, it is known that reduced E-cadherin levels are highly correlated with poor prognosis and decrease in survival in various cancers such as hepatocellular carcinoma, nonsmall cell lung, oral, esophageal, gastric, cervix and breast cancer, and bone and soft tissue sarcoma [87–95].

3.4. EMT in cancer metastasis: guilty or innocent?

Cancer metastasis is a complex multistep process with sequential molecular and cellular events that promote the transformation of cells, intravasation, survival and ultimately extravasation, implantation, growth, and colonization in a new and foreign tissue environment. As mentioned above, several evidences support that EMT has a major role in cancer metastasis. The EMT signifies the first step of the metastatic cascade. During EMT, cancer cells are able to invade adjacent cell layers following the loss of cell-to-cell adhesion and acquiring motility. Principally, the result of cellular motility is similar to the extensive cell migration and tissue reorganization that occurs during the embryogenesis and organogenesis; however, subsequent steps have different and complex events.

After a journey in the bloodstream, cancer cells that can escape from the immune system, extravasate from the circulation in order to implant and proliferate at the target organ, "*seed and soil theory*." Thereby, a colony of the primary tumor can regrow by inducing angiogenesis in a foreign and apparently "hostile" background. This process is induced by not only genetic/epigenetic factors but also by the nonneoplastic stromal cells [96]. *In vivo* studies demonstrated that this development is generally supplemented with partial or complete EMT. Therefore, the induction of EMT results in the acquisition of metastatic properties in different carcinoma cell lines. Main indicators for the acquisition of mesenchymal properties are the high level of mesenchyme-specific proteins [46]. In contrast to many studies, Tarin et al. reported that the acquirement of mesenchymal markers during tumor progression reflects genomic instability. Therefore, they advocated that EMT does not occur in carcinogenesis [97]. However, synchronized and complex gene-expression patterns are required to provide tumor cells with the mesenchymal properties. Moreover, genomic instability may have more important role in the regulation of EMT. For instance, SNAI1 regulates expression of EMT-associated genes in colorectal carcinoma [98].

A significant evidence for EMT during the metastatic process was presented by Yang et al. They reported that cancer cells were able to behave like mesenchymal cells and express α-SMA, FSP1, desmin, and vimentin [74]. Studies that include functional manipulations on EMT process also provide evidences. For instance, depletion of FSP1/S100A4-positive cells in tumors suppresses metastasis [73].

In adenomatous polyposis coli (APC) and β-catenin mutation-positive colorectal cancers, β-catenin levels are predominantly observed in tumor cells localized at invasion. Moreover, tumor cells with nuclear β-catenin seem to have undergone EMT [99]. Regardless of numerous studies, the major problem for the demonstration of the role of EMT in the metastatic cascade is the detection of cancer cells that have undergone EMT in primary human tumors.

The markers of EMT indicate epithelial phenotype or mesenchymal phenotype not the EMT in cancer metastasis. Therefore, *in vivo* studies with more sensitive indicators are required for understanding the role of EMT in cancer metastasis.

4. A new insight into the mechanisms of hypoxia-induced EMT

Hypoxia is a common situation in tumor microenvironment affecting cancer cell behavior, including progression and metastasis. Currently, it is clearly known that exposure to hypoxic conditions results in HIF-1α overexpression. As mentioned previously, overexpression of HIF-1a is related with promoting EMT for cancer cells. Additionally, it has been demonstrated that hypoxia-induced EMT includes the loss of cell adhesion and cell polarity. It has been observed that hypoxic conditions decrease the E-cadherin expression, but increase N-cadherin expression, a mesenchymal marker [100].

Azab et al. previously demonstrated that multiple myeloma cancer cells cultured in hypoxic conditions and injected into mice were able to spread to the new bone marrow faster than the cells cultured under normoxic conditions [101]. The hypoxia-induced EMT is mainly driven by stabilization and activation of HIF1α. It is controlled by epigenetic changes that result in a loss of tumor-suppressor functions and gain of oncogene functions (Ras, Raf, Src, mTOR, and Myc). Besides hypoxic conditions, the HIF pathway is also regulated by hypoxia-independent manner [102, 103]. Hypoxia-independent HIF-α stabilization and activation happens in response to cytokines, lipopolysaccharide (LPS), and growth factors in EMT mediated by PI3K/AKT/mTOR,29,30 MAPK,41 and NFκB pathways [104–106].

HIF-1α regulates hundreds of genes, and not only controls malignant and metastatic cancer cells but is also resistant to treatments. Thus, inhibition of hypoxia-induced EMT or HIF-1α may be promising as an anticancer therapy. Currently, there are many researches ongoing in this field. Besides targeting HIF-1α, another strategy is to block metastasis and target genes downstream of HIF-1α. Kaneko et al. have researched the hypoxia-induced EMT in oral cavity squamous cell carcinoma and showed that hypoxia-induced EMT in oral cavity cancer was improved by GSK3-β phosphorylation via PI3 K/Akt signaling [107]. Jiao and Nan showed that hypoxia-induced EMT and chemoresistance were supplemented with HIF-1α expression and Akt activation. Moreover, they demonstrated that PI3K/Akt and HIF-1α inhibition improved the therapeutic efficacy of hypoxic chemotherapy [108]. Lo Dico et al. reported that miR-675-5p promotes glioma growth through HIF-1α stabilization. Subsequently, they examined miR-675-5p specifically in colon cancer metastasis and demonstrated overexpression contributes to tumor progression through HIF-1α-induced EMT [109, 110].

5. Conclusion

Hypoxia is a hallmark of cells in the tumor microenvironment and has a major role in the carcinogenesis and metastasis processes. Hypoxia controls many crucial events such as tumor neovascularization, metabolism, cell survival, and cell death. Furthermore, hypoxia causes

EMT and CSC-like properties including resistance to treatment. Each step of the cancer adaptive process is regulated by HIF, NFκB, PI3K, and MAPK pathways. Understanding the impact of hypoxia and clarifying the hypoxia-induced responses and signaling modalities may pave the way to achieve important steps against cancer via hypoxia/HIF-targeted treatments.

Author details

Görkem Eskiizmir[1] and Erdoğan Özgür[2]*

*Address all correspondence to: erdoganozgur@mu.edu.tr

1 Department of Otorhinolaryngology, Head and Neck Surgery, Celal Bayar University, School of Medicine, Manisa, Turkey

2 Department of Otorhinolaryngology, Head and Neck Surgery, Muğla Sıtkı Koçman University, School of Medicine, Muğla, Turkey

References

[1] Chen F, Zhuang X, Lin L, Yu P, Wang Y, Shi Y, et al. New horizons in tumor microenvironment biology: challenges and opportunities. BMC Med. 2015;**13**:45

[2] Ran M, Witz IP. Tumor-associated immunoglobulins. Enhancement of syngeneic tumors by IgG2-containing tumor eluates. International Journal of Cancer. 1972;**9**:242-247

[3] Desmouliere A, Guyot C, Gabbiani G. The stroma reaction myofibroblast: a key player in the control of tumor cell behavior. International Journal of Developmental Biology. 2004;**48**:509-517

[4] Xing F, Saidou J, Watabe K. Cancer associated fibroblasts (CAFs) in tumor microenvironment. Frontiers in Bioscience. (Landmark Ed). 2010;**15**:166-179

[5] Wheeler SE, Shi H, Lin F, Dasari S, Bednash J, Thorne S, et al. Enhancement of head and neck squamous cell carcinoma proliferation, invasion, and metastasis by tumor-associated fibroblasts in preclinical models. Head Neck. 2014;**36**:385-392

[6] Ostman A, Augsten M. Cancer-associated fibroblasts and tumor growth--bystanders turning into key players. Current Opinion in Genetics & Development. 2009;**19**:67-73

[7] Birnie R, Bryce SD, Roome C, Dussupt V, Droop A, Lang SH, et al. Gene expression profiling of human prostate cancer stem cells reveals a pro-inflammatory phenotype and the importance of extracellular matrix interactions. Genome Biology. 2008;**9**:R83

[8] Birbrair A, Zhang T, Wang ZM, Messi ML, Olson JD, Mintz A, et al. Type-2 pericytes participate in normal and tumoral angiogenesis. American Journal of Physiology-Cell Physiology. 2014;**307**:C25-38

[9] McKeown SR. Defining normoxia, physoxia and hypoxia in tumours-implications for treatment response. The British Journal of Radiology. 2014;**87**:20130676

[10] Muz B, de la Puente P, Azab F, Azab AK. The role of hypoxia in cancer progression, angiogenesis, metastasis, and resistance to therapy. Hypoxia (Auckl). 2015;**3**:83-92

[11] Carreau A, El Hafny-Rahbi B, Matejuk A, Grillon C, Kieda C. Why is the partial oxygen pressure of human tissues a crucial parameter? Small molecules and hypoxia. Journal of Cellular and Molecular Medicine. 2011;**15**:1239-1253

[12] Vaupel P, Hockel M, Mayer A. Detection and characterization of tumor hypoxia using pO2 histography. Antioxid Redox Signal. 2007;**9**:1221-1235

[13] Vaupel P. Prognostic potential of the pre-therapeutic tumor oxygenation status. Advances in Experimental Medicine and Biology. 2009;**645**:241-246

[14] Dewhirst MW, Cao Y, Moeller B. Cycling hypoxia and free radicals regulate angiogenesis and radiotherapy response. Nature Reviews Cancer. 2008;**8**:425-437

[15] Guillemin K, Krasnow MA. The hypoxic response: huffing and HIFing. Cell. 1997;**89**:9-12

[16] Majmundar AJ, Wong WJ, Simon MC. Hypoxia-inducible factors and the response to hypoxic stress. Molecular Cell. 2010;**40**:294-309

[17] Wang GL, Jiang BH, Rue EA, Semenza GL. Hypoxia-inducible factor 1 is a basic-helix-loop-helix-PAS heterodimer regulated by cellular O2 tension. Proceedings of the National Academy of Sciences of the USA. 1995;**92**:5510-5514

[18] Ema M, Taya S, Yokotani N, Sogawa K, Matsuda Y, Fujii-Kuriyama Y. A novel bHLH-PAS factor with close sequence similarity to hypoxia-inducible factor 1alpha regulates the VEGF expression and is potentially involved in lung and vascular development. Proceedings of the National Academy of Sciences of the USA. 1997;**94**:4273-4278

[19] Flamme I, Frohlich T, von Reutern M, Kappel A, Damert A, Risau W. HRF, a putative basic helix-loop-helix-PAS-domain transcription factor is closely related to hypoxia-inducible factor-1 alpha and developmentally expressed in blood vessels. Mechanisms of Development. 1997;**63**:51-60

[20] Hogenesch JB, Chan WK, Jackiw VH, Brown RC, Gu YZ, Pray-Grant M, et al. Characterization of a subset of the basic-helix-loop-helix-PAS superfamily that interacts with components of the dioxin signaling pathway. Journal of Biological Chemistry. 1997;**272**:8581-8593

[21] Tian H, McKnight SL, Russell DW. Endothelial PAS domain protein 1 (EPAS1), a transcription factor selectively expressed in endothelial cells. Genes & Development. 1997;**11**:72-82

[22] Koh MY, Powis G. Passing the baton: the HIF switch. Trends in Biochemical Sciences.. 2012;**37**:364-372

[23] Holmquist-Mengelbier L, Fredlund E, Lofstedt T, Noguera R, Navarro S, Nilsson H, et al. Recruitment of HIF-1alpha and HIF-2alpha to common target genes is differentially

regulated in neuroblastoma: HIF-2alpha promotes an aggressive phenotype. Cancer Cell. 2006;**10**:413-423

[24] Pietras A, Gisselsson D, Ora I, Noguera R, Beckman S, Navarro S, et al. High levels of HIF-2alpha highlight an immature neural crest-like neuroblastoma cell cohort located in a perivascular niche. Journal of Pathology. 2008;**214**:482-488

[25] Pietras A, Hansford LM, Johnsson AS, Bridges E, Sjolund J, Gisselsson D, et al. HIF-2alpha maintains an undifferentiated state in neural crest-like human neuroblastoma tumor-initiating cells. Proceedings of the National Academy of Sciences of the USA. 2009;**106**:16805-16810

[26] Pietras A, Johnsson AS, Pahlman S. The HIF-2alpha-driven pseudo-hypoxic phenotype in tumor aggressiveness, differentiation, and vascularization. Current Topics in Microbiology and Immunology. 2010;**345**:1-20

[27] Makino Y, Kanopka A, Wilson WJ, Tanaka H, Poellinger L. Inhibitory PAS domain protein (IPAS) is a hypoxia-inducible splicing variant of the hypoxia-inducible factor-3alpha locus. Journal of Biological Chemistry. 2002;**277**:32405-32408

[28] Heikkila M, Pasanen A, Kivirikko KI, Myllyharju J. Roles of the human hypoxia-inducible factor (HIF)-3alpha variants in the hypoxia response. Cellular and Molecular Life Sciences. 2011;**68**:3885-3901

[29] Semenza GL. Targeting HIF-1 for cancer therapy. Nature Reviews Cancer. 2003;**3**:721-732

[30] Maxwell PH, Wiesener MS, Chang GW, Clifford SC, Vaux EC, Cockman ME, et al. The tumour suppressor protein VHL targets hypoxia-inducible factors for oxygen-dependent proteolysis. Nature. 1999;**399**:271-275

[31] An WG, Kanekal M, Simon MC, Maltepe E, Blagosklonny MV, Neckers LM. Stabilization of wild-type p53 by hypoxia-inducible factor 1alpha. Nature. 1998;**392**:405-408

[32] Dang CV, Kim JW, Gao P, Yustein J. The interplay between MYC and HIF in cancer. Nature Reviews Cancer. 2008;**8**:51-56

[33] Gordan JD, Bertout JA, Hu CJ, Diehl JA, Simon MC. HIF-2alpha promotes hypoxic cell proliferation by enhancing c-myc transcriptional activity. Cancer Cell. 2007;**11**:335-347

[34] Lavin MF, Gueven N. The complexity of p53 stabilization and activation. Cell Death & Differentiation. 2006;**13**:941-950

[35] Sengupta S, Peterson TR, Sabatini DM. Regulation of the mTOR complex 1 pathway by nutrients, growth factors, and stress. Molecular Cell. 2010;**40**:310-322

[36] Kumar V, Gabrilovich DI. Hypoxia-inducible factors in regulation of immune responses in tumour microenvironment. Immunology. 2014;**143**:512-519

[37] Bos R, Zhong H, Hanrahan CF, Mommers EC, Semenza GL, Pinedo HM, et al. Levels of hypoxia-inducible factor-1 alpha during breast carcinogenesis. Journal of the National Cancer Institute. 2001;**93**:309-314

[38] Zhong H, De Marzo AM, Laughner E, Lim M, Hilton DA, Zagzag D, et al. Overexpression of hypoxia-inducible factor 1alpha in common human cancers and their metastases. Cancer Research. 1999;**59**:5830-5835

[39] Bates RC, Mercurio AM. The epithelial-mesenchymal transition (EMT) and colorectal cancer progression. Cancer Biology & Therapy. 2005;**4**:365-370

[40] Abercrombie M, Heaysman JE. Observations on the social behaviour of cells in tissue culture. I. Speed of movement of chick heart fibroblasts in relation to their mutual contacts. Experimental Cell Research. 1953;**5**:111-131

[41] Abercrombie M, Heaysman JE. Observations on the social behaviour of cells in tissue culture. II. Monolayering of fibroblasts. Experimental Cell Research. 1954;**6**:293-306

[42] Abercrombie M, Heaysman JE. Invasiveness of sarcoma cells. Nature. 1954;**174**:697-698

[43] Abercrombie M, Heaysman JE, Karthauser HM. Social behaviour of cells in tissue culture. III. Mutual influence of sarcoma cells and fibroblasts. Experimental Cell Research. 1957;**13**:276-291

[44] Abercrombie M. Contact inhibition and malignancy. Nature. 1979;**281**:259-262

[45] Kalluri R, Neilson EG. Epithelial-mesenchymal transition and its implications for fibrosis. Journal of Clinical Investigation. 2003;**112**:1776-1784

[46] Lee JM, Dedhar S, Kalluri R, Thompson EW. The epithelial-mesenchymal transition: new insights in signaling, development, and disease. Journal of Cell Biology. 2006;**172**:973-981

[47] Locascio A, Nieto MA. Cell movements during vertebrate development: integrated tissue behaviour versus individual cell migration. Current Opinion in Genetics & Development. 2001;**11**:464-469

[48] Thiery JP. Epithelial-mesenchymal transitions in tumour progression. Nature Reviews Cancer. 2002;**2**:442-454

[49] Acloque H, Adams MS, Fishwick K, Bronner-Fraser M, Nieto MA. Epithelial-mesenchymal transitions: the importance of changing cell state in development and disease. Journal of Clinical Investigation. 2009;**119**:1438-1449

[50] Bischof P, Aplin JD, Bentin-Ley U, Brannstrom M, Casslen B, Castrillo JL, et al. Implantation of the human embryo: research lines and models. From the implantation research network 'Fruitful'. Gynecologic and Obstetric Investigation. 2006;**62**:206-216

[51] Vicovac L, Aplin JD. Epithelial-mesenchymal transition during trophoblast differentiation. Acta Anat (Basel). 1996;**156**:202-216

[52] Hay ED. Role of cell-matrix contacts in cell migration and epithelial-mesenchymal transformation. Cell Differentiation and Development. 1990;**32**:367-375

[53] Thiery JP, Sleeman JP. Complex networks orchestrate epithelial-mesenchymal transitions. Nature Reviews Molecular Cell Biology. 2006;**7**:131-142

[54] Liu P, Wakamiya M, Shea MJ, Albrecht U, Behringer RR, Bradley A. Requirement for Wnt3 in vertebrate axis formation. Nature Genetics. 1999;**22**:361-365

[55] Kalluri R, Weinberg RA. The basics of epithelial-mesenchymal transition. Journal of Clinical Investigation. 2009;**119**:1420-1428

[56] Chilosi M, Poletti V, Zamo A, Lestani M, Montagna L, Piccoli P, et al. Aberrant Wnt/beta-catenin pathway activation in idiopathic pulmonary fibrosis. American Journal of Pathology. 2003;**162**:1495-1502

[57] Ivanova L, Butt MJ, Matsell DG. Mesenchymal transition in kidney collecting duct epithelial cells. American Journal of Physiology-Renal Physiology. 2008;**294**:F1238-1248

[58] Okada H, Strutz F, Danoff TM, Kalluri R, Neilson EG. Possible mechanisms of renal fibrosis. Contributions to Nephrology. 1996;**118**:147-154

[59] Rastaldi MP, Ferrario F, Giardino L, Dell'Antonio G, Grillo C, Grillo P, et al. Epithelial-mesenchymal transition of tubular epithelial cells in human renal biopsies. Kidney International. 2002;**62**:137-146

[60] Strutz F, Zeisberg M, Ziyadeh FN, Yang CQ, Kalluri R, Muller GA, et al. Role of basic fibroblast growth factor-2 in epithelial-mesenchymal transformation. Kidney International. 2002;**61**:1714-1728

[61] Zeisberg M, Hanai J, Sugimoto H, Mammoto T, Charytan D, Strutz F, et al. BMP-7 counteracts TGF-beta1-induced epithelial-to-mesenchymal transition and reverses chronic renal injury. Nature Medicine. 2003;**9**:964-968

[62] Morrissey J, Hruska K, Guo G, Wang S, Chen Q, Klahr S. Bone morphogenetic protein-7 improves renal fibrosis and accelerates the return of renal function. Journal of the American Society of Nephrology. 2002;**13**(Suppl 1):S14-21

[63] Wiseman BS, Werb Z. Stromal effects on mammary gland development and breast cancer. Science. 2002;**296**:1046-1049

[64] Cunha GR, Hayward SW, Wang YZ. Role of stroma in carcinogenesis of the prostate. Differentiation. 2002;**70**:473-485

[65] Zajchowski DA, Bartholdi MF, Gong Y, Webster L, Liu HL, Munishkin A, et al. Identification of gene expression profiles that predict the aggressive behavior of breast cancer cells. Cancer Research. 2001;**61**:5168-5178

[66] Peinado H, Portillo F, Cano A. Transcriptional regulation of cadherins during development and carcinogenesis. The International Journal of Developmental Biology. 2004;**48**:365-375

[67] Tomita K, van Bokhoven A, van Leenders GJ, Ruijter ET, Jansen CF, Bussemakers MJ, et al. Cadherin switching in human prostate cancer progression. Cancer Research. 2000;**60**:3650-3654

[68] Hazan RB, Qiao R, Keren R, Badano I, Suyama K. Cadherin switch in tumor progression. Annals of the New York Academy of Sciences. 2004;**1014**:155-163

[69] Bryan RT, Tselepis C. Cadherin switching and bladder cancer. Journal of Urology. 2010;**184**:423-431

[70] Lade-Keller J, Riber-Hansen R, Guldberg P, Schmidt H, Hamilton-Dutoit SJ, Steiniche T. E- to N-cadherin switch in melanoma is associated with decreased expression of phosphatase and tensin homolog and cancer progression. British Journal of Dermatology. 2013;**169**:618-628

[71] Gilles C, Polette M, Piette J, Delvigne AC, Thompson EW, Foidart JM, et al. Vimentin expression in cervical carcinomas: association with invasive and migratory potential. The Journal of Pathology. 1996;**180**:175-180

[72] Ahmad A, Hanby A, Dublin E, Poulsom R, Smith P, Barnes D, et al. Stromelysin 3: an independent prognostic factor for relapse-free survival in node-positive breast cancer and demonstration of novel breast carcinoma cell expression. The American Journal of Pathology. 1998;**152**:721-728

[73] Xue C, Plieth D, Venkov C, Xu C, Neilson EG. The gatekeeper effect of epithelial-mesenchymal transition regulates the frequency of breast cancer metastasis. Cancer Research. 2003;**63**:3386-3394

[74] Yang J, Weinberg RA. Epithelial-mesenchymal transition: at the crossroads of development and tumor metastasis. Developmental Cell. 2008;**14**:818-829

[75] Brabletz T, Jung A, Kirchner T. Beta-catenin and the morphogenesis of colorectal cancer. Virchows Arch. 2002;**441**:1-11

[76] Bierie B, Moses HL. Tumour microenvironment: TGFbeta: the molecular Jekyll and Hyde of cancer. Nature Reviews Cancer. 2006;**6**:506-520

[77] Oft M, Heider KH, Beug H. TGFbeta signaling is necessary for carcinoma cell invasiveness and metastasis. Current Biology. 1998;**8**:1243-1252

[78] Piek E, Moustakas A, Kurisaki A, Heldin CH, ten Dijke P. TGF-(beta) type I receptor/ ALK-5 and Smad proteins mediate epithelial to mesenchymal transdifferentiation in NMuMG breast epithelial cells. J Cell Sci. 1999;**112**(Pt 24):4557-4568

[79] Derynck R, Akhurst RJ, Balmain A. TGF-beta signaling in tumor suppression and cancer progression. Nature Genetics. 2001;**29**:117-129

[80] Yang L, Lin C, Liu ZR. P68 RNA helicase mediates PDGF-induced epithelial mesenchymal transition by displacing Axin from beta-catenin. Cell. 2006;**127**:139-155

[81] Nawshad A, Lagamba D, Polad A, Hay ED. Transforming growth factor-beta signaling during epithelial-mesenchymal transformation: implications for embryogenesis and tumor metastasis. Cells Tissues Organs. 2005;**179**:11-23

[82] Edelman GM, Gallin WJ, Delouvee A, Cunningham BA, Thiery JP. Early epochal maps of two different cell adhesion molecules. Proceedings of the National Academy of Sciences of the USA. 1983;**80**:4384-4388

[83] Tepass U, Truong K, Godt D, Ikura M, Peifer M. Cadherins in embryonic and neural morphogenesis. Nature Reviews Molecular Cell Biology. 2000;**1**:91-100

[84] Eger A, Stockinger A, Schaffhauser B, Beug H, Foisner R. Epithelial mesenchymal transition by c-Fos estrogen receptor activation involves nuclear translocation of beta-catenin and upregulation of beta-catenin/lymphoid enhancer binding factor-1 transcriptional activity. Journal of Cell Biology. 2000;**148**:173-188

[85] Kim K, Lu Z, Hay ED. Direct evidence for a role of beta-catenin/LEF-1 signaling pathway in induction of EMT. Cell Biology International. 2002;**26**:463-476

[86] Scarpa E, Szabo A, Bibonne A, Theveneau E, Parsons M, Mayor R. Cadherin Switch during EMT in Neural Crest Cells Leads to Contact Inhibition of Locomotion via Repolarization of Forces. Developmental Cell. 2015;**34**:421-434

[87] Chen J, Zhao J, Ma R, Lin H, Liang X, Cai X. Prognostic significance of E-cadherin expression in hepatocellular carcinoma: a meta-analysis. PLoS One. 2014;**9**:e103952

[88] Hirohashi S. Inactivation of the E-cadherin-mediated cell adhesion system in human cancers. The American Journal of Pathology. 1998;**153**:333-339

[89] Li Z, Yin S, Zhang L, Liu W, Chen B. Prognostic value of reduced E-cadherin expression in breast cancer: a meta-analysis. Oncotarget. 2017;**8**:16445-16455

[90] Luo SL, Xie YG, Li Z, Ma JH, Xu X. E-cadherin expression and prognosis of oral cancer: a meta-analysis. Tumor Biology. 2014;**35**:5533-5537

[91] Peng J, Qi S, Wang P, Li W, Song L, Liu C, et al. Meta-analysis of downregulated E-cadherin as a poor prognostic biomarker for cervical cancer. Future Oncology. 2016;**12**:715-726

[92] Wang N, He YL, Pang LJ, Zou H, Liu CX, Zhao J, et al. Down-regulated E-cadherin expression is associated with poor five-year overall survival in bone and soft tissue sarcoma: results of a meta-analysis. PLoS One. 2015;**10**:e0121448

[93] Xing X, Tang YB, Yuan G, Wang Y, Wang J, Yang Y, et al. The prognostic value of E-cadherin in gastric cancer: a meta-analysis. International Journal of Cancer. 2013;**132**:2589-2596

[94] Xu XL, Ling ZQ, Chen SZ, Li B, Ji WH, Mao WM. The impact of E-cadherin expression on the prognosis of esophageal cancer: a meta-analysis. Dis Esophagus. 2014;**27**:79-86

[95] Yang YL, Chen MW, Xian L. Prognostic and clinicopathological significance of downregulated E-cadherin expression in patients with non-small cell lung cancer (NSCLC): a meta-analysis. PLoS One. 2014;**9**:e99763

[96] Valastyan S, Weinberg RA. Tumor metastasis: molecular insights and evolving paradigms. Cell. 2011;**147**:275-292

[97] Tarin D, Thompson EW, Newgreen DF. The fallacy of epithelial mesenchymal transition in neoplasia. Cancer Research. 2005;**65**:5996-6000; discussion 6000-5991

[98] De Craene B, Gilbert B, Stove C, Bruyneel E, van Roy F, Berx G. The transcription factor snail induces tumor cell invasion through modulation of the epithelial cell differentiation program. Cancer Research. 2005;**65**:6237-6244

[99] Fodde R, Brabletz T. Wnt/beta-catenin signaling in cancer stemness and malignant behavior. Current Opinion in Cell Biology. 2007;**19**:150-158

[100] Bao B, Ahmad A, Kong D, Ali S, Azmi AS, Li Y, et al. Hypoxia induced aggressiveness of prostate cancer cells is linked with deregulated expression of VEGF, IL-6 and miRNAs that are attenuated by CDF. PLoS One. 2012;**7**:e43726

[101] Azab AK, Hu J, Quang P, Azab F, Pitsillides C, Awwad R, et al. Hypoxia promotes dissemination of multiple myeloma through acquisition of epithelial to mesenchymal transition-like features. Blood. 2012;**119**:5782-5794

[102] Richard DE, Berra E, Gothie E, Roux D, Pouyssegur J. p42/p44 mitogen-activated protein kinases phosphorylate hypoxia-inducible factor 1alpha (HIF-1alpha) and enhance the transcriptional activity of HIF-1. Journal of Biological Chemistry. 1999;**274**:32631-32637

[103] van Uden P, Kenneth NS, Rocha S. Regulation of hypoxia-inducible factor-1alpha by NF-kappaB. Biochemical Journal. 2008;**412**:477-484

[104] Agani F, Jiang BH. Oxygen-independent regulation of HIF-1: novel involvement of PI3K/AKT/mTOR pathway in cancer. Current Cancer Drug Targets. 2013;**13**:245-251

[105] Kilic-Eren M, Boylu T, Tabor V. Targeting PI3K/Akt represses Hypoxia inducible factor-1alpha activation and sensitizes Rhabdomyosarcoma and Ewing's sarcoma cells for apoptosis. Cancer Cell International. 2013;**13**:36

[106] Seta KA, Spicer Z, Yuan Y, Lu G, Millhorn DE. Responding to hypoxia: lessons from a model cell line. Science's STKE. 2002;**2002**:re11

[107] Kaneko T, Dehari H, Sasaki T, Igarashi T, Ogi K, Okamoto JY, et al. Hypoxia-induced epithelial-mesenchymal transition is regulated by phosphorylation of GSK3-beta via PI3 K/Akt signaling in oral squamous cell carcinoma. Oral Surgery, Oral Medicine, Oral Pathology, and Oral Radiology. 2016;**122**:719-730

[108] Jiao M, Nan KJ. Activation of PI3 kinase/Akt/HIF-1alpha pathway contributes to hypoxia-induced epithelial-mesenchymal transition and chemoresistance in hepatocellular carcinoma. International Journal of Oncology. 2012;**40**:461-468

[109] Costa V, Lo Dico A, Rizzo A, Rajata F, Tripodi M, Alessandro R, et al. MiR-675-5p supports hypoxia induced epithelial to mesenchymal transition in colon cancer cells. Oncotarget. 2017;**8**:24292-24302

[110] Lo Dico A, Costa V, Martelli C, Diceglie C, Rajata F, Rizzo A, et al. MiR675-5p Acts on HIF-1alpha to Sustain Hypoxic Responses: A New Therapeutic Strategy for Glioma. Theranostics. 2016;**6**:1105-1118

6

Increased Air Pollution Causing Cancer and its Rapid Online Monitoring

Jianhai Sun, Jinhua Liu, Chunxiu Liu, Yanni Zhang, Xiaofeng Zhu, Jingjing Zhang and Zhanwu Ning

Abstract

Pollution of indoor and outdoor air has considerably been taken attention abroad as an important environmental problem, and there is sufficient evidence that exposure to outdoor air pollution causes lung cancer and other cancers. Therefore, the current situation of air pollution will be deeply discussed, and a portable environmental gas monitor integrated by a variety of highly sensitive sensors will be developed for rapidly monitoring air pollution, which is able to provide scientific data for environmental pollution control. By this way, human beings are able to be far away from cancer caused by environmental pollution and its suffering.

Keywords: air pollution, portable environmental gas monitor, volatile organic compounds, toxic gases, metal oxide sensor, particulate matters, photoionization detector

1. Introduction

Cancer is caused by changes in certain genes that alter the function of our cells. Some of these genetic changes occur naturally when DNA is replicated during the process of cell division. But others are the result of DNA damage caused by environmental exposure, and these exposures include toxic and harmful gases, repairable dust, chemicals, and radiation.

The air we breathe has been contaminated with a mixture of carcinogens [1–3]. We now know that outdoor or indoor air pollution has been acted as a major health risk [1–11] but also a leading environmental cause of cancer deaths. The risk of developing lung cancer is significantly increased in people exposed to air pollution. Air pollution is a gas (or a liquid or solid dispersed through ordinary air) released with a big-enough quantity to harm health of people or other animals, kill plants or stop them growing properly, damage or disrupt some other aspect of the environment (such as making buildings crumble), or cause some other kind of nuisance (reduced visibility, perhaps, or an unpleasant odor). Air pollution is predominantly caused by automobile exhaust, industrial and agricultural emissions, construction dust, chemical leakage, residential heating and cooking, as well as some pollution accidents (such as factory explosion, toxic runway and playground, etc.). It is uncertain to what degree air pollution contributes to cancer, but according to the largest study to date, more than 10% of lung cancers may be caused by air pollution. Moreover, experts have identified other ills caused by the air pollution, including an increased risk of asthma and heart disease.

It is generally known that a variety of harmful gases will be present in the air when air pollution occurs, and if the harmful gases reached a high enough concentration, the air becomes very harmful to human health. When we talk about the harmful gases, there are dozens of different pollution gases in the air. In practice, about several different substances cause most concern, and these harmful gases are mainly sulfur dioxide, carbon monoxide, carbon dioxide, nitrogen oxides, volatile organic compounds (VOCs), ozone [12, 13], particulates [13–18], and so on. Therefore, let us talk about the sources of these toxic gases and their major dangers.

Carbon monoxide (CO): CO is mainly come from the incomplete combustion of C, such as automobile exhaust, coal combustion (especially coal-fired power plants and coal-fired supply heating system, etc.), fuel-burning appliance, and so on. It is well known that CO with high concentrations can directly cause death.

Carbon dioxide (CO_2): CO_2 is one of basic component of the atmosphere, just as the N_2 and O_2, and this gas is central to everyday life and is not normally considered as a pollutant. We all produce it when we breathe out, and plants such as crops and trees need to "breathe" it in to grow. However, CO_2 with high concentrations can also directly cause suffocation or even death.

Sulfur dioxide: coal, petroleum, and other fuels are often impure and contain sulfur as well as organic compounds. When sulfur burns with oxygen from the air, sulfur dioxide (SO_2) is produced. In the atmosphere, sulfur dioxide can be oxidized to sulfuric acid fog or sulfate aerosol, which is an important precursor of environmental acidification. There is a potential impact on the human body when the concentration of sulfur dioxide in the atmosphere is above 0.5 ppm, most people will begin to feel stimulated when the concentration of SO_2 is over 1 ppm, and people suffer from ulcers and pulmonary edema and even death by asphyxiation when the concentration is over 400 ppm. Sulfur dioxide has synergistic effects with soot in the atmosphere. When the concentration of sulfur dioxide in the atmosphere is 0.21 ppm, the concentration of smoke and dust is greater than 0.3 mg/l, the incidence of respiratory diseases can be increased, and the condition of the patients with chronic diseases will deteriorate rapidly. Such as the London smog event, Maas Valley events, Donora smog, and other events were all caused by this synergistic effect.

Nitrogen oxides: nitrogen dioxide (NO_2) and nitrogen oxide (NO) are pollutants produced as an indirect result of combustion when nitrogen and oxygen from the air react together.

Nitrogen oxide pollution comes from automobile exhaust and power plants and plays an important role in the formation of acid rain, ozone, and smog. Nitrogen oxides are also "indirect greenhouse gases" because they contribute to global warming by producing ozone. Nitrogen oxides mainly damage the respiratory tract, and if people are living in this environment for a long time, people may suffer from delayed pulmonary edema and adult respiratory distress syndrome.

Volatile organic compounds (VOCs): these carbon-based (organic) chemicals evaporate easily at ordinary temperatures and pressures, so they readily become gases. That's precisely why they are used as solvents in many different household chemicals such as paints, waxes, and varnishes. Indoor VOCs which are greatly harmful emit mainly from building and building fitment materials. Unfortunately, VOCs are greatly harmful and have long-term effects on human health, and they also play a role in the formation of ozone and smog. Therefore, it is necessary to investigate emission of VOCs and its controlling method.

Particulates: the particles can be deposited in the respiratory tract, lung, and other parts due to small size. The smaller the particle size of the PM is, the deeper the PM enters into the respiratory tract. It is well known that the PM with 10 μm diameter is deposited in the upper respiratory tract, the PM with 5 μm diameter can enter into the deep part of the respiratory tract, and the PM with diameter less than 2 μm can be easily penetrated deep into bronchioles and alveoli, which was easy to cause cancer and other diseases. Therefore, it is of great significance to develop a rapid on-site detection technique for inhalable particles, which will be very conducive to the understanding of the formation mechanism of fog and haze. In cities, most particulates come from traffic fumes.

Ozone: some of the ozone near the ground comes from the upper layer of ozone, and some of the ozone comes from the soil, lightning, biological emissions, etc. These can be classified as "natural sources", already in nature. The main cause of ozone pollution is "anthropogenic sources". Coal, vehicle exhaust, petrochemical, and other pollutants (for example, NOx (nitrogen oxides)) will produce ozone and other NOx, which is called the two photochemical reaction. Studies have shown that only 23% total ozone pollution occurred each year in the near ground layer comes from the nature's own transport and as high as 48% total ozone comes from the photochemical reaction from NOx and other pollutants. It can be said that the concentration of ozone in urban areas depends mainly on the emission of motor vehicles exhaust. Ozone can cause great harm to the human body: ozone can damage lung function, stimulate respiratory tract, cause airway reaction, increase airway inflammation, and aggravate asthma. High levels of persistent ozone pollution may cause watering eyes, eye pain, headaches, and other symptoms, which can affect the respiratory and cardiovascular systems.

In this chapter, a portable gas monitor fabricated for rapidly monitoring air pollution was developed, and the systems consists of the following modules: an automated sampling device, multisensors-integrated sensing system, a signal acquisition, processing and display system, and a power supply. Finally, the proposed systems were used to monitor air pollution in various environmental sites, such as industrial chemical plan, pesticide plants, printing and dyeing plants, pesticide plants, and so on. These environmental pollution data will be provided to the local environmental monitoring department, and these data are very important for the purification and treatment of the environment, so that we are able to avoid the high-risk air pollution and the cancers caused by air pollution.

2. Experimental details

2.1. The schematic of the minienvironmental gas system

In order to effectively monitor toxic and harmful gas in the air, a multisensor integrated into the portable system is proposed, and its structure diagram was shown in **Figure 1**. The system mainly includes the following parts: (1) automatic injection system, (2) purification unit for sample, (3) gas sensing unit (4), signal acquisition, output, and display unit, and (5) power supply. The sampling section mainly includes a sampling pipe and a sampling pump, in which the sampling pipe was inserted into pollutant source or possible leakage spots, and then, the sample was pumped and transported into the purification unit. The purification unit consists of sample filtration and sample drying, by which the particulate matters are filtered through a filter membrane with pore size of 0.22 μm made by PTFE material, and at the same time, moisture was absorbed and removed by the purifying material packed in chamber of the purification unit. After the sample has been purified, the sample was then transported into the sensor unit for target identification and concentration identification. The sensing unit is the brain of the whole system, which consists of a variety of highly sensitive sensors, and each sensor can accurately identify a component and detect its concentration. Moreover, in the system, we can choose sensor combinations according to different application areas (different kinds of harmful gas) because the environmental gases contain some of the harmful gases, such as O_3, H_2S, CO, NO_2, NH_3, SO_2, formaldehyde, VOCs, and NO. Therefore, according to the different applications, some different high sensitive sensors were integrated into the system, such as mini PID sensor, H_2S sensor, SO_2 sensor, NO sensor, NO_2 sensor, NH_3 sensor, O_3 sensor, and so on. The signal processing system mainly includes signal acquisition, processing, transmission, and display. An output signal proportional to the concentration was obtained from the sensor, after the signal was processed by high-accurate AD converter

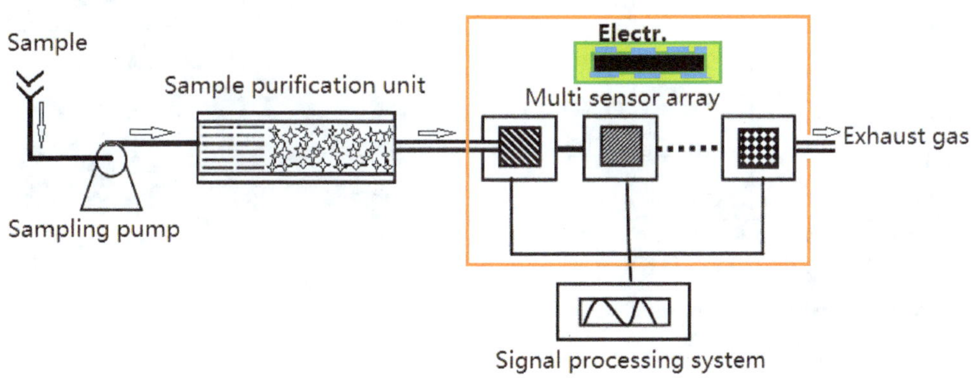

Figure 1. Schematic diagram of the portable gas monitor.

and MCU, the types and concentrations of this contaminated gas were displayed by a mini PC or liquid crystal display (LCD).

2.2. Highly sensitive sensors

2.2.1. High performance of mini PID

A photoionization detector (PID) uses an ultraviolet (UV) light source to ionize gas molecules to positive and negative ions that can be easily measured with a detector. The PID is commonly employed in the detection of volatile organic compounds (VOCs) such as alkanes, alkenes, oxygenated hydrocarbons, and halogenated hydrocarbons, etc. VOCs mainly come from the following aspects: industrial stationary source, vehicle exhaust emission source, and daily life source. The PID detectors are able to detect traces gas with concentration of ppb level and provide an instant reading indicating whether gas is present, which makes PID sensors useful in go/no-go situations, where personnel are unsure of what threats they face.

In this work, a mini PID detector has been developed, which can be used to detect volatile organic compounds in the environment with high sensitivity. In order to improve sensitivity of the PID, a little ionization chamber with volume of 10 μl, which was made of polytetrafluoroethylene (PTFE), was proposed. **Figure 2(a)** shows a side view of the ionization chamber and the fabricated mini PID. **Figure 2(b)** indicates photo of the fabricated PID. The characteristic of the fabricated PID was the little volume of the ionization chamber, dramatically reducing velocity of carrier gas (velocity of carrier gas was able to be reduced to less than 10 ml/min). The proposed PID demonstrated high-detection performance (refer to **Table 1**) by effectively reducing background noises, external electromagnetic interferences, and the ionization chamber volume.

In this work, in order to accurately detect the concentration of the VOCs come from pollution source, the fabricated PID was integrated into the monitoring system.

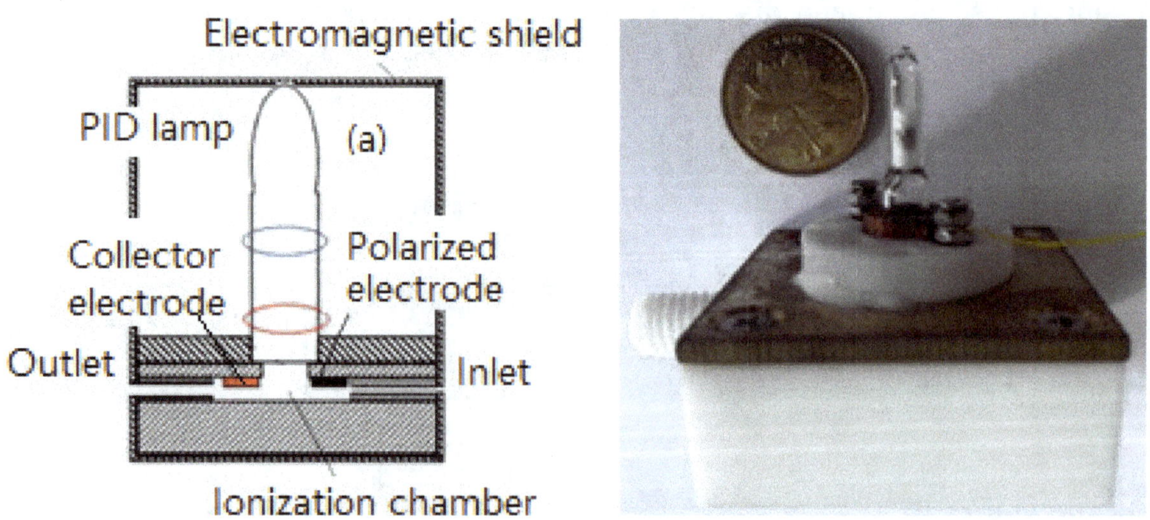

Figure 2. (a) Schematic of the fabricated mini PID, (b) photo of the fabricated PID.

Detection limit (for benzene)	1 ppb
Relative standard deviation (RSD)	0.5%
Baseline drift	1.0×10^{-13} A/30 min
Background noise	Less than 1.0×10^{-13} A
Linear range (for benzene)	10^5

Table 1. A summarized performance of the fabricated mini PID.

2.2.2. *High sensitivity sensors*

In order to effectively monitor these environmental harmful gases (such as O_3, H_2S, CO, NO_2, NH_3, SO_2, formaldehyde, VOCs, NO and so on), some highly sensitive sensors were selected to monitor these harmful gases, and the response characteristics of each sensor will be described as follows.

The H_2S sensor based on electrochemical principles is able to detect trace concentrations below 10 ppb, and **Figure 3** shows the responses to 200 ppb sample gases. The data indicate that the sensor has high resolution and good linearity, which is suitable for the analysis of trace gases in the environment.

The SO_2, NO, and O_3 sensor also based on electrochemical principles were able to detect trace concentrations, and **Figures 4–6** show the responses to sample gases. These experiment results show that these sensors have high sensitivity and can be used to detect various pollution sources in ambient air.

The formaldehyde sensor responds to formaldehyde that are electrochemically active, and the bias voltage of +300 mV is optimum for formaldehyde; however, the sensor also responds to other VOCs under other bias voltage. If the formaldehyde needs to be detected with high precision, TVOCs needs to be tested at once and then eliminate its impact. **Figure 7** shows the response of 3.8 ppm formaldehyde using the sensor.

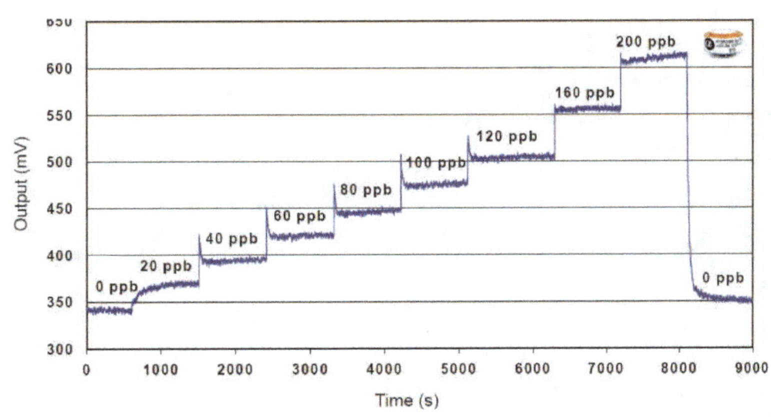

Figure 3. Response to 200 ppb H_2S using the H_2S sensor.

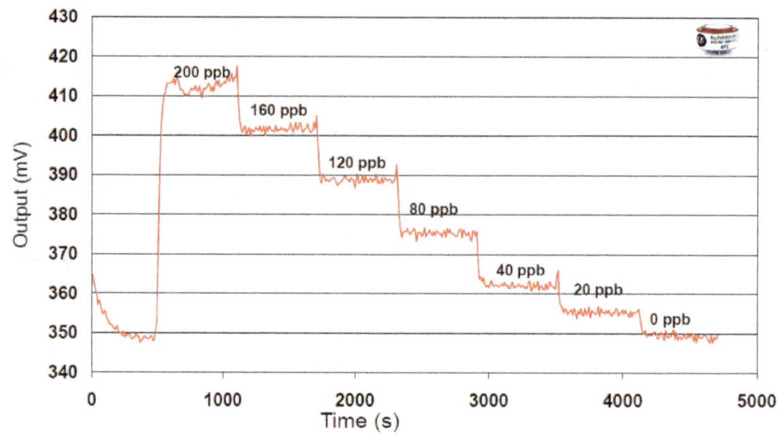

Figure 4. Response to 200 ppb SO_2 using the SO_2 sensor.

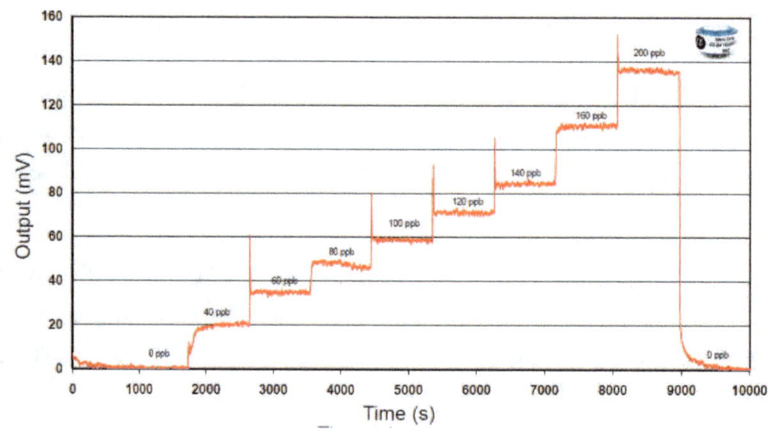

Figure 5. Response to 200 ppb NO using the NO sensor.

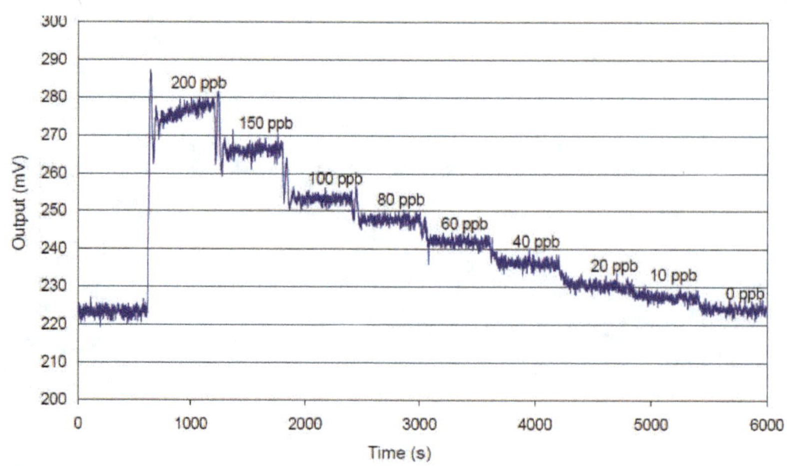

Figure 6. Response to 200 ppb O_3 using the O_3 sensor.

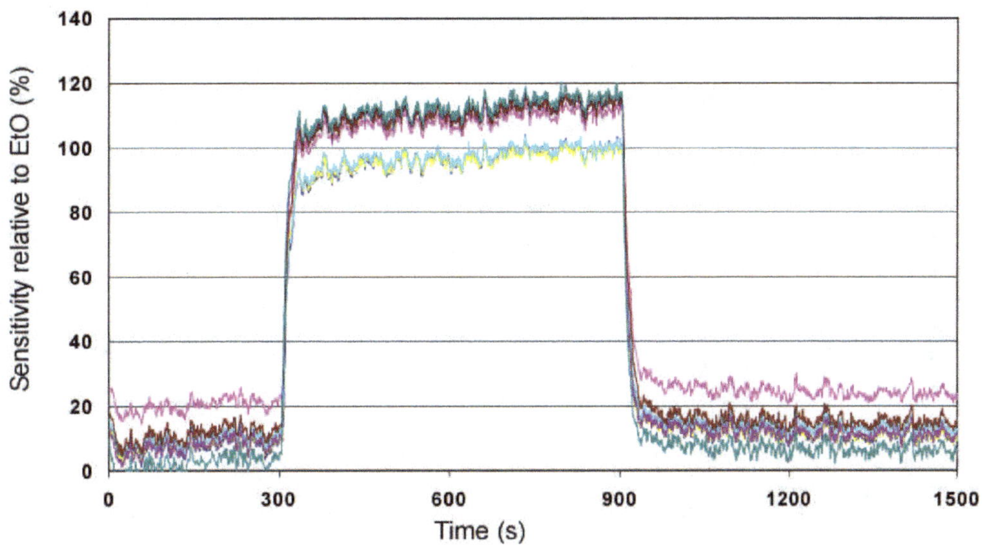

Figure 7. The response of 3.8 ppm formaldehyde.

Because of the basic principle of NDIR gas sensors, only the gas with asymmetric molecular structure can absorb strong infrared rays. Therefore, NDIR gas sensors can only measure SO_2, NO, CO_2, CO, CH_4, and other molecules with asymmetric molecular structure. For O_2, H_2, N_2, and other molecules with symmetrical molecular structure, the NDIR is incapable of action.

NDIR detectors are the industry standard method of measuring the concentration of carbon oxides (CO and CO_2). Each constituent gas in a sample will absorb some infrared at a particular frequency (**Figure 8** is the infrared absorption spectrum of CO_2). By shining an infrared beam through a sample chamber containing CO_2 and measuring the amount of infrared absorbed by the sample, the volumetric concentration of CO_2 in the sample can be reported. **Figure 9** shows the schematic diagram of the NDIR detector. In this work, a NDIR detector (Prime 2, purchased from Clairair Ltd.) was integrated for detecting the concentration of CO_2.

In this work, a microfabricated metal oxide (MOX) detector based on SnO/SnO_2/Au nanocomposite sensitive material was used to detect the CO gas. In order to increase conductivity of the sensitive material, SnO-doped sensitive material was proposed because of the low conductivity of SnO_2, which was able to greatly increase the activity of SnO_2 sensitive layer. The sensitive film (nano-metric thickness) was fabricated, and the process was defined as follows, and a schematic representation of the whole structure is depicted in **Figure 10**.

First of all, a layer of SnO and SnO_2 thin film deposited over the hotplate surface has been carried out by sputtering through a modified rheotaxial growth and thermal oxidation technique, and the thickness of the SnO and SnO_2 thin film was 50 nm and 150 nm, respectively. Then, an extremely thin Au film with thickness of 5 nm was deposited over its surface to act as a catalyst and consequently increase SnO_2 film selectivity. Finally, the release process (or suspension process) of the supported beam was shown as follows. A layer of photoresist with

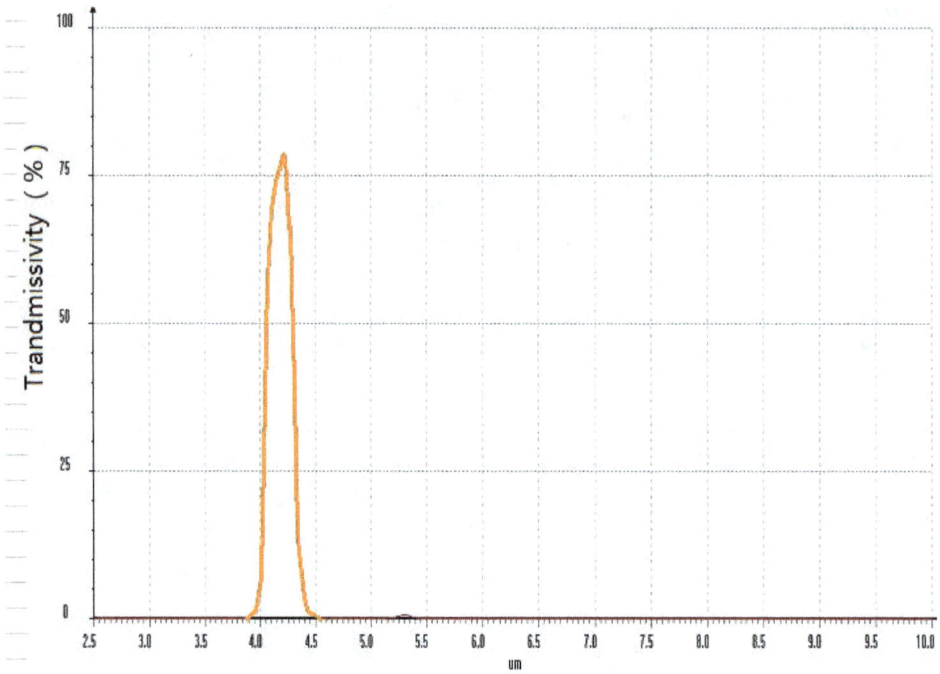

Figure 8. Infrared absorption spectrum of CO_2.

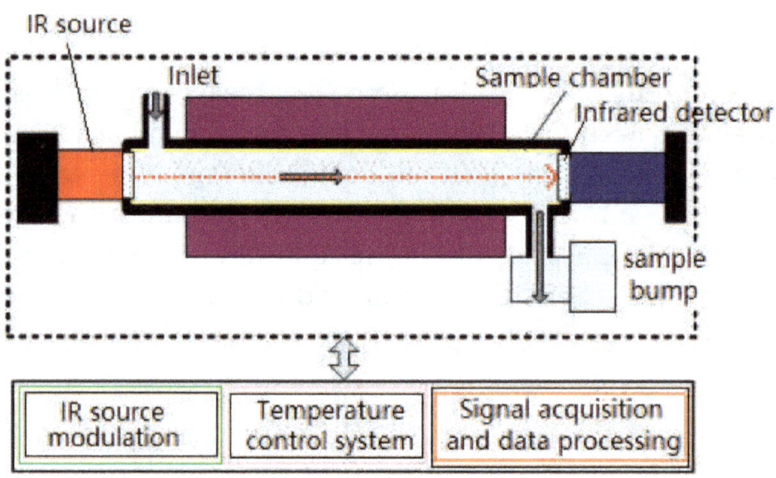

Figure 9. The schematic diagram of the NDIR detector.

thickness of 2 μm was coated and patterned as an etch mask for silicon nitride. After the two layers of the silicon nitride were etched by the reactive-ion etching (RIE) technology, a deep reactive-ion etching (DRIE) process was utilized to remove the diffusion of silicon in the micro channels. Then, the supported beam was released through a silicon etch (using 40 wt% KOH solution at 80°C for 70 min). The chip size (refer to **Figure 11**) is 8×10 mm^2 with an active area (for each of the four sensors) of 1×4 mm^2, consisting of platinum resistor acting as heater. The sensor can detect CO with a detection limit of 0.1 ppm, and the resolution of the sensor can be less than 1 ppm.

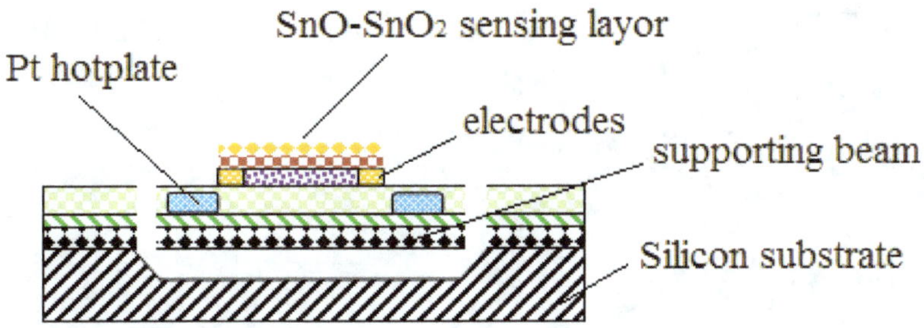

Figure 10. A schematic representation of the sensor.

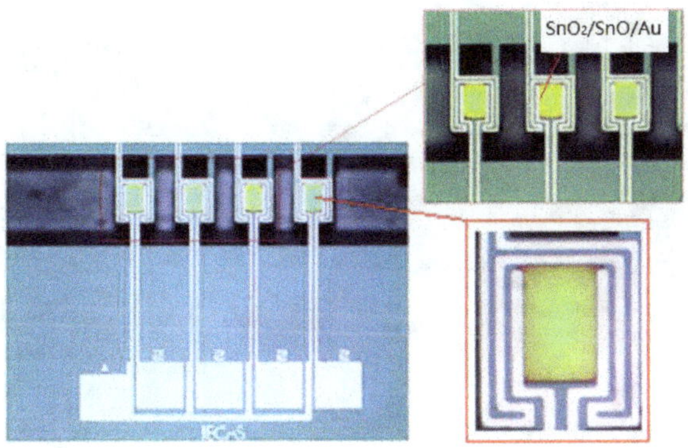

Figure 11. Photo of the MOX sensor based on SnO/SnO_2/Au nanocomposite sensitive material.

The particles can be deposited in the respiratory tract, lung, and other parts due to small size. The smaller the particle size of the PM is, the deeper the PM enters into the respiratory tract. PM is the leading cause of pneumoconiosis. Therefore, PM is especially harmful to humans, and its formation and monitoring should be paid special attention. In this work, optical method was used to monitor the PM, which monitors the change of light intensity to determine the average concentration of PM. **Figure 12** shows the photo of the PM sensor and the working schematic diagram.

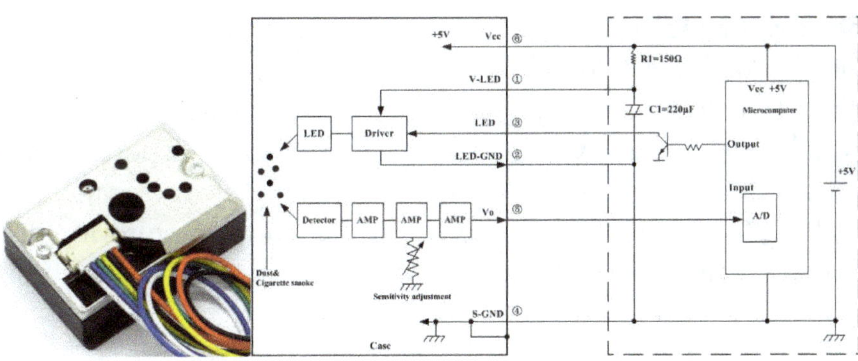

Figure 12. The PM sensor and the working schematic diagram.

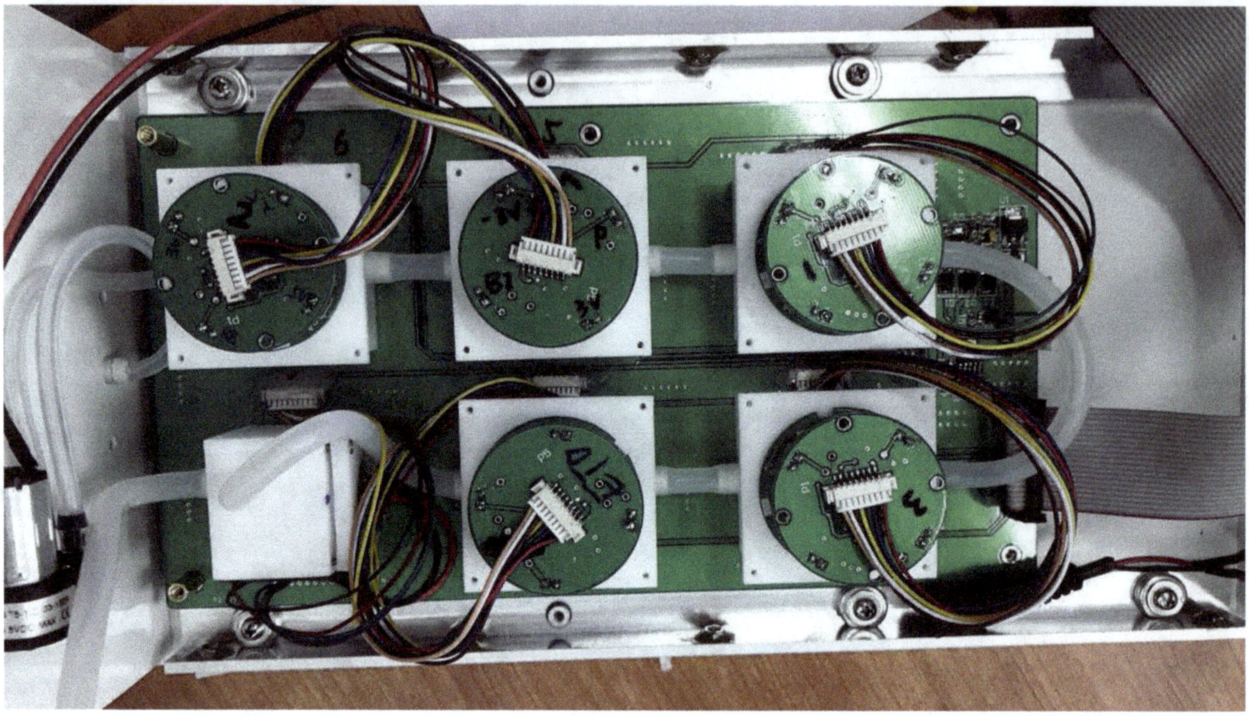

Figure 13. Portable environmental gas detection system.

2.3. Integration of monitoring system

In this work, the gas hoods using polytetrafluoroethylene (PTFE) for packaging these sensors were fabricated, and then these sensors were integrated into the system. **Figure 13** shows the photo of the portable system, in which the sample was transported by a mini pump and the power supply is a 12 V battery module. The data are processed through a high-resolution 24 bit AD (ADS1256) converter and displayed by a LCD. According to the application areas, we can easily change the sensor module.

3. Results and discussion

Air pollution has considerably been taken attention abroad as an important environmental problem, and there is sufficient evidence that exposure to air pollution causes lung cancer and other cancers. Therefore, it is necessary to develop highly sensitive systems to detect harmful gases. In this work, several different sensors were integrated into a portable system according to different application areas. For example, the proposed system integrated with TVOCs, H_2S, SO_2, CO, O_3, NO, CO_2, and formaldehyde sensor was used for monitoring pollution sources, such as the automobile coating industry, chemical processing industry, furniture manufacturing, oil refining, and chemical industry.

We selected a garage to monitor air pollution, it is well known that a lot of paint, gasoline, and lubricating oil was used at work, and a large amount of exhaust gas is emitted from the

	#1	#2	#3	#4	#5
TVOC (ppm)	5.524	5.461	5.556	5.270	5.353
H_2S (ppm)	0.564	0.556	0.578	0.489	0.486
SO_2 (ppm)	0.802	0.813	0.882	0.916	0.925
CO (ppm)	0.135	0.118	0.167	0.185	0.201
CO_2 (ppm)	578	586	592	597	620
O_3 (ppm)	0.225	0.186	0.175	0.216	0.228
NO (ppm)	0.102	0.125	0.118	0.102	0.128
Formaldehyde	1.068	1.025	1.086	1.164	1.125
PM 2.5 (μg/m^3)	230	243	241	236	230

Table 2. The concentration of each component in the garage detected by the monitor.

automobile; therefore, the component of the air is complex. In this work, the air pollution was monitored continuously using the proposed system. The testing cycle is every hour and 5 times in a row. **Table 2** indicates the concentration of each component of the garage detected by the monitor.

As we can see from the monitoring data, the concentration of TVOC, SO_2, H_2S, formaldehyde, O_3, NO, and PM are higher than their national standard in the auto repair factory. Obviously, these harmful gases will be harmful to health of workers if they work in such a "high pollution" environment for a long time, which will bring serious diseases and even cancer. In order to protect the health of workers, the air pollution need to be on-site monitored with high sensitive; at the same time, the harmful gases also need to be removed till their concentrations are reduced to the normal allowed level, which the workers can freely breathe the air.

4. Conclusion

The existence of a number of toxic and harmful gases has greatly damaged people's health. Therefore, real-time and high-precision detection of these gases is the primary basis for effective prevention of this pollution source, and the purpose of the elimination of these harmful gases can finally be achieved only through this high-precision detection technology. So that people can be away from cancer and be free breathing the air in the clean and blue sky.

Acknowledgements

The authors greatly acknowledge the financial support from National Key Research and Development Program of China under grant numbers: 2016YFF02045 and 2016YFC07006. The authors also greatly acknowledge the financial support from the National Science Foundation of China under grant numbers: 11574219, 61774157, and 61176112.

Author details

Jianhai Sun[1]*, Jinhua Liu[2], Chunxiu Liu[1], Yanni Zhang[2], Xiaofeng Zhu[2], Jingjing Zhang[1] and Zhanwu Ning[2]

*Address all correspondence to: jhsun@mail.ie.ac.cn

1 State Key Laboratory of Transducer Technology, Institute of Electronics, Chinese Academy of Sciences, Beijing, China

2 Beijing Municipal Institute of Labour Protection, Beijing, China

References

[1] Pekkanen J, Peter A, Hoek G, et al. Particulate air pollution and risk of ST-segment depression during repeated submaximal exercise tests among subjects with coronary heart disease. Circulation. 2002;**106**:933-938

[2] Peters A, Dockery DW, Muller JE, Mittleman MA. Increased particulate air pollution and the triggering of myocardial infaction. Circulation. 2001;**103**:2810-2815

[3] Ibald-Mulli A, Stieber J, Wichmann H, et al. Effects of air pollution on blood pressure a population-based approach. American Journal of Public Health. 2001;**91**:571-577

[4] Suwa T, Hogg JC, Quinlan KB, et al. Particulate air pollution induces progression of atherosclerosis. Journal of the American College of Cardiology. 2002;**39**:935-942

[5] Gold DR, Litonjua A, Schwartz J, et al. Ambient pollution and heart rate variability. Circulation. 2000;**101**:1267-1273

[6] Pope CA, Verrier RL, Lovett EG, et al. Heart rate variability associated with particulate air pollution. American Heart Journal. 1999;**138**:890-899

[7] Magari SR, Hauser R, Schwartz J, et al. Association of heart rate variability with occupational and environmental exposure to particulate air pollution. Circulation. 2001;**104**:986-991

[8] Stone PH, Godleski JJ. First steps toward understanding the pathophysiology between air pollution and cardiac mortality. American Heart Journal. 1999;**138**:804-807

[9] Peters A, Liu E, Verrier RL, Schwartz J, et al. Air pollution and incidence of cardiac arrhythmia. Epidemiology. 2000;**11**:11-17

[10] Ross R. Mechanisms of disease: Atherosclerosis an inflammatory disease. The New England Journal of Medicine. 1999;**340**:115-126

[11] Schachinger V, Britten MB, Zeiher AM. Prognostic impact of coronary vasodilator dysfunction on adverse long-term outcome of coronary heart disease. Circulation. 2000; **101**:1899-1906

[12] Brook RD, Brook JR, Urch B, et al. Inhalation of fine particulate air pollution and ozone causes acute arterial vasoconstriction in healthy adults. Circulation. 2002;**105**:1534-1536

[13] Bouthillier L, Vincent R, Geogan P, et al. Acute effects of inhaled urban particles and ozone. The American Journal of Pathology. 1998;**153**:1-12

[14] Quillen JE, Rossen JD, Oskarsson HJ, et al. Acute effect of cigarette smoking on the coronary circulation: Constriction of epicardial and resistance vessels. Journal of the American College of Cardiology. 1993;**22**:642-649

[15] Goerre S, Staehli C, Shaw S, et al. Effect of cigarette smoking and nicotine on plasma endothelin-1 levels. Journal of Cardiovascular Pharmacology. 1995;**26**:S236-S238

[16] Otsuka R, Watanabe H, Hirata K, et al. Acute effects of passive smoking on the coronary circulation in healthy young adults. Journal of the American Medical Association. 2001;**286**:436-441

[17] Ikeda M, Watarai K, Suzuki M, et al. Mechanism of pathophysiological effects of diesel exhaust particles on endothelial cells. Environmental Toxicology and Pharmacology. 1998;**6**:117-123

[18] Ghio AJ, Kim C, Devlin RB. Concentrated ambient air particles induce mild pulmonary inflammation in healthy human volunteers. American Journal of Respiratory and Critical Care Medicine. 2000;**162**(3):981-988

7

Ovarian Clear Cell Carcinoma: Metastatic Pathways

Chrisostomos Sofoudis

Abstract

Ovarian carcinoma reflects the biggest challenge among the field of gynecologic oncology. It represents the most common death cause of genital carcinomas throughout years. The major classification consists of epithelial and non-epithelial types. Due to the histologic origin, epithelial types of ovarian carcinoma are endometrioid, serous-mucinous, and clear cell types. Due to intense metastatic infiltration and rapid tumor spread, clear cell ovarian carcinoma constitutes type of lesion with the most poor prognosis, decreased overall survival, decreased free survival, and poor quality of life of the patient. The metastatic infiltration is strongly accompanied with all significant prognostic factors. All biochemical pathways at the time of the infiltration are correlated with tumor size, lymphatic spread, staging of the lesion, histologic type, and grade of differentiation of the lesion.

Keywords: clear cell, chemotherapy, debulking, metastasis, ovarian carcinoma

1. Introduction

According to current literature, ovarian cancer represents a high mortality neoplasm in gynecologic malignancy. The 2017 incidence estimates 22,400 new cases in the United States [1]. The increased mortality rate is strongly accompanied with staging of the lesion at the time of the diagnosis. Many predisposition factors influence the therapeutic mapping. Age of the patient, parity, staging, cluster of differentiation, surgical margins, and lymphatic infiltration consist the gold standard of therapeutic strategy (**Figure 1**).

The frequency of the lesion increases in ages between 55 and 65 years old. There are also studies implicating younger or older patients. The lesion is more frequent in developed countries of the Western World and less in Asian countries [2]. Ovarian neoplasms express

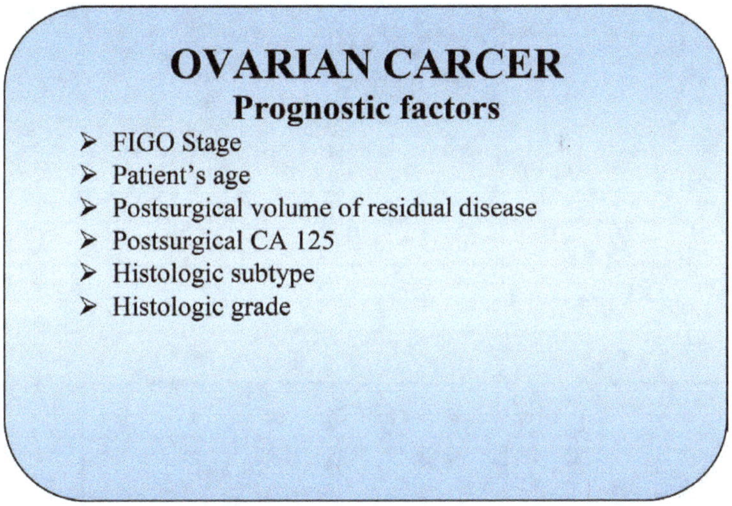

Figure 1. Prognostic factors in ovarian cancer. Ozols RF et al. Cancer Principles and Practice of Oncology. 5th ed. 1997;1510.

a wide variety. The most practical and useful classification depends on the histogenetic origin. Histological classification represents an autonomic entity with independent subtypes, disease-free survival, and quality of life of the patient (**Figure 2**).

On the other hand, depiction of histopathology, immunohistochemistry, and molecular genetic analysis reveal five basic types of ovarian carcinoma: high-grade serous carcinoma (HGSC 70%), endometrioid carcinoma (EC 10%), clear cell carcinoma (CCC 10%), mucinous carcinoma (MC 3%), and low-grade serous carcinoma (LGSC <5%) [3] (**Table 1**).

All recent conducted studies with classification parameter of the histogenetic origin express in 90% of cases the epithelial type as the most common type of ovarian carcinoma. Many useful tools, such as physical examination, transvaginal ultrasonography, Ca-125 levels, abdominal CT, or MRI, are mandatory in order to establish a more accurate clinical diagnosis [4]. Depending on clinical diagnosis, proper therapeutic mapping can be performed.

Among histologic subtypes of epithelial ovarian carcinoma, the most significant type with chemoresistance and poor prognosis consists clear cell ovarian carcinoma (CCC).

Clear cell carcinoma represents a distinct entity of epithelial ovarian carcinoma with an incidence less than 5% of all ovarian lesions [5]. Gold standard concerning therapeutic strategy of epithelial ovarian cancer and, respectively, of clear cell carcinoma is based on abdominal total hysterectomy, bilateral salpingo-oophorectomy, partial omentectomy with peritoneal sampling, and lymphadenectomy, adding cytoreductive surgery in advanced cases.

In many cases, surgical mapping for clear cell carcinoma remains a controversial issue. Many studies underline the decreased impact of adjuvant chemotherapy in patients with stage I clear cell carcinoma and the relation of the lesion with overall survival [6]. The ultimate scope of cytoreductive surgery in patients with clear cell carcinoma reflects the acknowledgment of high-risk patients correlated with recurrence of the lesion.

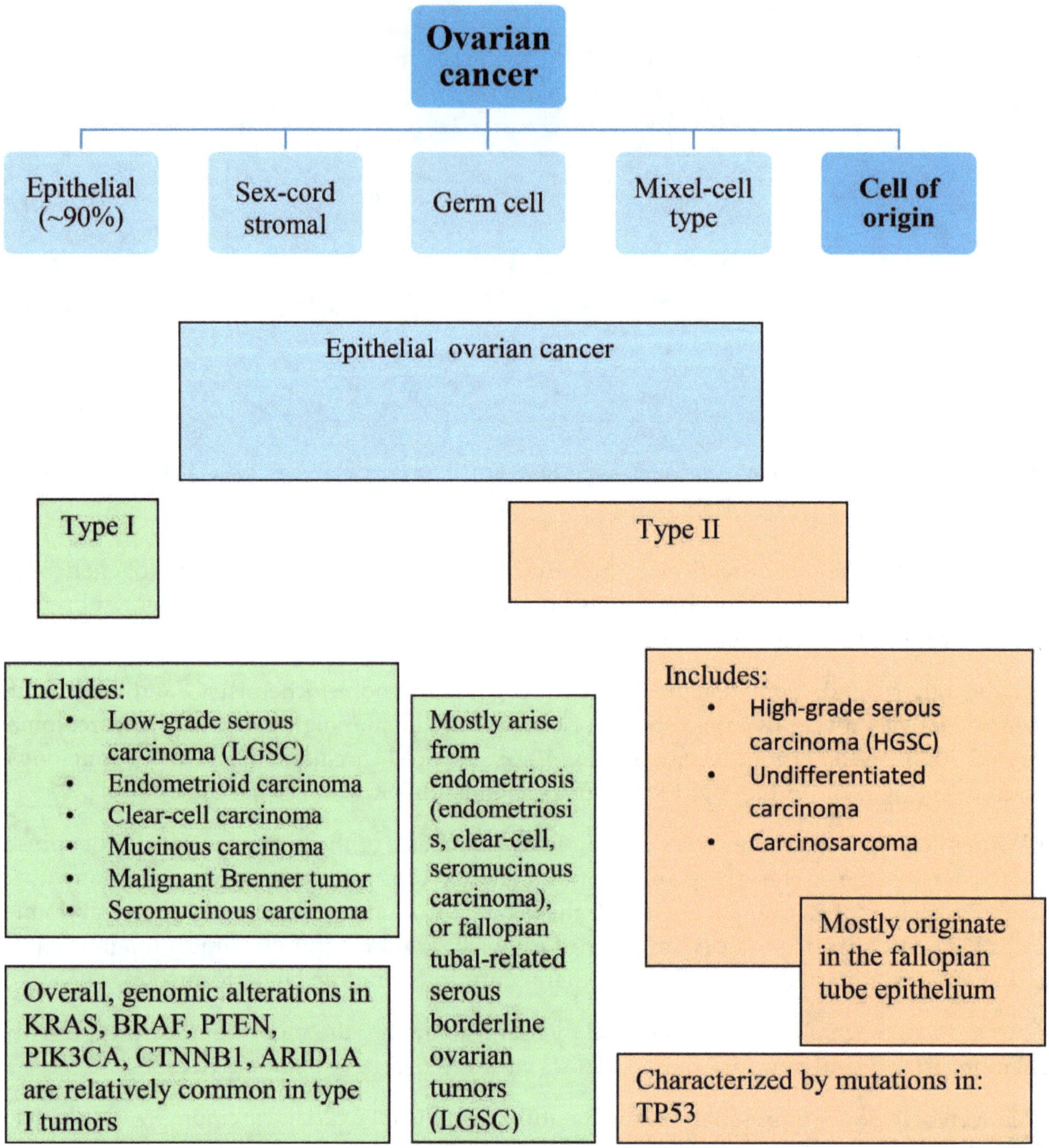

Figure 2. (A) Histological subtypes of ovarian cancer and (B) widely accepted epithelial ovarian cancer classification paradigm based on clinic, pathologic, and molecular evidence that type I and type II tumors develop through different pathways. *Indicates rare tumor. †Mucinous and malignant Brenner tumors are considered to be possible exceptions that may arise from transitional cells at or close to the junction of the fallopian tube and the peritoneum. Kurman RJ, Shih Ie M. The dualistic model of ovarian carcinogenesis: Revisited, revised, and expanded. Am. J. Pathol. 2016, 186, 733–747.

The significant role to metastatic pathways of clear cell carcinoma and the therapeutic mapping reflects the histologic configuration of the lesion. Histologic figures of clear cell carcinomas express clear cytoplasm with large nuclei and prominent nucleoli and a partial hobnail appearance (**Figure 3**).

	HGSC	LGSC	MC	EC	CCC
Risk factors	BRCA1/BRCA2	?	?	HNPCC[2]	?
Precursor lesions	Tubal intraepithelial carcinoma	Serous borderline tumor	Cystadenoma/ borderline tumor?	Atypical endometriosis	Atypical endometriosis
Pattern of spread	Very early transcoelomic spread	Transcoelomic spread	Usually confined to the ovary	Usually confined to the pelvis	Usually confined to the pelvis
Molecular abnormalities	BRCA, p53	BRAF, KRAS	KRAS, HER2	PTEN, ARIDIA	HNF1, ARIDIA
Chemosensitivity	High	Intermediate	Low	High	Low
Prognosis	Poor	Intermediate	Favorable	Favorable	Intermediate

Rat J. New insights into ovarian cancer pathology. Annals of Oncology 23 (Supplement 10): x111-x117, 2012.

HGSC, high-grade serous carcinoma; LGSC, low-grade serous carcinoma; MC, mucinous carcinoma; EC, endometrioid carcinoma; CCC, clear cell carcinoma. [a]Hereditary nonpolyposis colorectal carcinoma.

Table 1. Ovarian carcinoma: clinical and molecular features of the five most common types.

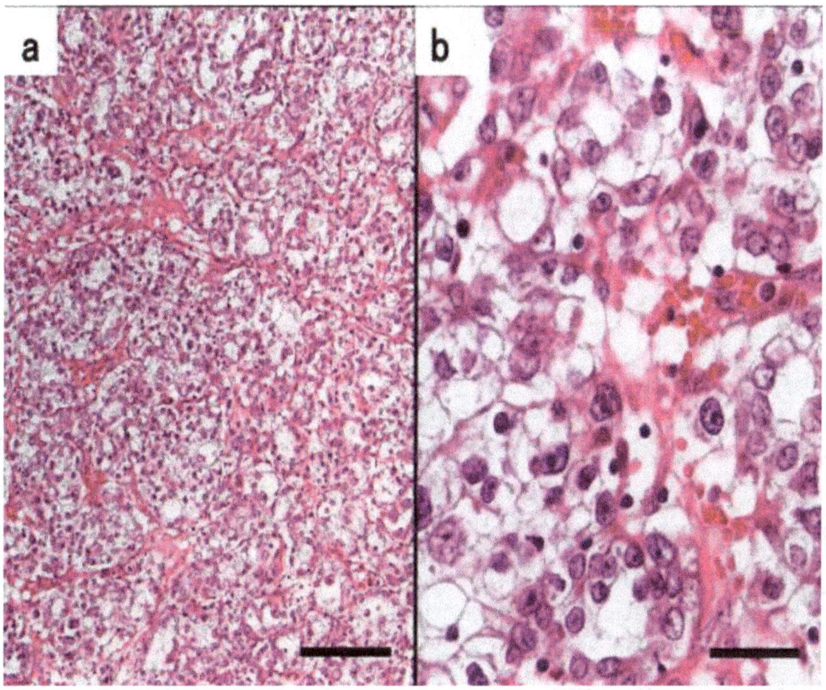

Figure 3. Histology of the original tumor. The left ovarian tumor is a clear cell carcinoma, with cells harboring clear cytoplasm and a partial hobnail appearance, as shown by hematoxylin and eosin (HE) staining ((a) bar = 200 μm; (b) bar = 50 μm). Yamada T et al. Characterization of a Novel Cell Line (HCH-3) Derived from a Human Ovarian Clear Cell Carcinoma. Yamada et al., J Carcinogene Mutagene 2017.

2. Discussion

Despite poor prognosis, overall survival, and quality of life of the patient, all conducted studies are focusing on the pathologic and metastatic pathways of the lesion. This issue remains controversial.

Szubert et al. described the correlation of endometriosis and clear cell ovarian carcinoma [7]. All the efforts lead to correlate the risk factors of endometriosis and clear cell carcinoma. We must never forget the role of endometriosis as trigger point and prominent risk factor of ovarian cancer. On the other point, many conducted studies depict the opposite statistic conclusion, gaining the impression of controversial issue. Zafrakas et al. correlated all the current data without an informative meta-analysis [8]. More conducted studies were mandatory in order to establish such a hypothesis.

Critical points of clear cell ovarian carcinoma remain the understanding of carcinogenesis, the genetic changes of the lesion, and most of all the mechanisms of target therapy.

Mabuchi et al. described and correlated all the critical genetic changes in clear cell carcinoma [9] (**Table 2**). Focusing on gene mutation, pathway bridge, and following tumor implications, we can explain the carcinogenesis of clear cell carcinoma.

Focusing on tumor angiogenesis, many conducted studies described targeted antibodies as therapeutic shield toward the production of tumor vessels [10]. Classical examples of target therapy consist monoclonal antibodies against vascular endothelial growth factor (VEGF), platelet-derived growth factor (PDGF), fibroblast growth factor (PDGF), and angiopoietin/Tie2 receptor complex [11]. Therapeutic philosophy depends on adjunction of monoclonal antibodies with growth factors, in order to prohibit tumor angiogenesis and infiltration. The emphasis in this procedure reflects the significant chemoresistance and poor prognosis of the lesion. The results of this target therapy remain controversial, justifying the significance of therapeutic strategy (**Figure 4**).

All therapeutic strategies consisted of overall survival, patient's quality of life and, in young ages with early stage lesion, the fertility-sparing surgery [12]. There are extreme selected indications, performing this surgical dissection.

Nasioudis et al. using the National Cancer Institute's Surveillance Epidemiology and End Results (SEER) database managed to perform the safety of fertility-sparing surgery in stages IA and IC of ovarian clear cell carcinoma [13]. The comparison, in patients with stage I ovarian clear cell carcinoma with preservation of the uterus and ovaries with general survival outcome, did not lead to statistical conclusion. However, further conducted studies are mandatory, in order to establish this type of surgical strategy in young female patients with stage IA or IC ovarian clear cell carcinoma.

Besides understanding the carcinogenesis of the lesion, the biochemical pathways, and the effort of fertility-sparing surgery in young female patients, we must mention the advanced metastatic opportunity of the lesion.

Lymphatic, hematogenic, and endoperitoneal infiltration of the lesion can lead to advanced metastatic possibilities. First of all, the lesion can penetrate the local anatomic organs: the salpinx, round ligament, uterus, peritoneal wall, colon, or even the omentum [14].

The most common, premature, and characteristic route of infiltration consists of the endoperitoneal [15]. All neoplasmatic cells are deafened, entering the peritoneal cavity. Through respiratory movements, endoperitoneal fluid with neoplasmatic cells finally reaches all epithelial

Gene	Gene type	Change	Pathways affected	Roles in tumor development
ARID1A	Tumor suppressor	Mutation in ~50%	SWI/SNF chromatin complex	Modulate accessibility of transcription factors to promoters
PIKECA	Oncogenic	Mutation in ~40%	PI3K/AKT/mTOR	Proliferation/survival
PPP2R1A	Oncogenic	Mutation in 7%	AKT/MAPK	Proliferation/survival
KRAS	Oncogenic	Mutation in 5%	AKT/MAPK	Proliferation/survival
BRCA1/BRCA2	Tumor suppressor	Mutation in 6%	DNA repair	Genomic instability
PTEN	Tumor suppressor	Mutation in 5%	PI3K/AKT/mTOR	Proliferation/survival
CDKN2A/CDKN2B	Tumor suppressor	Deletion in 9%	CDK inhibitors (p15/p16)	Cell cycle progression
ZNF217	Oncogenic	Amplification in 36%	ZNF217	Antiapoptosis
PPM1D	Oncogenic	Amplification in 10%	P53-mediated apoptosis	Antiapoptosis
AKT2	Oncogenic	Amplification in 14%	AKT/mTOR	Proliferation/survival
MET	Oncogenic	Amplification in 37%	AKT/MARK	Proliferation/survival

ARID1A, AT-rich interactive domain 1A; BRCA, breast cancer; CDK, cyclin-dependent kinase; CDKN, cyclin-dependent kinase inhibitor; MAPK, mitogen-activated protein kinases; mTOR, mammalian target of rapamycin; PIK3CA, phosphatidylinositol-45-bisphosphate 3-kinase catalytic subunit alpha; PI3K, phosphatidylinositol 3-kinase; PPM1D, protein phosphatase 1D; PPP2R1A, protein phosphatase 2 regulatory subunits 1A; PTEN, phosphatase and tensin homolog; SWI/SNF, SWItch/sucrose non-fermentable; ZNF217, zinc finger protein 217.

Table 2. Mabuchi S, Sugiyama T, Kimura T. Clear cell carcinoma of the ovary: molecular insights and future therapeutic perspectives. J Gynecol Oncol. 2016May; 27(3); e31.

areas and especially the hemidiaphragms. Final result, building of metastatic lesions as metastatic plaque or in advanced lesion as neoplasmatic "cake" (**Figure 5**). Through the right hemidiaphragm, the lesion can be spread in the pleura area, provoking hydrothorax or reaching the subclavian lymph nodes.

Usual distant organs with signs of infiltration are liver, lungs, and lymph nodes beyond the pelvic and para-aortic chains. Lymphatic spread of this lesion is common. The spread route follows the lymphatic vessels of ligamentum teres uteri or the lymphatic vessels of the right hemidiaphragm. The most common areas are pelvic lymph nodes with less frequent inguinal, axillary, or subclavian lymph nodes.

Hematogenic infiltration is strongly connected with advanced stages of the lesion. In these cases, the most common is liver and lung infiltration. In extreme advanced stages of the lesion, there are cases of skin or brain infiltration.

Nam et al. reported skin metastases in ovarian clear cell carcinoma as severe advanced metastatic area of the lesion [16]. Infiltration of these organs reflects severe decrease of disease-free survival, overall survival, and quality of life of the patient.

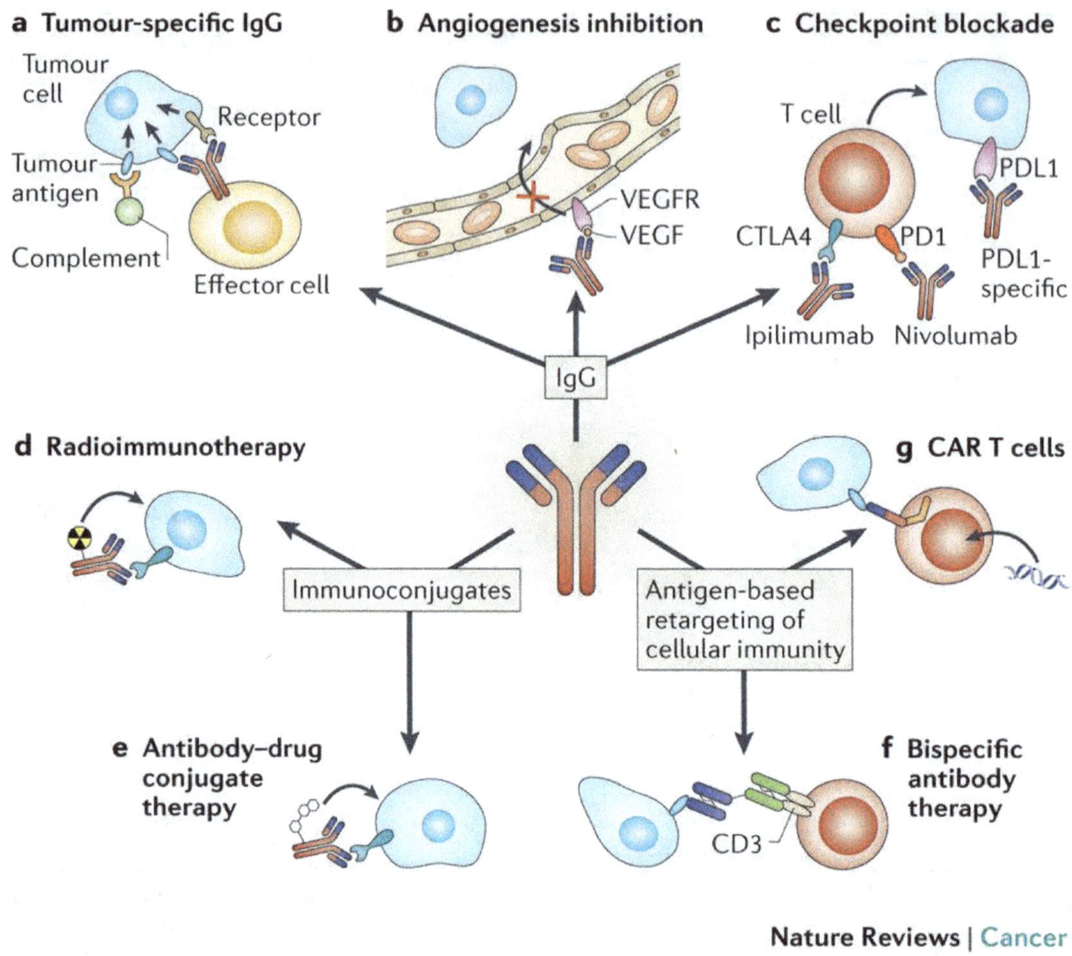

Figure 4. Weiner Building better monoclonal antibody-based therapeutics. Nature Reviews Cancer 15,361–370 (2015).

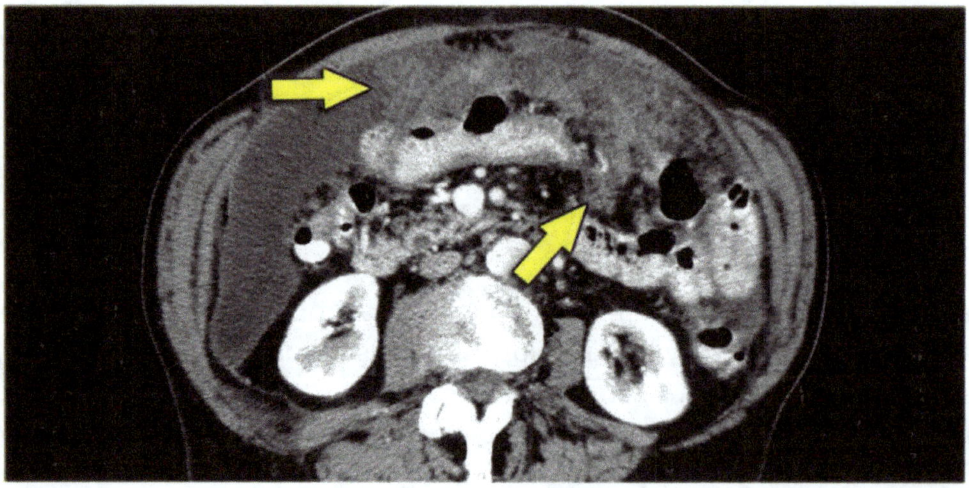

Figure 5. Omental cake (arrows) and ascites in a patient with peritoneal metastases derived from ovarian cancer. Levy Angela. Chief Gastrointestinal Radiology, Department of Radiologic Pathology, Armed Forces Institute of Pathology, Washington DC, Associate Professor of Radiology, Uniformed Services University of the Health Sciences, Bethesda, MD.

Postoperative treatment of clear cell ovarian carcinoma deviates, representing a distinct entity from other epithelial ovarian carcinomas. Reflecting a chemoresistant phenotype, the final prognosis of the lesion is poor, decreasing the quality of life of the patient. In cases of clear cell carcinoma, gold standard combination with paclitaxel and carboplatin consists a not promising therapeutic strategy. Irinotecan hydrochloride, a topoisomerase I inhibitor, reflects an alternative solution regarding the postoperative treatment of clear cell carcinoma [17] (first-line chemotherapy for clear cell carcinoma) (**Table 3**).

Many conducted studies managed to express the synergic effects of the combined therapeutic strategy of irinotecan and cisplatin (**Table 4**).

In cases of recurrent clear cell carcinoma, therapeutic mapping is very disappointed. Even in cases of sensitive platinum disease, the use of antineoplasmatic agents offers a response rate not up to 10% [18] (second-line chemotherapy for clear cell carcinoma).

Regimen	Author	Year	Response/number of patient, response rate
Conventional platinum based	Goff (28)	1996	1/6, 17%
	Sugiyama (29)	2000	3/27, 11%
	Ho (30)	2004	4/15, 27%
	Takano (9)	2006	5/30, 17%
Taxane-platinum	Ecomoto (31)	2003	2/9, 22%
	Ho (30)	2004	9/16, 56%
	Utsunomiya (32)	2006	8/15, 53%
	Takano (9)	2006	9/28, 32%
Irinotecan-cisplatin	Takano (9)	2006	3/10, 30%

Takano et al. Clear cell carcinoma of the ovary: Is there a role of histology-specific treatment? Journal of Experimental & Clinical Cancer Research 2012, 31:53

Table 3. Response rates of primary chemotherapy for clear cell carcinoma.

Regimen	Author	Year	Response/number of patient, response rate
Megestrol acetate	Malailak (45)	2001	2/10, 20%
Cyclophosphamide + cisplatin	Takano (46)	2008	1/9, 11%
Irinotecan + platinum	Sugiyama (29)	1998	1/3, 33%
	Takano (46)	2008	2/15, 13%
Etoposide + platinum	Takano (46)	2008	2/13, 15%
Paclitaxel + carboplatin	Utsunomiya (32)	2006	3/13, 23%
	Crotzer (43)	2007	2/7, 29%
Gemcitabine	Crotzer (43)	2007	1/9, 11%
	Yoshino (47)	2012	1/5, 20%
Docetaxel + irinotecan	Yoshino (47)	2012	1/11, 9%
Temsirolimus	Takano (46)	2011	1/5, 20%

Takano et al. Clear cell carcinoma of the ovary: Is there a role of histology-specific treatment? Journal of Experimental & Clinical Cancer Research 2012, 31:53.

Table 4. Response rates of salvage chemotherapy for recurrent or refractory clear cell carcinoma.

The main objective of the previous study was the presentation and implementation of an epithelial-type ovarian carcinoma with specific metastatic pathways, prohibiting especially episodes of target therapy. New scientific keys, in the near future, will unlock unknown biochemical mechanisms and give answers to many questions, concerning the understanding of carcinogenesis of this lesion.

3. Conclusion

Ovarian clear cell carcinoma represents a rare histological entity with extreme chemoresistance and poor prognosis in correlation with overall survival and quality of life of the patient. Better understanding of metastatic and biochemical pathways of the lesion could schedule a proper therapeutic mapping. Further conducted studies are needed, in order to establish such strategy.

Conflict of interest

The author declares any financial interest with respect to this manuscript.

Author details

Chrisostomos Sofoudis

Address all correspondence to: chrisostomos.sofoudis@gmail.com

Department of Obstetrics and Gynecology, Konstandopoulio General Hospital, Athens, Greece

References

[1] Siegel PL, Miller KD, Jemal A. Cancer statistics, 2017. CA: A Cancer Journal for Clinicians. 2017;**67**:7-30

[2] Benedet JL, Bender HJ, et al. FIGO staging classifications and clinical practice guidelines in the management of gynecological cancers. International Journal of Gynecology & Obstetrics. 2000;**70**(2):209-262

[3] Prat J. Ovarian carcinomas: Five distinct diseases with different origins, genetic alterations, and clinicopathological features. Virchows Archiv. 2012;**460**:237-249

[4] Forstner R. Radiological staging of ovarian cancer: Imaging findings and contribution of CT or MRI. European Radiology. 2007;**17**(12):3223-3235

[5] Crozier MA, Copeland LJ, Silva EG, et al. Clear cell carcinoma of the ovary: A study of 59 cases. Gynecologic Oncology. 1989;**35**:199-203

[6] Takano M, Sugiyama T, Yaegashi N, et al. Less impact of adjuvant chemotherapy for stage I clear cell carcinoma of the ovary: A retrospective Japan Clear Cell Carcinoma Study. International Journal of Gynecological Cancer. 2010;**20**:1506-1510

[7] Szubert M, Suzin J, Obirek K, et al. Clear cell carcinoma and endometriosis: Is there a relationship? Menopause Review. 2016;**15**(2):85-89

[8] Zafrakas M, Gribizis G, Timoglou A, Tarlatzis BC. Endometriosis and ovarian cancer risk: A systematic review of epidemiological studies. Frontiers in Surgery. 2014;**8**:14

[9] Mabuchi S, Sugiyama T, Kimura T. Clear cell carcinoma of the ovary: Molecular insights and future therapeutic perspectives. Journal of Gynecologic Oncology. 2016;**27**(3):e31

[10] Mabuchi S, Kawase C, Altomare DA, et al. Vascular endothelial growth factor is a promising therapeutic target for the treatment of clear cell carcinoma of the ovary. Molecular Cancer Therapeutics. 2010;**9**(8):2411-2422

[11] Stany MP, Vathipadiekal V, Ozbun L, et al. Identification of novel therapeutic targets in microdissected clear cell ovarian cancers. PLoS One. 2011;**6**(7):e21121

[12] Park JY. Safety of fertility-sparing surgery for stage I ovarian clear cell carcinoma. Journal of Gynecologic Oncology. 2017;**28**(6):e91

[13] Nasioudis D, Chapman-Davis E, Frey MK, Witkin SS, Holcomb K. Could fertility-sparing surgery be consisted for women with early stage ovarian clear cell carcinoma? Journal of Gynecologic Oncology. 2017;**28**:e71

[14] Gass I, Li A, Runowicz C, et al. Pattern of lymph node metastases in clinically unilateral stage I invasive epithelial ovarian carcinomas. Gynecologic Oncology. 2001;**80**:56-61

[15] Dauplant J, Hacker NF, Neiberg RK, Berek JS, Rose TP, Sagae S. Distant metastasis in epithelial ovarian carcinoma. Cancer. 1987;**60**:1561-1566

[16] Nam G, Lim Y, Cho MS, Lee J, Kim YH. Skin metastases in ovarian clear cell carcinoma: A case report and review of the literature. Obstetrics & Gynecology Science. 2017;**60**(6):593-597

[17] Sugiyama T, Yakushiji M, Nishida T, et al. Irinotecan (CPT-11) combined with cisplatin in patients with refractory or recurrent ovarian cancer. Cancer. 1998;**128**:211-218

[18] Takano M, Sugiyama T, Yeagashi N, et al. Low response rate of second-line chemotherapy for recurrent or refractory clear cell carcinoma of the ovary: A retrospective Japan Clear Cell Carcinoma Study. International Journal of Gynecological Cancer. 2008;**18**:937-942

8

Heavy Metals and Cancer

Austin Carver and Vincent S. Gallicchio

Abstract

There has been increased concern surrounding exposure to heavy metals due to the evolving understanding of their role in the development of cancer. This review highlights research related to the impact that heavy metals aluminum, arsenic, beryllium, cadmium, lead, mercury, nickel and radium have on human health. Research was collected through PubMed, and it was compiled to assess the current knowledge of exposure sources, types of cancers induced and therapeutic measures for these metals. Furthermore, it was designed to assist in guiding future research efforts with respect to heavy metals and cancer.

Keywords: heavy metals, carcinogenesis, exposure, treatment

1. Introduction

Exposure to heavy metals represents significant health concerns in the human population. These elements have the ability to induce a number of adverse health effects, but one of their more serious actions is their role in carcinogenesis. There exists a plethora of information on the research database, PubMed, regarding various exposure patterns and cancers induced by these heavy metals. However, this information has remained largely disconnected at this point, which necessitates the consolidation of this research. Our work reviews studies for how humans are exposed to heavy metals as well as what specific body systems are targeted.

2. Aluminum

Aluminum is a unique heavy metal with numerous pathways of exposure. Exposure to this element has been documented in contaminated food, vaccines to elicit a more powerful immune response and aluminum salts used in industrial processes and commercial products [1, 2].

Specific commercial products containing aluminum salts include certain antacids and antiperspirant deodorants [1–3].

Aluminum exposure has been strongly correlated with carcinogenesis in the breast tissue. Mice subjected to $AlCl_3$, the same aluminum salt used in antiperspirant deodorants, displayed malignant growth of mammary gland epithelial cells [1]. This same result was observed in studies performed on samples of human breast cells [1–3]. This heavy metal was also hypothesized to have a role in the development of sarcomas [4]. Additionally, in one patient, it was proposed that the chronic exposure of aluminum containing heavy metal salts resulted in the development of an atypical neuroectodermal tumor [4].

There have been several determined mechanisms for the carcinogenic activity of aluminum. After exposing samples of human breast cells to this element, one study observed diminished concentrations of mRNA for the recognized tumor suppressor gene BRCA1 in addition to mRNA concentrations for other essential DNA maintenance genes [3]. Another study determined that subjecting human breast cells to aluminum had the potential to induce uncontrolled growth [2]. In this study, aluminum was observed to act as a metalloestrogen, which behaves as an agonist for estrogen receptors, and represents a known risk for carcinogenesis in the breast [2]. In another area of the body, analyzed samples of bladder carcinomas displayed statistically higher levels of aluminum, among other heavy metals [5]. Although a mechanism has not been established currently, this evidence suggests that this metal plays at least a supportive role in malignant growth in the bladder [5]. Standard therapy following aluminum poisoning has been the use of chelators. Aluminum in the human body has been demonstrated to bioaccumulate in soft and skeletal tissues, which are target areas for the removal of aluminum [6]. The common chelator used therapeutically has been desferrioxamine [6]. This chelator has proven effective in eliminating aluminum from the body; however, there are a number of toxic side effects associated with its use [6]. There have been several promising candidates to replace desferrioxamine, but none have proved to be as effective thus far [6]. The most successful method in limiting the toxic effects of aluminum is to reduce exposure to the metal. One potential solution for reducing public exposure is the use of reverse osmosis filtration. This technology has demonstrated the ability to remove significant levels of aluminum from copper mining waste at the experimental stage [7].

3. Arsenic

Arsenic is a cytotoxic element, and exposure to this metal presents serious risks to human health. Contact with arsenic generally results from ingesting contaminated food and water, occupational exposure and environmental pollution [8–11] Common occupations where arsenic exposure is common include smelting and arsenic based pesticide industries [12]. One noted source of environmental exposure to this heavy metal is contact with contaminated soil, which has the potential to enter the human food chain [13].

This heavy metal has been detected in an extensive variety of malignant growths. Research strongly supports role of arsenic in the development of lung, bladder and skin cancer [8, 11, 12]. Another study determined a strong positive association between exposure and mortality rates of cancers including colon, gastric, kidney, lung and nasopharyngeal [13]. Epidemiological studies have also suggested an association between chronic low-level exposure to arsenic and development of pancreatic cancer and non-Hodgkin's lymphoma [14, 15].

Well-documented carcinogenic mechanisms for this heavy metal include generation of reactive oxygen species (ROS), epigenetic alterations and damage to the dynamic DNA maintenance system [8, 9, 12]. Key epigenetic changes induced by arsenic include alterations to the status of DNA methylation, histones, and miRNA, which are all changes that have the potential to cause malignant growth [9, 12]. Another study found that this toxic metal could induce inappropriate growth cycles for macrophages in addition to lung epithelial cells [16]. Furthermore, it was observed that macrophages exposed to ROS generated by arsenic responded by activating through the M2 phase, which is correlated with potential lung carcinogenesis [16]. Arsenic displayed a specific mechanism of action against human lung epithelial cells. This heavy metal was determined to alter the expression of the p53 protein, which resulted in decreased expression of p21, one downstream target [17]. The observed inappropriate proliferation was attributed to this mechanism [17]. Further examination of arsenic revealed its ability to reduce intracellular concentrations of glutathione, a natural antioxidant [18]. This carries the potential for carcinogenic activity by subjecting the cell to oxidative stress [18]. An additional carcinogenic mechanism proposed for this heavy metal lies in its ability to influence base excision repair [19]. The enzyme DNA polymerase beta was involved with this repair system, and arsenic was observed to inhibit its activity at high concentrations [19]. Another novel pathway for tumorigenic activity was discovered in human bladder cells. This study determined that chronic arsenic exposure had the potential to induce morphology changes and alter gene expression for proteins that regulate proliferation [20]. The use of chelators has remained the most effective way to eliminate arsenic from the body. Rac-2,3-dimercaptopropanol, or British anti-lewisite, contains two thiol functional groups, and it is one prominent chelator for this metal [21]. Although lacking clinical data at this point, 2,3-dimercaptopropane-1-sulphonate was used in one individual with acute arsenic poisoning [22]. This therapy resulted in successful treatment with limited side effects, which suggests the importance of future study [22]. Following arsenic exposure, dietary antioxidants have been recommended to mitigate carcinogenic effects of this metal, such as oxidative stress [23]. Developing novel prevention methods is essential for limiting human exposure. Rice and apple juice have been recognized as two common sources of exposure [24]. Safety standards of 5 μg/L of arsenic have been recommended for apple juice, due to its extensive ingestion by children [24]. Current research to limit its presence in rice includes genetic modifications to inhibit arsenic uptake, and the use of microbes that compete for arsenic in the environment [24]. It has also been observed that the use of sprinkler irrigation has the potential to significantly reduce the concentration of arsenic in rice by inducing its precipitation [24, 25].

4. Beryllium

Beryllium is a heavy metal that has uses in industrial processes and technology production. The primary environmental contamination source for this element is thought to be power plants, which leech beryllium in the form of dust [26, 27]. Due to inhalation being the general method of exposure for this contaminant, current research is investigating its role in lung carcinogenesis [27–29]. There are mixed reviews supporting the extent of the role for beryllium in lung cancer, but recent research has determined a more significant correlation between the two [28–30]. Furthermore, an increased risk of lung cancer was observed in individuals exposed to exceptionally high concentrations of beryllium, which suggests that this element does induce some carcinogenic mechanism [29]. The use of beryllium in the dental industry creates additional occupational risk for exposure [29]. It was determined that the use of protective equipment significantly reduced the level of exposure in individuals [31]. Additionally, elevated concentrations of beryllium were detected in patients with stage III breast cancer [32]. However, beryllium was one of several heavy metals detected, so a defined role has not been identified at this point [32]. Exposure to beryllium is also recognized as a risk for the potential development of osteosarcomas [33].

Currently, there has not been much research relevant to beryllium's carcinogenic mechanisms. Most literature that exists now is related to action against the lungs. For instance, one potentially carcinogenic mechanism identified was its role in inducing a higher level of tumor necrosis factor alpha (TNF-α) cytokine secretion from CD4+ T-cells in the lungs [30, 34]. Both of these proteins have a role in the inflammation process, and their elevated presence was suspected to have action in chronic inflammation [30, 34]. Beryllium also has the potential to induce inappropriate genetic changes. For instance, this heavy metal was observed to methylate the *p16* gene, a known tumor suppressor gene, and induce its inactivation [30]. Chelators are common forms of therapy used to eliminate beryllium from the body and reduce its toxic effects. Relevant chelators include 4,-dihydroxy-1,3-benzene disulphonic acid disodium salt (Tiron) and D-penicillamine (DPA), which proved to be effective when tested in animals [35–37]. Also, the chelator meso-2,3-dimercaptosuccinic acid (DMSA) was used in a case study to successfully save a child suffering from heavy metal poisoning [38]. This result suggested potential clinical significance and requires further investigation [38]. There have been significant efforts to reduce exposure to this metal, especially occupational exposure [39, 40]. These efforts include company programs instituted to screen blood samples for beryllium sensitization during employment as well as providing refined ventilation and dust control to processes where exposure is common [40]. Attention was also given to educating employees about the importance of using protective equipment, and illuminating the potential risks involved with chronic beryllium exposure [39, 40].

5. Cadmium

Cadmium is an immensely toxic heavy metal, and it is associated with significant health implications as an environmental contaminant. Cadmium contamination generally results from emissions from industries that utilize this element including mining, metal research, development of certain batteries and preventing precipitation in pigments [41]. Soil pollution is a serious issue from cadmium emissions, and human exposure typically occurs from inhalation, smoking and ingesting contaminated food and water [41, 42]. Another source of environmental contamination is landfills, which have been observed to contain levels of cadmium exceeding safety standards in certain cases [43]. Additionally, ingesting this metal from contaminated food has been noted as a typical source of exposure [14, 44].

Exposure to cadmium has been associated with carcinogenesis in multiple tissues including breast, esophagus, stomach, intestines, prostate, lungs and testes [41, 45, 46]. Cadmium also has a proposed role in the development of cancer in the gallbladder. The composition of gallstones, which are recognized as a risk factor for carcinogenesis, were analyzed from patients with this type of cancer [47]. Statistically higher concentrations of cadmium, along with other heavy metals, were observed [47]. Although a causal link involving cadmium was not observed, it does suggest a potential role in malignant growth of the bladder [47]. Cadmium has also demonstrated carcinogenic activity on liver cells in a laboratory setting [44]. Additionally, increased concentrations of cadmium were detected in patients with malignant gliomas, suggesting a potential role of carcinogenesis in the brain [48]. Another organ where cadmium is suggested to exert carcinogenic influence is the pancreas [15, 49]. This metal also has a suspected association with the development of chronic myeloid and lymphoblastic leukemia. It was determined that, when compared to controls, patients with these forms of leukemia displayed significantly elevated concentrations of cadmium and lower levels of magnesium in blood and serum samples [50]. Further work with this metal determined that increased concentration of cadmium in urine was strongly correlated with risk of developing gastrointestinal cancer [51].

Similar to other heavy metals, carcinogenic mechanisms associated with cadmium include generation of ROS, epigenetic alterations, inhibiting DNA repair processes and apoptosis [41, 46, 52, 53]. It has been demonstrated that both chronic and acute cadmium exposure has the ability to induce changes in gene regulation, which generates an increased risk for malignant growth [44]. Key proteins that displayed upregulated expression include DNAJB9, a protein involved in regulating cell destruction, and metallothioneins [44]. Important regulatory proteins also displayed downregulated expression, such as EGR-1, a protein involved in regulating transcription [44]. There are not currently any standard therapeutic measures for the treatment of cadmium poisoning [54]. However, there is ongoing research to develop compounds that reduce the toxic effects of this metal. For example there has been research to develop unique peptoid ligands with selective affinity for cadmium [54]. It has also been determined that flavonoids, compounds present in most plants, have antioxidant properties and can chelate cadmium atoms [55]. Further study is recommended to determine how the structure of flavonoids relates to its action on cadmium [55]. There is also investigation into the use of stem cells as a therapeutic measure for cadmium induced damage. For one study, rat testes were subjected to damaging levels of cadmium [56]. Upon treatment with bone marrow mesenchymal stem cells, it was observed that the rat testes displayed more appropriate levels of proteins related to apoptosis regulation [56]. Additionally, these cells were determined to restore damaged testes tissue, and it was suggested that a possible mechanism is associated with mitochondrial apoptosis [56].

6. Lead

Lead is a toxic heavy metal and exposure constitutes significant risks to health. One common source of environmental pollution has been found in the soil, which can enter the human food cycle through contaminated produce [57–59]. Despite being banned from use in commercially available gasoline in 1995, lead is still added to aviation fuel [59]. This source of environmental pollution has been determined to contribute high emission levels of lead [59]. It was also determined that smokers contained elevated levels of blood lead, representing an additional source of environmental exposure [60]. Certain occupations also play a role in lead exposure, such as mining [57].

Various epidemiological studies have been performed to determine if increased lead exposure is associated with any forms of cancer. Additionally, current research has indicated at this point that lead may not have a causal role in cancer, but it may play a more supportive role [61]. Along with cadmium, lead was detected in significantly higher concentrations in glioma patients, suggesting these two metals combined may produce excessively toxic effects [48]. One study has determined strong correlation between lead exposure and the development of kidney cancer [58]. Another study concluded that patients with higher levels of blood lead had an increased risk of developing renal cell carcinoma [60]. Lead was one of several heavy metals observed in statistically higher concentrations in gallstones [47]. This suggests exposure to this metal represents an increased risk of malignant growth in the gallbladder [47]. In a study performed on lead exposed workers, positive correlation was observed between exposure to this heavy metal and increased risk of carcinogenesis in lung tissue and marginal positive correlation for malignant growth in brain, larynx and bladder tissues [62]. Along with several additional heavy metals, lead was reportedly detected in elevated levels in individuals with exocrine pancreatic cancer, suggesting an unknown mechanism in the development of this cancer [15].

Current literature has not displayed a comprehensive understanding of carcinogenic mechanisms of lead; however, plausible mechanisms have been proposed. Based on the present understanding of lead, it was hypothesized to support the carcinogenic process by disrupting cellular tumor regulation genes, the DNA repair system and inducing DNA damage [63]. In a study performed on mice, there was evidence to support lead's role in generating ROS and altering chromosomal structure and sequence [63]. It was also determined that lead had the potential to disrupt the transcription process by replacing zinc in certain proteins that regulate this system [63]. In an epidemiological study, it was determined that elevated levels of serum calcium were correlated with lower risk of developing renal cell carcinoma, which suggested the need for a clinical trial to determine significance [60]. Chelation therapy is the recommended course of action for individuals with lead poisoning [64]. Common chelators for reducing levels of lead in the body include British, Anti-Lewisite, calcium disodium ethylenediaminetetraacetic acid, D-penicillamine and Meso-2,3-dimercaptosuccinic acid, and use of a specific chelator depends on the situation of the individual [64]. There has also been research into the effectiveness of less toxic therapies. For instance, when garlic was administered in a clinical setting, it was found to reduce blood lead levels in non-severe lead poisoning and alleviate symptoms [64]. The most effective strategy for keeping blood concentration of lead low is prevention of exposure [58]. This includes ensuring that industries that generate significant levels of lead emissions and employees follow safety guidelines for limiting exposure [64]. It has also been suggested that identification of lead contamination sources, followed by removal or avoidance, constitutes the ideal solution to reduce exposure to this heavy metal [64].

7. Mercury

Mercury is another toxic heavy metal with the potential for serious health complications. Although this element can be found in trace amounts in mineral form, most present in the environment is due to human induced pollution from processed mercury [65]. Mercury has a wide range of uses that result in occupational and environmental contamination. Several sources of this heavy metal have been identified as thermometers, fossil fuel emissions, dental fillings, certain batteries and burning medical waste [65, 66]. Mercury compounds have the potential to be vaporized and enter the atmosphere or leech into soil or water systems [65, 67]. Consuming large quantities of seafood has been identified as a primary method for environmental exposure to methyl mercury [65]. Although the pathway through which mercury enters the ecosystem has not been discovered, bioaccumulation of this heavy metal has been observed in shellfish and tuna [65, 68, 69].

Although a causal role has not been established at this time, it has been proposed that mercury exposure may be associated with renal cancer due to this organ being a target for this element [65]. Another study observed that increased mercury exposure has been correlated with liver cancer, and it also has the carcinogenic potential to induce gastric cancer [70]. Mercury was another heavy metal detected in gallstones in statistically higher concentrations from patients with gallbladder cancer [47]. A causal association was not observed with this metal, but a role in carcinogenic development was hypothesized [47].

Comparable to most of the other heavy metals discussed in this study, mercury has the potential to induce malignant growth through several specific mechanisms. These include the ability to generate free radicals as well as disrupt DNA molecular structure and the maintenance system [66]. However, there have been several proposed carcinogenic mechanisms of mercury that are either unique to this metal or not observed in most heavy metals. One mechanism that enhances the carcinogenicity of mercury is its role in reducing the body's concentration of glutathione, a natural antioxidant [71]. This could potentially contribute to increasing susceptibility of essential cellular components to oxidative stress. Oxidative stress on cells has been shown to elevate rates of lipid peroxidation, another mechanism associated with carcinogenesis [65]. It has also been proposed that mercury can affect the microtubules in cells, which, among other processes, can disrupt cellular division [66]. The use of chelators is the common therapeutic strategy for eliminating mercury from the body. It has been determined that the two most effective chelators in a clinical setting are dimercaptosuccinic acid (DMSA) and dimercaptopropane sulfonate (DMPS) [72, 73]. There has also been research to investigate untested chelators for their effectiveness against mercury. For instance, deferasirox and deferiprone were combined and tested on rats [74]. It was observed that this combination was able to successfully chelate mercury and reduced toxic effects of mercury [74]. One unique experimental chelator was thiol-modified nanoporous silica material [75]. Following animal testing, it was observed that this material displayed tremendous potential for eliminating mercury, along with several other heavy metals, with marginal toxicity [75].

8. Nickel

Nickel, a heavy metal present in Earth's core, has garnered research attention due to increased understanding of carcinogenic properties. This metal can produce toxic effects upon exposure in an environmental or occupational setting. Several industries involving potential occupational exposure to nickel include mining, metal alloys and the refinement of nickel [76–78]. Pollution of this heavy metal can enter the environment and bioaccumulate in organisms that enter the human food chain, such as fish [79]. Contaminated soil represents another method of contacting this toxic metal [76]. Emissions from oil refineries have also been established as a significant source of nickel pollution, creating risk for environmental exposure to residents in close proximity [80].

There are a variety of cancers that have been associated with nickel exposure. Epidemiological studies have revealed a significant correlation between exposure and the incidence of carcinogenesis in lung, nasal and sinus tissues [13, 77, 81, 82]. In another study, high levels of serum nickel were determined to be statistically significant in patients with breast cancer, suggesting that exposure has potentially carcinogenic consequences [83]. Exposure to this heavy metal has also been associated with the development of acute myeloid and lymphoblastic leukemia. It was determined that urine contained higher levels of nickel and 8-hydroxy-2′-deoxyguanosine in children with this leukemia [84]. These results suggested a role of nickel in acute leukemia by inducing oxidative damage as a mechanism of action [84]. Research has also revealed the presence of elevated nickel concentrations in individuals with exocrine pancreatic cancer [15]. Although there were other heavy metals present, these findings suggest carcinogenic action from nickel [15]. Another study proposed a link between chronic allergic stimulation from several heavy metals, including nickel, and the development of cutaneous T-cell lymphoma [85]. Furthermore, significant correlation was observed between exposure and mortality rates of liver cancer [13].

Nickel has an extensive range of carcinogenic mechanisms. One such mechanism involves its role in affecting the expression of specific long noncoding RNAs. It has been determined that nickel possesses the ability to induce the downregulation of maternally expressed gene 3 (MEG3) through the methylation of its related promoter [81]. This process was shown to inhibit expression of PHLPP1 and upregulate hypoxia-inducible factor-1α, two proteins recognized for their role in carcinogenesis [81]. It has also been demonstrated that nickel can generate free radicals, which contributes to the carcinogenic process [86]. Exposure to this heavy metal also has the ability to alter the regulation status for the transcription of various mRNAs and microRNAs [78]. The expression of these transcripts has roles in immunity as well as inflammation, which both have proposed roles in the development of malignant growth [78].

The role of nickel in chronic inflammation was investigated in animals and samples of human cells. It was concluded that exposure elevated expression of proteins SQSTM1 and TNF, which have roles in maintaining levels of inflammation, and induced carcinogenesis [82]. Like other heavy metals, nickel has the potential to induce epigenetic changes such as alterations in DNA methylation. For instance, it was observed that nickel ions (Ni2+) had the potential to induce the tri-methylation of histone H3K4 [87]. This process has been correlated with inappropriate transcriptional activation, which suggests another carcinogenic mechanism for nickel [87]. Compared to other heavy metals, the use of chelators involving nickel has been markedly different. Sodium diethyldithiocarbamate has proven to be an effective chelator in response to nickel carbonyl, but a chelator associated with nickel cancer has not been recommended at this point [88]. Despite this fact, there has been research into the use of chelators to remove nickel from the environment. For instance, it was observed that ethylene diamine tetraacetic acid (EDTA) induces the uptake of nickel from contaminated soil in *Arundo donax* L. [89]. This carries tremendous potential for use in areas where nickel is present in dangerous concentrations. It was also determined that CaNa(2) EDTA reverses the damage induced by nickel chloride as well as eliminate the metal from Cirrhinus mrigala [90].

9. Radium

Radium is a radioactive heavy metal that can negatively impact health. This ionizing radiation results from radium decaying into toxic radon gas [91]. Occupational and environmental presence of radium generates opportunities for exposure to ionizing radiation. Coal mining has been noted as one of the most relevant occupations with risk for exposure [92]. Wastewater drained from mines also carries potential for environmental radium contamination [92]. Radium presents further occupational hazards from exposure sources that include soil, building materials and water systems [93]. A study performed in Italy suggested radon gas tends to concentrate in confined spaces of buildings, such as basements or storage areas [91]. Due to radon's ability to bind to cigarette smoke, it was observed that this act increased the accumulation of radon inside buildings [93]. This suggests that smoking increases radium's impact as an environmental contaminant.

Radium is a known carcinogen that is associated with several cancers. Since a primary method of exposure to radon gas has been identified as inhalation, radium has been strongly correlated with the development of lung cancer [91]. Due to the radioactive nature of this metal, chelators are generally not necessary. Nevertheless, it has been determined to have several unique uses. For example, radium has been used as a therapy for patients with ankylosing spondylitis. However, injection of this metal was determined to be associated with increased risk of various forms of leukemia [94]. Injection of mice with radium was determined to cause the generation of osteosarcomas [94]. In another particular case, it was proposed that a patient developed a cutaneous squamous cell carcinoma in response to treatment with radium-223 that extravasated [95]. This study suggested that patients with extravasated radioactive substances require the oversight of a dermatologist [95].

10. Conclusion

Heavy metals exhibit an immense range of toxic effects in humans with regard to carcinogenesis. The research available at this point has illuminated several areas of emphasis for future work. It is clear that a refined understanding of carcinogenic mechanisms is necessary. This could help generate personalized therapeutic or prevention measures for specific heavy metals. Continued consolidation of information is another essential factor moving forward. Effective educational programs are also needed in high-risk areas to raise awareness of the risks associated with exposure to heavy metals.

Author details

Austin Carver and Vincent S. Gallicchio*

*Address all correspondence to: vsgall@clemson.edu

Department of Biological Sciences, College of Science, Clemson University, Clemson, South Carolina, United States of America

References

[1] Mandriota SJ, Tenan M, Ferrari P, Sappino AP. Aluminium chloride promotes tumorigenesis and metastasis in normal murine mammary gland epithelial cells. International Journal of Cancer. 2016;**139**(12):2781-2790. DOI: 10.1002/ijc.30393

[2] Darbre PD. Aluminium and the human breast. Morphologie. 2016;**100**(329):65-74. DOI: 10.1016/j.morpho.2016.02.001

[3] Farasani A, Darbre PD. Effects of aluminium chloride and aluminium chlorohydrate on DNA repair in MCF10A immortalised non-transformed human breast epithelial cells. Journal of Inorganic Biochemistry. 2015;**152**:186-189. DOI: 10.1016/j.jinorgbio.2015.08.003

[4] Roncati L, Gatti AM, Capitani F, Barbolini G, Maiorana A, Palmieri B. Heavy metal bioaccumulation in an atypical primitive neuroectodermal tumor of the abdominal wall. Ultrastructural Pathology. 2015;**39**(4):286-292. DOI: 10.3109/01913123.2015.1013655

[5] Abdel-Gawad M, Elsobky E, Shalaby MM, Abd-Elhameed M, Abdel-Rahim M, Ali-El-Dein B. Quantitative evaluation of heavy metals and trace elements in the urinary bladder: Comparison between cancerous, adjacent non-cancerous and normal cadaveric tissue. Biological Trace Element Research. 2016;**174**(2):280-286. DOI: 10.1007/s12011-016-0764-6

[6] Yokel RA. Aluminum chelation: Chemistry, clinical, and experimental studies and the search for alternatives to desferrioxamine. Journal of Toxicology and Environmental Health. 1994;**41**(2):131-174. DOI: 10.1080/15287399409531834

[7] Ambiado K, Bustos C, Schwarz A, Bórquez R. Membrane technology applied to acid mine drainage from copper mining. Water Science and Technology. 2016;**75**(3):705-715. DOI: 10.2166/wst.2016.556

[8] Martinez VD, Vucic EA, Becker-Santos DD, Gil L, Lam WL. Arsenic exposure and the induction of human cancers. Journal of Toxicology. 2011;**2011**:1-13. DOI: 10.1155/2011/431287

[9] Bjørklund G, Aaseth J, Chirumbolo S, Urbina MA, Uddin R. Effects of arsenic toxicity beyond epigenetic modifications. Environmental Geochemistry and Health. 2017;**39**:1-11 DOI: 10.1007/s10653-017-9967-9

[10] Chakraborti D, Das B, Rahman MM, Nayak B, Pal A, Sengupta MK, Ahamed S, Hossain MA, Chowdhury UK, Biswas BK, Saha KC, Dutta RN. Arsenic in groundwater of the Kolkata Municipal Corporation (KMC), India: Critical review and modes of mitigation. Chemosphere. 2017;**180**:437-447. DOI: 10.1016/j.chemosphere.2017.04.051

[11] Nachman KE, Ginsberg GL, Miller MD, Murray CJ, Nigra AE, Pendergrast CB. Mitigating dietary arsenic exposure: Current status in the United States and recommendations for an improved path forward. Science of the Total Environment. 2017;**581-582**:221-236. DOI: 10.1016/j.scitotenv.2016.12.112

[12] Pershagen G. The carcinogenicity of arsenic. Environmental Health Perspectives. 1981;**40**:93-100. DOI: 10.2307/3429223

[13] Chen K, Liao QL, Ma ZW, Jin Y, Hua M, Bi J, Huang L. Association of soil arsenic and nickel exposure with cancer mortality rates, a town-scale ecological study in Suzhou, China. Environmental Science and Pollution Research. 2014;**22**(7):5395-5404. DOI: 10.1007/s11356-014-3790-y

[14] Satarug S, Vesey DA, Gobe GC. Kidney cadmium toxicity, diabetes and high blood pressure: The perfect storm. The Tohoku Journal of Experimental Medicine. 2017;**241**(1):65-87. DOI: 10.1620/tjem.241.65

[15] Amaral AF, Porta M, Silverman DT, Milne RL, Kogevinas M, Rothman N, Cantor KP, Jackson BP, Pumarega JA, López T, Carrato A, Guarner L, Real FX, Malats N. Pancreatic cancer risk and levels of trace elements. Gut. 2011;**61**(11):1583-1588. DOI: 10.1620/tjem.241.65

[16] Cui J, Xu W, Chen J, Li H, Dai L, Frank JA, Peng S, Wang S, Chen G. M2 polarization of macrophages facilitates arsenic-induced cell transformation of lung epithelial cells. Oncotarget. 2017;**8**(13):21398-21409. DOI: 10.18632/oncotarget.15232

[17] Park YH, Kim D, Dai J, Zhang Z. Human bronchial epithelial BEAS-2B cells, an appropriate in vitro model to study heavy metals induced carcinogenesis. Toxicology and Applied Pharmacology. 2015;**287**(3):240-245. DOI: 10.1016/j.taap.2015.06.008

[18] Hall MN, Niedzwiecki M, Liu X, Harper KN, Alam S, Slavkovich V, Ilievski V, Levy D, Siddique S, Parvez F, Mey JL, van Geen A, Graziano J, Gamble MV. Chronic arsenic exposure and blood glutathione and glutathione disulfide concentrations in

Bangladeshi adults. Environmental Health Perspectives. 2013;**121**(9):1068-1074. DOI: 10.1289/ehp.1205727

[19] Sykora P, Snow ET. Modulation of DNA polymerase beta-dependent base excision repair in cultured human cells after low dose exposure to arsenite. Toxicology and Applied Pharmacology. 2008;**228**(3):385-394. DOI: 10.1016/j.taap.2007.12.019

[20] He J, Wang F, Luo F, Chen X, Jiang W, Huang Z, Lei J, Shan F, Xu X. Effects of long term low- and high-dose sodium arsenite exposure in human transitional cells. American Journal of Translational Research. 2017;**9**(2):416-428

[21] Harper LK, Bayse CA. Modeling the chelation of As(III) in lewisite by dithiols using density functional theory and solvent-assisted proton exchange. Journal of Inorganic Biochemistry. 2015;**153**:60-67. DOI: 10.1016/j.jinorgbio.2015.10.004

[22] Lu PH, Tseng JC, Chen CK, Chen CH. Survival without peripheral neuropathy after massive acute arsenic poisoning: Treated by 2,3-dimercaptopropane-1-sulphonate. Journal of Clinical Pharmacy and Therapeutics. 2017;**42**(4):506-508. DOI: 10.1111/jcpt.12538

[23] Mandal P. Molecular insight of arsenic-induced carcinogenesis and its prevention. Naunyn-Schmiedeberg's Archives of Pharmacology. 2017;**390**(5):443-455. DOI: 10.1007/s00210-017-1351-x

[24] Stanton BA, Caldwell K, Congdon CB, Disney J, Donahue M, Ferguson E, Flemings E, Golden M, Guerinot ML, Highman J, James K, Kim C, Lantz RC, Marvinney RG, Mayer G, Miller D, Navas-Acien A, Nordstrom DK, Postema S, Rardin L, Rosen B, Sengupta A, Shaw J, Stanton E, Susca P. MDI biological laboratory arsenic summit: Approaches to limiting human exposure to arsenic. Current Environmental Health Reports. 2015;**2**(3):329-337. DOI: 10.1007/s40572-015-0057-9

[25] Spanu A, Daga L, Orlandoni AM, Sanna G. The role of irrigation techniques in arsenic bioaccumulation in rice (*Oryza sativa* L.). Environmental Science & Technology. 2012;**46**(15):8333-8340. DOI: 10.1021/es300636d

[26] Nogaj E, Kwapulinski J, Misiołek M, Golusiński W, Kowol J, Wiechuła D. Beryllium concentration in pharyngeal tonsils in children. Annals of Agricultural and Environmental Medicine. 2014;**21**(2):267-271. DOI: 10.5604/1232-1966.1108589

[27] Shay E, De Gandiaga E, Madl AK. Considerations for the development of healthbased surface dust cleanup criteria for beryllium. Critical Reviews in Toxicology. 2013;**43**(3):220-243. DOI: 10.3109/10408444.2013.767308

[28] Boffetta P, Fryzek JP, Mandel JS. Occupational exposure to beryllium and cancer risk: A review of the epidemiologic evidence. Critical Reviews in Toxicology. 2012;**42**(2):107-118. DOI: 10.3109/10408444.2011.631898

[29] Hollins DM, McKinley MA, Williams C, Wiman A, Fillos D, Chapman PS, Madl AK. Beryllium and lung cancer: A weight of evidence evaluation of the toxicological and epidemiological literature. Critical Reviews in Toxicology. 2009;**39**(1):1-32. DOI: 10.1080/10408440902837967

[30] Beryllium and Beryllium Compounds. International Agency for Research on Cancer. 2012;**100C**:95-120

[31] Stark M, Lerman Y, Kapel A, Pardo A, Schwarz Y, Newman L, Maier L, Fireman E. Biological exposure metrics of beryllium-exposed dental technicians. Archives of Environmental & Occupational Health. 2013;**69**(2):89-99. DOI: 10.1080/19338244.2012.744736

[32] Benderli Cihan Y, Sözen S, Oztürk Yıldırım S. Trace elements and heavy metals in hair of stage III breast cancer patients. Biological Trace Element Research. 2011;**144**(1-3):360-379. DOI: 10.1007/s12011-011-9104-z

[33] Sandhu R, Lal H, Kundu ZS, Kharb S. Serum fluoride and sialic acid levels in osteosarcoma. Biological Trace Element Research. 2009;**144**(1-3):1-5. DOI: 10.1007/s12011-009-8382-1

[34] Radauceanu A, Grzebyk M, Edmé JL, Chérot-Kornobis N, Rousset D, Dziurla M, De Broucker V, Hédelin G, Sobaszek A, Hulo S. Effects of occupational exposure to poorly soluble forms of beryllium on biomarkers of pulmonary response in exhaled breath of workers in machining industries. Toxicology Letters. 2016;**263**:26-33. DOI: 10.1016/j.toxlet.2016.10.013

[35] Shukla S, Sharma P, Johri S, Mathur R. Influence of chelating agents on the toxicity and distribution of beryllium in rats. Journal of Applied Toxicology. 1998;**18**(5):331-335. DOI: 10.1002/(SICI)1099-1263(1998090)18:5<331::AID-JAT517>3.0.CO;2-0

[36] Johri S, Shukla S, Sharma P. Role of chelating agents and antioxidants in beryllium induced toxicity. Indian Journal of Experimental Biology. 2002;**40**(5):575-582

[37] Sharma P, Johri S, Shukla S. Beryllium-induced toxicity and its prevention by treatment with chelating agents. Journal of Applied Toxicology. 2000;**20**(4):313-318. DOI: 10.1002/1099-1263(200007/08)20:4<313::AID-JAT660>3.0.CO;2-J

[38] Crinnion WJ, Tran JQ. Case report: Heavy metal burden presenting as Bartter syndrome. Alternative Medicine Review. 2010;**15**(4):303-310

[39] Mayer AS, Brazile WJ, Erb SA, Barker EA, Miller CM, Mroz MM, Maier LA, Van Dyke MV. Developing effective health and safety training materials for workers in beryllium-using industries. Journal of Occupational and Environmental Medicine. 2013;**55**(7):746-751. DOI: 10.1097/JOM.0b013e3182972f1b

[40] Thomas CA, Deubner DC, Stanton ML, Kreiss K, Schuler CR. Long-term efficacy of a program to prevent beryllium disease. American Journal of Industrial Medicine. 2013;**56**(7):733-741. DOI: 10.1002/ajim.22175

[41] Bertin G, Averbeck D. Cadmium: Cellular effects, modifications of biomolecules, modulation of DNA repair and genotoxic consequences (a review). Biochimie. 2006;**88**(11):1549-1559. DOI: 10.1016/j.biochi.2006.10.001

[42] Chunhabundit R. Cadmium exposure and potential health risk from foods in contaminated area, Thailand. Toxicological Research. 2016;**32**(1):65-72. DOI: 10.5487/TR.2016.32.1.065

[43] Alimba CG, Gandhi D, Sivanesan S, Bhanarkar MD, Naoghare PK, Bakare AA, Krishnamurthi K. Chemical characterization of simulated landfill soil leachates from Nigeria and India and their cytotoxicity and DNA damage inductions on three human cell lines. Chemosphere. 2016;**164**:469-479. DOI: 10.1016/j.chemosphere.2016.08.093

[44] Cartularo L, Laulicht F, Sun H, Kluz T, Freedman JH, Costa M. Gene expression and pathway analysis of human hepatocellular carcinoma cells treated with cadmium. Toxicology and Applied Pharmacology. 2015;**288**(3):399-408. DOI: 10.1016/j.taap.2015.08.011

[45] Larsson SC, Orsini N, Wolk A. Urinary cadmium concentration and risk of breast cancer: A systematic review and dose-response meta-analysis. American Journal of Epidemiology. 2015;**182**(5):375-380. DOI: 10.1093/aje/kwv085

[46] Bishak YK, Payahoo L, Osatdrahimi A, Nourazarian A. Mechanisms of cadmium carcinogenicity in the gastrointestinal tract. Asian Pacific Journal of Cancer Prevention. 2015;**16**(1):9-21. DOI: 10.7314/APJCP.2015.16.1.9

[47] Mondal B, Maulik D, Mandal M, Sarkar GN, Sengupta S, Ghosh D. Analysis of carcinogenic heavy metals in gallstones and its role in gallbladder carcinogenesis. Journal of Gastrointestinal Cancer. 2016;1-8. DOI: 10.1007/s12029-016-9898-1

[48] Arslan M, Demir H, Arslan H, Gokalp AS, Demir C. Trace elements, heavy metals and other biochemical parameters in malignant glioma patients. Asian Pacific Journal of Cancer Prevention. 2011;**12**(2):447-451

[49] García-Esquinas E, Pollan M, Tellez-Plaza M, Francesconi KA, Goessler W, Guallar E, Umans JG, Yeh J, Best LG, Navas-Acien A. Cadmium exposure and cancer mortality in a prospective cohort: The strong heart study. Environmental Health Perspectives. 2014;**122**(4):363-370. DOI: 10.1289/ehp.1306587

[50] Khan N, Afridi HI, Kazi TG, Arain MB, Bilal M, Akhtar A, Khan M. Correlation of cadmium and magnesium in the blood and serum samples of smokers and nonsmokers chronic leukemia patients. Biological Trace Element Research. 2016;**176**(1):81-88. DOI: 10.1007/s12011-016-0816-y

[51] Ostadrahimi A, Payahoo L, Somi MH, Khajebishak Y. The association between urinary cadmium levels and dietary habits with risk of gastrointestinal cancer in Tabriz, Northwest of Iran. Biological Trace Element Research. 2016;**175**(1):72-78. DOI: 10.1007/s12011-016-0764-6

[52] Xiao CL, Liu Y, Tu W, Xia YJ, Tian KM, Zhou X. Research progress of the mechanisms underlying cadmium-induced carcinogenesis. Zhonghua Yu Fang Yi Xue Za Zhi. 2016;**50**(4):380-384. DOI: 10.3760/cma.j.issn.0253-9624.2016.04.021

[53] Inglot P, Lewinska A, Potocki L, Oklejewicz B, Tabecka-Lonczynska A, Koziorowski M, Bugno-Poniewierska M, Bartosz G, Wnuk M. Cadmium-induced changes in genomic DNA-methylation status increase aneuploidy events in a pig Robertsonian translocation model. Mutation Research/Genetic Toxicology and Environmental Mutagenesis. 2012;**747**(2):182-189. DOI: 10.1016/j.mrgentox.2012.05.007

[54] Knight AS, Zhou EY, Francis MB. Development of peptoid-based ligands for the removal of cadmium from biological media. Chemical Science. 2015;**6**(7):4042-4048. DOI: 10.1039/C5SC00676G

[55] Li X, Jiang X, Sun J, Zhu C, Li X, Tian L, Liu L, Bai W. Cytoprotective effects of dietary flavonoids against cadmium-induced toxicity. Annals of the New York Academy of Sciences. 2017;**1398**:5-19. DOI: 10.1111/nyas.13344

[56] Wang YJ, Yan J, Zou XL, Guo KJ, Zhao Y, Meng CY, Yin F, Guo L. Bone marrow mesenchymal stem cells repair cadmium-induced rat testis injury by inhibiting mitochondrial apoptosis. Chemico-Biological Interactions. 2017;**271**:39-47. DOI: 10.1016/j.cbi.2017.04.024

[57] Orisakwe OE, Dagur EA, Mbagwu HO, Udowelle NA. Lead levels in vegetables from artisanal mining sites of Dilimi River, Bukuru and Barkin Ladi North Central Nigeria: Cancer and non-cancer risk assessment. Asian Pacific Journal of Cancer Prevention. 2017;**18**(3):621-627. DOI: 10.22034/APJCP.2017.18.3.621

[58] Rashidi M, Alavipanah S. Relation between kidney cancer and soil leads in Isfahan Province, Iran between 2007 and 2009. Journal of Cancer Research and Therapeutics. 2016;**12**(2):716-720. DOI: 10.4103/0973-1482.154936

[59] McCumber A, Strevett KA. A geospatial analysis of soil lead concentrations around regional Oklahoma Airports. Chemosphere. 2017;**167**:62-70. DOI: 10.1016/j.chemosphere.2016.09.127

[60] Southard EB, Roff A, Fortugno T, Richie JP, Kaag M, Chinchilli VM, Virtamo J, Albanes D, Weinstein S, Wilson RT. Lead, calcium uptake, and related genetic variants in association with renal cell carcinoma risk in a cohort of male Finnish smokers. Cancer Epidemiology Biomarkers & Prevention. 2011;**21**(1):191-201. DOI: 10.1158/1055-9965.EPI-11-0670

[61] Silbergeld EK. Facilitative mechanisms of lead as a carcinogen. Mutation Research/Fundamental and Molecular Mechanisms of Mutagenesis. 2003;**533**(1-2):121-133. DOI: 10.1016/j.mrfmmm.2003.07.010

[62] Steenland K, Barry V, Anttila A, Sallmén M, Mcelvenny D, Todd AC, Straif K. A cohort mortality study of lead-exposed workers in the USA, Finland and the UK. Occupational and Environmental Medicine. 2017;May 2017. DOI: 10.1136/oemed-2017-104311

[63] Silbergeld EK, Waalkes M, Rice JM. Lead as a carcinogen: Experimental evidence and mechanisms of action. American Journal of Industrial Medicine. 2000;**38**(3):316-323. DOI: 10.1002/1097-0274(200009)38:3<316::AID-AJIM11>3.0.CO;2-P

[64] Kianoush S, Sadegehi M, Balali-Mood M. Recent advances in the clinical management of lead poisoning. Acta Medica Iranica. 2015;**53**(6):327-336

[65] Rice KM, Walker EM, Wu M, Gillette C, Blough ER. Environmental mercury and its toxic effects. Journal of Preventive Medicine & Public Health. 2014;**47**(2):74-83. DOI: 10.3961/jpmph.2014.47.2.74

[66] Crespo-López ME, Macêdo GL, Pereira SI, Arrifano GP, Picanço-Diniz DL, do Nascimento JL, Herculano AM. Mercury and human genotoxicity: Critical considerations and possible molecular mechanisms. Pharmacological Research. 2009;**60**(4):212-220. DOI: 10.1016/j.phrs.2009.02.011

[67] Branco V, Caito S, Farina M, Rocha J, Aschner M, Carvalho C. Biomarkers of mercury toxicity: Past, present, and future trends. Journal of Toxicology and Environmental Health, Part B. 2017;**20**(3):119-154. DOI: 10.1080/10937404.2017.1289834

[68] Junqué E, Garí M, Arce A, Torrent M, Sunyer J, Grimalt JO. Integrated assessment of infant exposure to persistent organic pollutants and mercury via dietary intake in a central western Mediterranean site (Menorca Island). Environmental Research. 2017;**156**:714-724. DOI: 10.1016/j.envres.2017.04.030

[69] Alcala-Orozco M, Morillo-Garcia Y, Caballero-Gallardo K, Olivero-Verbel J. Mercury in canned tuna marketed in Cartagena, Colombia and estimation of human exposure. Food Additives & Contaminants: Part B. 2017;**10**:1-7. DOI: 10.1080/19393210.2017.1323803

[70] Yuan W, Yang N, Li X. Advances in understanding how heavy metal pollution triggers gastric cancer. BioMed Research International. 2016;**2016**:1-10. DOI: 10.1155/2016/7825432

[71] Valko M, Morris H, Cronin MT. Metals, toxicity and oxidative stress. Current Medicinal Chemistry. 2005;**12**(10):1161-1208. DOI: 10.2174/0929867053764635

[72] Kosnett MJ. The role of chelation in the treatment of arsenic and mercury poisoning. Journal of Medical Toxicology. 2013;**9**(4):347-354.DOI: 10.1007/s13181-013-0344-5

[73] Sears, ME. Chelation: Harnessing and enhancing heavy metal detoxification—A review. The Scientific World Journal. 2013;**2013**:1-13. DOI: 10.1155/2013/219840

[74] Iranmanesh M, Fatemi SJ, Golbafan MR, Balooch FD. Treatment of mercury vapor toxicity by combining deferasirox and deferiprone in rats. BioMetals. 2013;**26**(5):783-788. DOI: 10.1007/s10534-013-9656-9

[75] Sangvanich T, Morry J, Fox C, Ngamcherdtrakul W, Goodyear S, Castro D, Fryxell GE, Addleman RS, Summers AO, Yantasee W. Novel oral detoxification of mercury, cadmium, and lead with thiol-modified nanoporous silica. ACS Applied Materials & Interfaces. 2014;**6**(8):5483-5493. DOI: 10.1021/am5007707

[76] Ngole-Jeme VM, Fantke P. Ecological and human health risks associated with abandoned gold mine tailings contaminated soil. Plos One. 2017;**12**(2). DOI: 10.1371/journal.pone.0172517

[77] Pavela M, Uitti J, Pukkala E. Cancer incidence among copper smelting and nickel refining workers in Finland. American Journal of Industrial Medicine. 2016;**60**(1):87-95. DOI: 10.1002/ajim.22662

[78] Gölz L, Buerfent BC, Hofmann A, Rühl H, Fricker N, Stamminger W, Oldenburg J, Deschner J, Hoerauf A, Nöthen MM, Schumacher J, Hübner MP, Jäger A. Genome-wide transcriptome induced by nickel in human monocytes. Acta Biomaterialia. 2016;**43**:369-382. DOI: 10.1016/j.actbio.2016.07.047

[79] Plavan G, Jitar O, Teodosiu C, Nicoara M, Micu D, Strungaru SA. Toxic metals in tissues of fishes from the Black Sea and associated human health risk exposure. Environmental Science and Pollution Research. 2017;**24**(8):7776-7787. DOI: 10.1007/s11356-017-8442-6

[80] Harari R, Harari F, Forastiere F. Environmental nickel exposure from oil refinery emissions: A case study in Ecuador. Annali dell'Istituto Superiore di Sanità. 2016;**52**(4):495-499. DOI: 10.4415/ANN_16_04_06

[81] Zhou C, Huang C, Wang J, Huang H, Li J, Xie Q, Liu Y, Zhu J, Li Y, Zhang D, Zhu Q. LncRNA MEG3 downregulation mediated by DNMT3b contributes to nickel malignant transformation of human bronchial epithelial cells via modulating PHLPP1 transcription and HIF-1α translation. Oncogene. 2017;**36**:3878-3889. DOI: 10.1038/onc.2017.14

[82] Huang H, Zhu J, Li Y, Zhang L, Gu J, Xie Q, Jin H, Che X, Li J, Huang C, Chen LC, Lyu J, Gao J, Huang C. Upregulation of SQSTM1/p62 contributes to nickel-induced malignant transformation of human bronchial epithelial cells. Autophagy. 2016;**12**(10):1687-1703. DOI: 10.1080/15548627.2016.1196313

[83] Yu M, Zhang J. Serum and hair nickel levels and breast cancer: Systematic review and meta-analysis. Biological Trace Element Research. 2017:**175**(2):1-7. DOI: 10.1007/s12011-017-0949-7

[84] Yang Y, Jin X, Yan C, Tian Y, Tang J, Shen X. Urinary level of nickel and acute leukaemia in Chinese children. Toxicology and Industrial Health. 2008;**24**(9):603-610. DOI: 10.1177/0748233708100091

[85] Tilakaratne D, Sidhu S. Heavy metal (monoclonal) bands: A link between cutaneous T-cell lymphoma and contact allergy to potassium dichromate, nickel and cobalt? Australasian Journal of Dermatology. 2014;**56**(1):59-63. DOI: 10.1111/ajd.12182

[86] Zambelli B, Uversky VN, Ciurli S. Nickel impact on human health: An intrinsic disorder perspective. Biochimica Et Biophysica Acta (BBA) – Proteins and Proteomics. 2016;**1864**(12):1714-1731. DOI: 10.1016/j.bbapap.2016.09.008

[87] Ma L, Bai Y, Pu H, Gou F, Dai M, Wang H, He J, Zheng T, Cheng N. Histone methylation in nickel-smelting industrial workers. Plos One. 2015;**10**(10). DOI: 10.1371/journal.pone.0140339

[88] Sunderman FW. Chelation therapy in nickel poisoning. Annals of Clinical and Laboratory Science. 1981;**11**(1):1-8

[89] Atma W, Larouci M, Meddah B, Benabdeli K, Sonnet P. Evaluation of the phytoremediation potential of *Arundo donax* L. for nickel-contaminated soil. International Journal of Phytoremediation. 2017;**19**(4):377-386. DOI: 10.1080/15226514.2016.1225291

[90] Gopal R, Narmada S, Vijayakumar R, Jaleel CA. Chelating efficacy of CaNa2 EDTA on nickel-induced toxicity in Cirrhinus mrigala (Ham.) through its effects on glutathione peroxidase, reduced glutathione and lipid peroxidation. Comptes Rendus Biologies. 2009;**332**(8):685-696. DOI: 10.1016/j.crvi.2009.03.004

[91] Di Loreto G, Sacco A, Felicioli G. Radon in workplaces, a review. Giornale Italiano Di Medicina Del Lavoro Ed Ergonomia. 2010;**32**(4):251-254

[92] Chałupnik S, Wysocka M, Janson E, Chmielewska I, Wiesner M. Long term changes in the concentration of radium in sischarge waters of coal mines and Upper Silesian rivers. Journal of Environmental Radioactivity. 2017;**171**:117-123. DOI: 10.1016/j.jenvrad.2017.02.007

[93] Abdel Ghany HA. Enhancement of radon exposure in smoking areas. Environmental Geochemistry and Health. 2007;**29**(3):249-255. DOI: 10.1007/s10653-007-9082-4

[94] Wick RR, Nekolla EA, Gaubitz M, Schulte TL. Increased risk of myeloid leukaemia in patients with ankylosing spondylitis following treatment with radium-224. Rheumatology. 2008;**47**(6):855-859. DOI: 10.1093/rheumatology/ken060

[95] Benejegerdes KE, Brown SC, Housewright CD. Focal cutaneous squamous cell carcinoma following radium-223 extravasation. Proceedings (Baylor University Medical Center). 2017;**30**(1):78-79

9

Genetic Mutations and Ubiquitination in Melanoma Growth and Metastasis

Anushka Dikshit and Jennifer Zhang

Abstract

Upon neoplastic transformation, melanoma is intrinsically prone to metastasis, which marks the most dangerous aspect of the disease and dubs it one of the most challenging cancers to treat. BRAF/MEK oncokinase inhibitors and immunotherapies have shown considerable promise in some patients, but the clinical benefits are often short-lived due to rapid development of resistance. Recently, ubiquitination enzymes have emerged as potential therapeutic targets. These enzymes can be targeted to increase expression of tumor suppressors and impede activation of oncogenic signaling pathways mediating cell proliferation and tissue invasion. This chapter describes some of the common genetic mutations in melanoma, ubiquitinating and deubiquitinating enzymes that are linked to melanoma progression, metastasis, and therapeutic resistance.

Keywords: A20, BAP1, BRAF, CDKN2A, CYLD, DUB, E-cadherin, ERK, melanoma, N-cadherin, Snail1, TRAF6, UBE2S, ubiquitination, USP

1. Introduction

Melanoma is the most aggressive form of skin cancer. The 5-year survival rate for metastatic melanoma is less than 20%. The incidence of melanoma is on the rise especially among the young population. The NIH SEER program estimated that 87,110 people were diagnosed with melanoma in the United States in 2017, accounting for 5.2% of all new cases of cancer, which is 1.2% higher than the melanoma cases reported in 2007. About 11% of the newly diagnosed patients would succumb to the disease due to uncontrollable metastatic tumor growth [1, 2]. This chapter describes the common genetic mutations and posttranslational modifications crucial for melanoma growth, survival and dissemination, with a particular focus on enzymes regulating ubiquitination.

2. Melanoma staging and diagnosis

Melanoma treatment plans are designed based on the stage of the disease. In 2017, the American Joint Committee on Cancer (AJCC) published the 8th edition of the tumor, lymph node, and metastasis (**TNM**) system. The **T** recognizes tumor thickness or the depth of the cancer in the skin and characterizes the tumor as being ulcerated or non-ulcerated. The **N** is used to establish whether the cancer has spread to the proximal lymph nodes and finally, the **M** stands for metastasis and gives information if the cancer has spread to distant lymph nodes or other organs [3]. Using the TNM numbers along with elaborate clinical and pathological assessments, the cancer is assigned a stage. Further histological analyses allow pathologists to assign a 'grade' to the tumor which is an indication of the abnormality of the tumor cells. Both staging and grading are crucial to determine the course of treatment and give an overall prognosis for the disease. Although it is under debate whether a linear progression is the primary theme, cutaneous melanomas can progress from a precursor lesion, namely benign nevi which becomes dysplastic, to melanoma in situ, and finally to invasive melanoma. A nevus is a benign aggregation of melanocytes that is formed at the junction of the dermis and epidermis or within the dermis. When the nevus shows signs of cytological atypia and change in growth, it becomes dysplastic. Melanoma in situ, also called as the stage (0) melanoma, is when the transformed melanocytes are still within the epidermis or the dermal/epidermal junction. Lastly, when the transformed melanocytes invade the dermis and gain access to other cell tissues and/or the vascular system, they turn into metastatic melanoma [4]. The development of melanoma involves multifactorial and heterogeneous biologic processes that are controlled at the genetic, transcriptional, and posttranslational levels [5, 6].

3. Genetic mutations

3.1. Germline mutations in melanoma

Certain genetic changes predispose an individual to an increased risk of melanoma. These changes include point mutations, amplifications, deletions or translocations. CDKN2A is one of the first genes linked to the familial atypical mole melanoma (FAMM). Deletion or loss of heterozygosity of CDKN2A increases patient susceptibility to developing melanoma [7]. Consistently, germline deletion of Cdkn2a in mice sensitizes animals to developing cutaneous melanoma when coupled with an activating HRAS mutation in the melanocytes [8]. While the CDKN2A gene codes for two proteins, p16 INK4A and p15 ARF, p16 INK4A loss-of-function is responsible for spontaneous and carcinogen induced melanoma [9]. CDK4 and RB1 are two other genes with germlines mutations linked to familial susceptibility to melanoma. CDK4, a kinase involved in regulating cell cycle, is amplified or mutated in human melanomas with some studies showing 100% of all the affected family members harboring a specific CDK4 mutation [10, 11]. Inactivation of RB1 tumor suppressor causes hereditary retinoblastoma and increases the risk of developing melanoma by about 80-fold [12]. Variants of the melanocortin-1 receptor (MC1R) are associated with fair pigmentation and melanoma risk [13]. The presence of a CDKN2A mutation gave a hazard ratio of 13.35, and the MC1R variants increase the hazard ratio by 3.72-fold [14].

3.2. Somatic mutations in melanoma

Ultraviolet (UV) radiation induces somatic gene mutations and is the major risk factor for melanoma [6, 15]. The RAS/RAF/MEK/ERK signaling pathway is commonly mutated in melanoma. Among the RAS GTPase family members, NRAS is the most frequently mutated protein with activating mutations detected in up to 56% of benign nevi and 26% of metastatic melanoma [16, 17]. Activating mutations of BRAF are found in about 70% of cutaneous melanomas, and 90% of these mutations are of the BRAF(V600E) (valine to glutamic acid substitution) [18, 19]. There is a well-established correlation between sun-exposure and the development of BRAF mutations [15, 20]. BRAF(V600E) mutation is observed in the benign melanocytic nevi, indicating that this mutation alone is not sufficient for malignant transformation [19, 21]. Other genetic changes such as CDKN2B loss are required for the progression from benign melanocytic nevus to melanoma [22]. Random mutagenesis screens have revealed that ERK point mutations impart resistance to RAF and MEK inhibitors, although such mutations are infrequent [23].

4. Melanocyte origin and its intrinsic effects on melanoma metastasis

Melanoma is intrinsically prone to metastasis [4]. Melanocyte precursors are derived from highly migratory neural crest cells, which give rise to a number of differentiated cells including the melanocytes. During this process, they express several canonical neural crest markers such as SOX8, SOX9, SOX10, Snail1, and Snail2. The strong metastatic potential of melanoma can be attributed to the plethora of mutations acquired over the development of the disease and to the aberrant reactivation of some of the transcriptional factors such as Sox5, Sox10, and Snail1 that are crucial for the melanocyte differentiation program [24–26].

The Wnt signaling pathway plays a major role in melanocyte differentiation and migration mainly through the activation of the microphthalmia-associated transcription factor (MITF) [27]. MITF promotes melanocyte differentiation and melanin production, in addition, MITF is often upregulated in melanomas associated with poor prognosis [28]. β-catenin dependent MITF activation induces proliferation of melanoma cells and inhibition of β-catenin leads to a cell cycle arrest along with downregulation of MITF [29]. Hyperactivated Wnt signaling has been reported in about 30% of melanoma samples [30] and is shown to promote melanomagenesis. On the other hand, there are also reports that demonstrate loss of β-catenin decreases melanoma cell proliferation, but promotes invasion and predicts poor prognosis [31]. This discrepancy is predominantly because the Wnt proteins utilize three distinct signaling pathways with different mediators [29]. The canonical Wnt signaling pathway entails activation of the frizzled surface receptors by the Wnt ligand, leading to the formation of a vast protein complex on the cell surface. This leads to a cascade of events, resulting in the nuclear translocation of β-catenin which then acts as a co-activator to regulate target gene expression [32]. A non-canonical Wnt signaling pathway involves activation of GTPases such as RAC1 and

RHOA, and MAP kinase such as JNK, downstream of the frizzled receptor. A second non-canonical pathway includes activation of phospholipase C (PLC) that promotes the release of intracellular Ca^{2+}, leading to the expression of target genes involved in cell migration and inflammation [33]. The noncanonical Wnt signaling is shown to stimulate cytoskeletal remodeling, increase cell survival, and promote invasive characteristics [34, 35]. Both the canonical and the noncanonical Wnt signaling pathways are involved in the promotion of melanoma cell proliferation and epithelial-mesenchymal translation (EMT) [29, 36].

5. Ubiquitination in melanoma

Posttranslational modification (PTM) is a reversible and dynamic process that regulates protein function at a posttranslational level and plays crucial roles in signal transduction, gene regulation, vesicle transportation, and protein degradation. PTMs include phosphorylation, ubiquitination, sumoylation, methylation, acetylation, glycosylation and N-nitrosylation. Dysregulation of PTM results in pathogenesis including cancer [37]. Phosphorylation is catalyzed by protein kinases and is the core mediator of signal transduction. Oncogenic mutations of the protein kinases, most notably BRAF(V600E), result in constitutive phosphorylation and activation of the downstream targets such as the MEK and ERK kinases [38]. Kinase-mediated signals are also regulated by other PTMs including ubiquitination.

Ubiquitination (Ub) is a rather complex process involving a substantial series of variable components. Mono-Ub involves a covalent attachment of a 76 amino acid ubiquitin polypeptide to a lysine residue of a target protein. Poly-Ub involves attachment of additional ubiquitin moieties to one of the seven lysine (K) residues (K6, K11, K27, K29, K33, K48 and K63) or the methionine residue (M1) of the proceeding ubiquitin, forming structurally and functionally distinct polymers. If more than one K-residues are involved, it is called a heteropolymeric chain and, if a single K-residue is involved, it is called as a homopolymeric chain, such as K48-Ub and K63-Ub [39]. Different Ubs carry out distinct functions, ensuring the robust control of essentially every cellular process spanning from signal transduction, DNA-repair, vesicle transportation, cell division, differentiation, and migration [40]. While K48-Ub generally marks protein for proteasomal degradation, K63-Ub regulates signal transduction, RNA splicing, protein sorting, DNA repair and immune response [41–43].

Ubiquitination generally requires a three-step process: the E1 enzyme catalyzes the first step by activating an ubiquitin moiety in the presence of ATP and the E2 conjugase carries the ubiquitin via covalent bonding, and works together with an E3 ligase to complete ubiquitin ligation with the target protein [44]. There are two known E1 enzymes, UBA1 and UBA6 [45]. The canonical UBA1 is characterized as a potential target for the treatment of hematologic malignancies [46]. The noncanonical UBA6 suppresses epithelial-mesenchymal transition of mammary epithelial cells [47]. The role of UBA1 and UBA6 in melanoma is not well-understood.

5.1. Ubiquitin conjugases in melanoma

There are about 50 known E2 conjugating enzymes. Each of them contains a conserved cysteine residue that accepts the ubiquitin molecule activated by the E1 enzyme. A number of E2 enzymes have been implicated in melanoma. For example, Rad6 promotes melanoma development and progression by inducing nuclear translocation of β-catenin [48]. Overexpression of E2-EPF UCP (ubiquitin carrier protein) promotes melanoma metastasis, while its downregulation decreases tumor invasion [49]. UBE2S targets VHL protein for proteasomal degradation via a K48-Ub-mediated process. UBE2S is overexpressed in metastatic melanoma cell lines and mediates the degradation of VHL and a consequent upregulation of HIF-1α and VEGF proteins to promote distant metastasis and angiogenesis [50].

5.2. Ubiquitin ligases in melanoma

There are over 600 putative E3 Ubiquitin ligases in the human genome. These enzymes display substrate specificity, and have attracted tremendous attention for therapeutic targeting. The SCF ubiquitin ligases constitute the largest family of E3 ligase enzymes characterized by an F-box component that interacts with the substrate. Among the SCF family members, β-TrCP (beta transducing repeats containing protein) is upregulated in melanomas with BRAF(V600E) mutation and a corresponding increase of NF-κB activity [51]. Another SCF family member, SCF-Skp2 is shown to promote melanoma cell cycle progression by degradation of CDK inhibitors such as p27 and p57 [52]. FBXW7, a component of the SCF-FBW7 E3 complex, is mutated in 8.1% of melanoma patients and some of these mutations interfere with its substrate binding, leading to oncogenic activation of substrates including Notch1 [53, 54]. FBXW7 inactivating mutations are detected in melanomas without the typical BRAF(V600E) and NRAS(G12D/G13R/Q61K/L/S) mutations [55]. Knockdown of FBXW7 in melanoma cell lines leads to the upregulation of NOTCH1, HEY1, and the downstream effectors Cyclin E, Aurora A and Myc, resulting in increased tumorigenesis [56–58].

The E3 ligase MDM2 regulates p53 and its expression in melanoma correlates with increased malignancy, tumor thickness and invasion [59]. TRAF6 is a K63-Ub ligase overexpressed in primary and metastatic melanoma, and it promotes tissue invasion by stimulating MMP9 activation [60]. TRAF6 recruitment and activation is regulated by EGFR through the oncoprotein, DCBLD2 (discoidin, CUB, and LCCL domain-containing protein) in a number of cancers including melanoma [61]. TRAF6 together with p62 also regulates mTOR activation via K63-Ub which is important for the mTORC1 and mTORC2 complex formation [62]. TRAF2 mediates K63-Ub of GβL (mTOR LST8 homolog) thereby preventing mTORC1 complex formation. Mutations in the K63-Ub site of GβL are shown to promote chemoresistance of melanoma cells in vitro and in the xenograft mouse model [63].

The E3 ubiquitin ligase RNF125 negatively regulates the retinoic acid-inducible gene I (RIG-I) signaling pathway by targeting RIG-I for proteasomal degradation [64]. It also regulates p53 and innate immune adaptor protein TRIM14 [65, 66]. Deletion and missense mutations in RNF125 are linked to the overgrowth syndrome [67]. RNF125 is regulated by MITF and SOX10 transcription factors and its downregulation elevates JAK1 and EGFR signaling, and underlies resistance of melanoma cells to the BRAF inhibitor, vemurafenib [68].

Oncogenic RAS and BRAF mutants drive tumor growth through hyperactivation of ERK1/2 kinases and concomitantly induce ERK-dependent negative feedback. Relief of this feedback inhibition by RAF inhibitors contributes to the attenuation of the therapeutic potency in BRAF mutant melanomas [69]. Ubiquitination-dependent degradation of BRAF constitutes for one of the negative feedback mechanisms [70]. The $APC^{/C}$ E3 ligase complex activator FZR1 but not FBXW7 tumor suppressor controls BRAF oncogene function [70, 71]. FZR1 as a direct target of ERK and CyclinD1/CDK4 kinases and its phosphorylation inhibits APC^{FZR1}, leading to increased expression of a cohort of oncogenic APC^{FZR1} substrates important for melanomagenesis [71].

The E3 ubiquitin ligase Trim7 is activated by the Ras/RAF/MEK/ERK pathway via MSK1-mediated phosphorylation, and consequently mediates K63-Ub of the AP-1 co-activator RACO-1, leading to RACO-1 protein stabilization and increased AP-1-dependent gene expression [72]. The c-Jun/RHOB/AKT pathway confers resistance to BRAF mutant melanoma cells from BRAF and MEK inhibitors [73]. Trim7 may represent a potential target for combination therapies to mitigate therapeutic resistance.

5.3. Deubiquitinating enzymes in melanoma

Ubiquitination is a reversible process and a group of enzymes called the deubiquitinases (DUBs) cleave the isopeptide linkage between the polyubiquitin chains and the target proteins. There are five major families of deubiquitinases: ubiquitin-specific proteases (USP), ubiquitin carboxyl-terminal hydrolases (UCH), Jab1/MPN domain associated metalloisopeptidase domain proteins, Machado-Joseph Domain (Josephin domain) containing proteins (MJD) and Otubain/Ovarian tumor domain containing proteins (OTU) [74]. Major functions of DUBs involve rescuing incorrectly ubiquitinated proteins from degradation and modulating target protein function. DUBs play important roles in DNA repair, apoptosis, cell proliferation, kinase activation, and chromatin remodeling, and they can function as tumor suppressors as well as oncogenes [75].

5.3.1. Deubiquitinating enzymes acting as tumor suppressor

***5.3.1 a* BAP1** (BRCA-associated protein 1) is a deubiquitinase belonging to the ubiquitin C-terminal hydrolases family (UHCs). BAP1 binds to BRCA1, and acts a tumor suppressor. Loss of function of BAP1 due to germline mutations leads to the tumor predisposition syndrome which increases the risks of uveal and cutaneous melanomas, and malignant mesotheliomas. Individuals who carry the mutated BAP1 gene develop melanocytic lesions later in their life and some of those benign lesions can transform into cutaneous melanomas [76]. In addition to its deubiquitinase function, BAP1 possess a nuclear localization signal that allows it to translocate to the nucleus and interact with proteins such as HCF-1 to regulate cell growth [77].

***5.3.1 b* A20** (TNFAIP3) is a deubiquitinase commonly induced by inflammatory cytokines via NF-κB. It has an innate deubiquitinating activity imparted by the OUT zinc finger domain that allows it to interact with ubiquitinated substrates and maintain specificity. A20 inhibits auto-ubiquitination of the K63-Ub E3 ligase TRAF6, and consequently inhibits IKK/NF-κB activation [78]. Independent of its deubiquitinating functions, A20 disrupts the interaction between the E2 conjugase (UBE2N) and the E3 ligase (TRAF2/TRAF6), and consequently promotes K48-Ub and proteasomal degradation of these enzymes [79]. A20 is characterized as a potent tumor suppressor in non-Hodgkin's lymphomas including diffuse large cell lymphoma, mantel cell lymphoma and ocular marginal zone B-cell lymphoma [80], but its role in melanoma is not at all clear. Increased expression of A20 in $CD8^+$ T cells results in impaired anti-tumor immunity in a melanoma animal model, while knockdown of A20 in $CD8^+$ T cells increases cytokine production and decreases melanoma tumor burden [81].

5.3.1 c **CYLD** is a deubiquitinase that preferentially removes K63-Ub and M1-Ub from target proteins [82, 83]. CYLD has been identified as a tumor suppressor on account of its loss-of-function correlating to a number of cancers including melanoma [53, 84]. In addition to gene deletion and mutation, CYLD is downregulated by Snail1 at the transcriptional level and by microRNAs including mir-186 and mir-767 at the post-transcriptional level [85, 86]. Furthermore, CYLD is subject to proteolytic inactivation by MALT1, a paracaspase known to promote melanoma growth and metastasis through JNK/c-Jun signaling pathway [87]. CYLD exhibits anti-oncogenic effects by regulating cell proliferation, angiogenesis, and tumor cell differentiation [88].

CYLD inhibits K63-Ub of a plethora of target proteins. Among these are Bcl3, TRAF2/6, Tak1, plk1, lck, HDAC6, Dvl, and c-Jun/c-Fos AP1 subunits [89–93]. In the absence of CYLD, Bcl3 along with NF-κB is recruited to the Cyclin D1 promoter to facilitate its transcription to induce G1 to S cell cycle progression. CYLD inhibits JNK activation and expression of the β1-integrin in non-melanoma and melanoma cells with a corresponding decrease in cell proliferation and increase in apoptosis [88, 89]. On the other hand, CYLD regulates cell motility via inhibition of HDAC6-mediated deacetylation of tubulin and cortactin, by directly binding to the catalytic domain of HDAC6 [94, 95].

EMT and metastasis are orchestrated by an array of gene regulators, such as TWIST1/2, SNAIL1/2, ZEB1/2 and FOXC2 [96]. Snail1-mediated suppression of CYLD is crucial for melanoma progression and metastasis [97]. CYLD regulates EMT by facilitating the maintenance of E-Cadherin expression and inhibiting N-Cadherin expression in melanoma [84]. E-cadherin is a crucial protein facilitating cell-cell adhesion, maintaining cytoskeletal stability and regulating cell polarization. Germline mutations in E-cadherin predispose individuals to a higher risk of breast and gastric cancers [98]. E-cadherin appeared downregulated in melanoma predominantly due to the alterations in the tumor microenvironment rather than genetic mutations as reported in some gynecological cancers [99]. Loss of E-cadherin expression/function increases melanocyte proliferation due to impaired interaction with keratinocytes [100]. When melanocytes are cultured in vitro, in the absence of the basal keratinocytes, they not only display increase in doubling time but also begin expression of melanoma-related markers such as β3-integrin, MUC18, melanotransferrin, and other growth factor receptors. These melanocytes regain their normal phenotype when co-cultured with keratinocytes [100]. E-cadherin also regulates the activation of β-catenin, c-Myc and Cyclin D1.

N-cadherin is expressed in melanoblasts during embryonic development, which helps cell migration from the neural crest to the epidermis by the way of interacting with fibroblasts and endothelial cells. In adults, upregulation of N-cadherin potentiates the ability of melanoma cells to invade through the stroma and interact with the vascular endothelial cells and fibroblasts, which facilitates migration of cancer cells. N-cadherin has also been demonstrated to stabilize β-catenin thereby promoting anti-apoptotic proteins and inhibiting pro-apoptotic proteins such as Bad [101]. Normal melanocytes do not express N-Cadherin, while melanoma cells display moderate to strong expression of N-cadherin with a corresponding decrease in the expression of E-cadherin. This phenomenon termed as the 'cadherin switching' is a hallmark of EMT [102].

Snail1 also regulates the expression of Notch-4, MMP-2, TIMP-1, SPARC, and T-PA, among others, in melanoma cells [103]. Notch4 and SPARC expression can be directly regulated by Snail or indirectly via E-cadherin [103]. MMP-2 is a matrix metalloprotease that is involved in remodeling of the extracellular matrix through degradation of cell adhesion proteins and in turn facilitating tumor cell migration and invasion [104]. SPARC is a potent inducer of MMP-2, and downregulation of Snail1 decreases the expression of MMP-2 and SPARC [103, 104], as well as T-PA, a protease that converts plasminogen to active zymogen [105], leading to reduced degradation of the extracellular matrix and subsequent invasion. Notch signaling mediates melanoma-endothelial cell and melanoma-keratinocyte communications, facilitating melanoma cell migration and metastasis [106, 107]. Notch 4 expression in melanoma is stimulated by Snail, independent of the repression of E-cadherin [103]. Notch inhibition enhances the efficacy of ERK and ERBB inhibitors for melanoma growth arrest [108, 109].

5.3.2. Deubiquitinating enzymes required for melanoma growth and metastasis

Deubiquitinases (DUB) have a role in stem cell maintenance and tumor growth [110]. Among the 89 DUBs examined in over 300 different tumor samples of breast, colon, lung, stomach, kidney, prostate, non-Hodgkin's lymphoma, and melanoma, 22 DUBs are significantly dysregulated in at least one tumor type [111]. Specifically, three DUBs, USP10 (ubiquitin specific peptidase 10), USP11 and USP22, are expressed significantly higher in metastatic melanoma compared to benign nevi and primary tumor. In addition, expression of USP10 and USP22 is significantly correlated to the presence of ulceration and the Breslow index, a prognostic parameter indicating the depth of tumor invasion. USP10, USP11 and USP22 regulate deubiquitination of target proteins crucial for melanoma transformation and metastasis [111]. For example, USP22 deubiquitinates chromosomal binding proteins H2A-Ub1 and H2A-Ub2, and consequently activates transcription factors and induces epigenetic modifications favorable for cancer growth and metastasis [112].

USP7 mediates degradation of tumor suppressors such as p53, MDM2, FOXO and PTEN [110]. USP14 is expressed at increased levels in melanoma cells compared to melanocytes, and its high expression correlates with melanoma progression and poorer survival. Knockdown or pharmacological inhibition of USP14 impairs viability of melanoma cells irrespective of the mutational status of BRAF, NRAS and TP53, and overcomes resistance to MAPK inhibitors. This was accompanied by accumulation of poly-ubiquitinated proteins, mitochondrial dysfunction, ER stress, and a ROS production [113].

USP9X, another member of the USP family, is responsible for attenuating the degradation of Mcl-1, an anti-apoptotic protein in melanoma and other cancers [53]. USP9X deubiquitinates, and stabilizes ETS-1, a transcription factor involved in regulation of angiogenesis, cell migration, proliferation and cellular differentiation in melanoma [114]. Phenethyl ITC, an inhibitor of USP9X, is currently in a Phase I trial for the treatment of melanoma and leukemia and Phase II trials for oral and lung cancer [53]. WP1130 (degrasyn) is another agent that inhibits USP9X and promotes the accumulation of protein-ubiquitin conjugates, leading to formation of aggresomes and apoptosis. This agent is shown to decrease melanoma cell growth both in vitro and in vivo melanoma models [115].

6. Conclusion

Melanoma is an aggressive disease intrinsically prone to metastasis. Germline and sporadic mutations are responsible for the initiation and progression of the disease and PTMs such as ubiquitination play dominant roles in melanoma growth and metastasis, and offer wealth of opportunities for therapeutic targeting. With better mechanistic understating of specific functions of the ubiquitinating enzymes as well as the deubiquitinases, new targeted therapies are expected to emerge in the foreseeable feature.

Author details

Anushka Dikshit and Jennifer Zhang*

*Address all correspondence to: jennifer.zhang@duke.edu

Department of Dermatology, Duke University Medical Center, Durham, NC, USA

References

[1] Howlader N NA, Krapcho M, Miller D, Bishop K, Kosary CL, Yu M, Ruhl J, Tatalovich Z, Mariotto A, Lewis DR, Chen HS, Feuer EJ, Cronin KA (eds). https://seercancergov/csr/1975_2014/, based on November 2016 SEER data submission, posted to the SEER web site, April 2017

[2] Horner M, Ries L, Krapcho M, Neyman N, Aminou R, Howlader N, et al. SEER Cancer Statistics Review, 1975-2006. Bethesda, MD: National Cancer Institute. 2009

[3] Amin MB, Greene FL, Edge SB, Compton CC, Gershenwald JE, Brookland RK, Meyer L, Gress DM, Byrd DR, Winchester DP. The eighth edition AJCC Cancer staging manual: Continuing to build a bridge from a population-based to a more "personalized" approach to cancer staging. CA: a Cancer Journal for Clinicians. 2017;**67**(2):93-99

[4] Shain AH, Bastian BC. From melanocytes to melanomas. Nature Reviews. Cancer. 2016;**16**(6):345

[5] Roh MR, Eliades P, Gupta S, Tsao H. Genetics of melanocytic nevi. Pigment Cell & Melanoma Research. 2015;**28**(6):661-672

[6] Lo JA, Fisher DE. The melanoma revolution: From UV carcinogenesis to a new era in therapeutics. Science (New York, New York). 2014;**346**(6212):945-949

[7] Aoude LG, Wadt KAW, Pritchard AL, Hayward NK. Genetics of familial melanoma: 20 years after CDKN2A. Pigment Cell & Melanoma Research. 2015;**28**(2):148-160

[8] Chin L, Garraway LA, Fisher DE. Malignant melanoma: Genetics and therapeutics in the genomic era. Genes & Development. 2006;**20**(16):2149-2182

[9] Chin L. The genetics of malignant melanoma: Lessons from mouse and man. Nature Reviews. Cancer. 2003;**3**(8):559

[10] Fletcher O, Easton D, Anderson K, Gilham C, Jay M, Peto J. Lifetime risks of common cancers among retinoblastoma survivors. Journal of the National Cancer Institute. 2004;**96**(5):357-363

[11] Muthusamy V, Hobbs C, Nogueira C, Cordon-Cardo C, McKee PH, Chin L, Bosenberg MW. Amplification of CDK4 and MDM2 in malignant melanoma. Genes, Chromosomes and Cancer. 2006;**45**(5):447-454

[12] Eng C, Li FP, Abramson DH, Ellsworth RM, Wong FL, Goldman MB, Seddon J, Tarbell N, Boice JD Jr. Mortality from second tumors among long-term survivors of retinoblastoma. Journal of the National Cancer Institute. 1993;**85**(14):1121-1128

[13] Valverde P, Healy E, Sikkink S, Haldane F, Thody AJ, Carothers A, Jackson IJ, Rees JL. The Asp84Glu variant of the melanocortin 1 receptor (MC1R) is associated with melanoma. Human Molecular Genetics. 1996;**5**(10):1663-1666

[14] Box NF, Duffy DL, Chen W, Stark M, Martin NG, Sturm RA, Hayward NK. MC1R genotype modifies risk of melanoma in families segregating CDKN2A mutations. American Journal of Human Genetics. 2001;**69**(4):765-773

[15] Maldonado JL, Fridlyand J, Patel H, Jain AN, Busam K, Kageshita T, Ono T, Albertson DG, Pinkel D, Bastian BC. Determinants of BRAF mutations in primary melanomas. Journal of the National Cancer Institute. 2003;**95**(24):1878-1890

[16] Stas M, Degreef H, Demunter A, De Wolf-Peeters C, van den Oord JJ. Analysis of N-and K-ras mutations in the distinctive tumor progression phases of melanoma. The Journal of Investigative Dermatology. 2001;**117**(6):1483-1489

[17] Papp T, Pemsel H, Zimmermann R, Bastrop R, Weiss DG, Schiffmann D. Mutational analysis of the N-ras, p53, p16INK4a, CDK4, and MC1R genes in human congenital melanocytic naevi. Journal of Medical Genetics. 1999;**36**(8):610-614

[18] Libra M, Malaponte G, Navolanic PM, Gangemi P, Bevelacqua V, Proietti L, Bruni B, Stivala F, Mazzarino MC, Travali S. Analysis of BRAF mutation in primary and metastatic melanoma. Cell Cycle. 2005;**4**(10):1382-1384

[19] Pollock PM, Harper UL, Hansen KS, Yudt LM, Stark M, Robbins CM, Moses TY, Hostetter G, Wagner U, Kakareka J. High frequency of BRAF mutations in nevi. Nature Genetics. 2003;**33**(1):19-20

[20] Edwards R, Ward M, Wu H, Medina C, Brose M, Volpe P, Nussen-Lee S, Haupt H, Martin A, Herlyn M. Absence of BRAF mutations in UV-protected mucosal melanomas. Journal of Medical Genetics. 2004;**41**(4):270-272

[21] Yazdi AS, Palmedo G, Flaig MJ, Puchta U, Reckwerth A, Rütten A, Mentzel T, Hügel H, Hantschke M, Schmid-Wendtner M-H. Mutations of the BRAF gene in benign and malignant melanocytic lesions. The Journal of Investigative Dermatology. 2003;**121**(5): 1160-1162

[22] McNeal AS, Liu K, Nakhate V, Natale CA, Duperret EK, Capell BC, Dentchev T, Berger SL, Herlyn M, Seykora JT, et al. CDKN2B loss promotes progression from benign melanocytic nevus to melanoma. Cancer Discovery. 2015;**5**(10):1072-1085

[23] Goetz EM, Ghandi M, Treacy DJ, Wagle N, Garraway LA. ERK mutations confer resistance to mitogen-activated protein kinase pathway inhibitors. Cancer Research. 2014;**74**(23):7079-7089

[24] Dong C, Wilhelm D, Koopman P. Sox genes and cancer. Cytogenetic and Genome Research. 2004;**105**(2-4):442-447

[25] Ernfors P. Cellular origin and developmental mechanisms during the formation of skin melanocytes. Experimental Cell Research. 2010;**316**(8):1397-1407

[26] Gupta PB, Kuperwasser C, Brunet J-P, Ramaswamy S, Kuo W-L, Gray JW, Naber SP, Weinberg RA. The melanocyte differentiation program predisposes to metastasis after neoplastic transformation. Nature Genetics. 2005;**37**(10):1047

[27] Ploper D, Taelman VF, Robert L, Perez BS, Titz B, Chen H-W, Graeber TG, von Euw E, Ribas A, De Robertis EM. MITF drives endolysosomal biogenesis and potentiates Wnt signaling in melanoma cells. Proceedings of the National Academy of Sciences. 2015;**112**(5):E420-E4E9

[28] Hartman ML, Czyz M. Pro-survival role of MITF in melanoma. The Journal of Investigative Dermatology. 2015;**135**(2):352-358

[29] Xue G, Romano E, Massi D, Mandalà M. Wnt/β-catenin signaling in melanoma: Preclinical rationale and novel therapeutic insights. Cancer Treatment Reviews. 2016;**49**:1-12

[30] Larue L, Delmas V. 5.2. 3.1. LEF 5.2. 3.2. ICAT 5.2. 3.3. Proven targets of beta-catenin in melanocytes and melanoma 5.2. 3.3. 1. Mitf-M 5.2. 3.3. 2. Dct. Frontiers in Bioscience. 2006;**11**:733-742

[31] Arozarena I, Bischof H, Gilby D, Belloni B, Dummer R, Wellbrock C. In melanoma, beta-catenin is a suppressor of invasion. Oncogene. 2011;**30**(45):4531

[32] Brugmann SA, Goodnough LH, Gregorieff A, Leucht P, ten Berge D, Fuerer C, Clevers H, Nusse R, Helms JA. Wnt signaling mediates regional specification in the vertebrate face. Development. 2007;**134**(18):3283-3295

[33] Gómez-Orte E, Sáenz-Narciso B, Moreno S, Cabello J. Multiple functions of the noncanonical Wnt pathway. Trends in Genetics. 2013;**29**(9):545-553

[34] Iden S, Collard JG. Crosstalk between small GTPases and polarity proteins in cell polarization. Nature Reviews. Molecular Cell Biology. 2008;**9**(11):846

[35] Sahai E, Marshall CJ. RHO–GTPases and cancer. Nature Reviews. Cancer. 2002;**2**(2):133

[36] Kovacs D, Migliano E, Muscardin L, Silipo V, Catricalà C, Picardo M, Bellei B. The role of Wnt/β-catenin signaling pathway in melanoma epithelial-to-mesenchymal-like switching: Evidences from patients-derived cell lines. Oncotarget. 2016;**7**(28):43295

[37] Krueger KE, Srivastava S. Posttranslational protein modifications current implications for cancer detection, prevention, and therapeutics. Molecular & Cellular Proteomics. 2006;**5**(10):1799-1810

[38] Jørgensen K, Holm R, Mælandsmo GM, Flørenes VA. Expression of activated extracellular signal-regulated kinases 1/2 in malignant melanomas: Relationship with clinical outcome. Clinical Cancer Research. 2003;**9**(14):5325-5331

[39] Komander D, Rape M. The ubiquitin code. Annual Review of Biochemistry. 2012;**81**: 203-229

[40] Yau R, Rape M. The increasing complexity of the ubiquitin code. Nature Cell Biology. 2016;**18**(6):579-586

[41] Doil C, Mailand N, Bekker-Jensen S, Menard P, Larsen DH, Pepperkok R, Ellenberg J, Panier S, Durocher D, Bartek J. RNF168 binds and amplifies ubiquitin conjugates on damaged chromosomes to allow accumulation of repair proteins. Cell. 2009;**136**(3):435-446

[42] Lauwers E, Jacob C, André B. K63-linked ubiquitin chains as a specific signal for protein sorting into the multivesicular body pathway. The Journal of Cell Biology. 2009;**185**(3):493-502

[43] Deng L, Wang C, Spencer E, Yang L, Braun A, You J, Slaughter C, Pickart C, Chen ZJ. Activation of the IκB kinase complex by TRAF6 requires a dimeric ubiquitin-conjugating enzyme complex and a unique polyubiquitin chain. Cell. 2000;**103**(2):351-361

[44] Deng L, Wang C, Spencer E, Yang L, Braun A, You J, Slaughter C, Pickart C, Chen ZJ. Activation of the IkappaB kinase complex by TRAF6 requires a dimeric ubiquitin-conjugating enzyme complex and a unique polyubiquitin chain. Cell. 2000;**103**(2):351-361

[45] Groettrup M, Pelzer C, Schmidtke G, Hofmann K. Activating the ubiquitin family: UBA6 challenges the field. Trends in Biochemical Sciences. 2008;**33**(5):230-237

[46] Xu GW, Ali M, Wood TE, Wong D, Maclean N, Wang X, Gronda M, Skrtic M, Li X, Hurren R. The ubiquitin-activating enzyme E1 as a therapeutic target for the treatment of leukemia and multiple myeloma. Blood. 2010;**115**(11):2251-2259

[47] Liu X, Sun L, Gursel DB, Cheng C, Huang S, Rademaker AW, Khan SA, Yin J, Kiyokawa H. The non-canonical ubiquitin activating enzyme UBA6 suppresses epithelial-mesenchymal transition of mammary epithelial cells. Oncotarget. 2017;**8**(50):87480-87493

[48] Rosner K, Mehregan DR, Kirou E, Abrams J, Kim S, Campbell M, Frieder J, Lawrence K, Haynes B, Shekhar MP. Melanoma development and progression are associated with Rad6 upregulation and β-catenin relocation to the cell membrane. Journal of Skin Cancer. 2014;**2014**:10. Article ID:` 439205. https://doi.org/10.1155/2014/439205

[49] Ohh M. pVHL's kryptonite: E2-EPF UCP. Cancer Cell. 2006;**10**(2):95-97

[50] Jung C-R, Hwang K-S, Yoo J, Cho W-K, Kim J-M, Kim WH, Im D-S. E2-EPF UCP targets pVHL for degradation and associates with tumor growth and metastasis. Nature Medicine. 2006;**12**(7):809

[51] Liu S, Yamauchi H. p27-associated G1 arrest induced by hinokitiol in human malignant melanoma cells is mediated via down-regulation of pRb, Skp2 ubiquitin ligase, and impairment of Cdk2 function. Cancer Letters. 2009;**286**(2):240-249

[52] Hershko DD. Oncogenic properties and prognostic implications of the ubiquitin ligase Skp2 in cancer. Cancer. 2008;**112**(7):1415-1424

[53] Ma J, Guo W, Li C. Ubiquitination in melanoma pathogenesis and treatment. Cancer Medicine. 2017

[54] Gregori L, Poosch MS, Cousins G, Chau V. A uniform isopeptide-linked multiubiquitin chain is sufficient to target substrate for degradation in ubiquitin-mediated proteolysis. The Journal of Biological Chemistry. 1990;**265**(15):8354-8357

[55] Aydin IT, Melamed RD, Adams SJ, Castillo-Martin M, Demir A, Bryk D, Brunner G, Cordon-Cardo C, Osman I, Rabadan R, et al. FBXW7 mutations in melanoma and a new therapeutic paradigm. Journal of the National Cancer Institute. 2014;**106**(6):dju107

[56] Sato M, Rodriguez-Barrueco R, Yu J, Do C, Silva JM, Gautier J. MYC is a critical target of FBXW7. Oncotarget. 2015;**6**(5):3292-3305

[57] Fujii Y, Yada M, Nishiyama M, Kamura T, Takahashi H, Tsunematsu R, Susaki E, Nakagawa T, Matsumoto A, Nakayama KI. Fbxw7 contributes to tumor suppression by targeting multiple proteins for ubiquitin-dependent degradation. Cancer Science. 2006;**97**(8):729-736

[58] Richards MW, Burgess SG, Poon E, Carstensen A, Eilers M, Chesler L, Bayliss R. Structural basis of N-Myc binding by aurora-A and its destabilization by kinase inhibitors. Proceedings of the National Academy of Sciences of the United States of America. 2016;**113**(48):13726-13731

[59] Rajabi P, Karimian P, Heidarpour M. The relationship between MDM2 expression and tumor thickness and invasion in primary cutaneous malignant melanoma. Journal of research in medical sciences: the official journal of Isfahan University of Medical. Sciences. 2012;**17**(5):452

[60] Luo Z, Zhang X, Zeng W, Su J, Yang K, Lu L, Lim CB, Tang W, Wu L, Zhao S. TRAF6 regulates melanoma invasion and metastasis through ubiquitination of Basigin. Oncotarget. 2016;**7**(6):7179

[61] Feng H, Lopez GY, Kim CK, Alvarez A, Duncan CG, Nishikawa R, Nagane M, A-JA S, Auron PE, Hedberg ML. EGFR phosphorylation of DCBLD2 recruits TRAF6 and stimulates AKT-promoted tumorigenesis. The Journal of Clinical Investigation. 2014; **124**(9):3741-3756

[62] Linares JF, Duran A, Yajima T, Pasparakis M, Moscat J, Diaz-Meco MT. K63 polyubiquitination and activation of mTOR by the p62-TRAF6 complex in nutrient-activated cells. Molecular Cell. 2013;**51**(3):283-296

[63] Wang B, Jie Z, Joo D, Ordureau A, Liu P, Gan W, Guo J, Zhang J, North BJ, Dai X. TRAF2 and OTUD7B govern a ubiquitin-dependent switch that regulates mTORC2 signalling. Nature. 2017;**545**(7654):365

[64] Arimoto K, Takahashi H, Hishiki T, Konishi H, Fujita T, Shimotohno K. Negative regulation of the RIG-I signaling by the ubiquitin ligase RNF125. Proceedings of the National Academy of Sciences of the United States of America. 2007;**104**(18):7500-7505

[65] Yang L, Zhou B, Li X, Lu Z, Li W, Huo X, Miao Z. RNF125 is a ubiquitin-protein ligase that promotes p53 degradation. Cellular Physiology and Biochemistry. 2015;**35**(1):237-245

[66] Jia X, Zhou H, Wu C, Wu Q, Ma S, Wei C, Cao Y, Song J, Zhong H, Zhou Z, et al. The ubiquitin ligase RNF125 targets innate immune adaptor protein TRIM14 for ubiquitination and degradation. Journal of Immunology. 2017;**198**(12):4652-4658

[67] Tenorio J, Mansilla A, Valencia M, Martinez-Glez V, Romanelli V, Arias P, Castrejon N, Poletta F, Guillen-Navarro E, Gordo G, et al. A new overgrowth syndrome is due to mutations in RNF125. Human Mutation. 2014;**35**(12):1436-1441

[68] Kim H, Frederick DT, Levesque MP, Cooper ZA, Feng Y, Krepler C, Brill L, Samuels Y, Hayward NK, Perlina A, et al. Downregulation of the ubiquitin ligase RNF125 underlies resistance of melanoma cells to BRAF inhibitors via JAK1 deregulation. Cell Reports. 2015;**11**(9):1458-1473

[69] Lito P, Pratilas CA, Joseph EW, Tadi M, Halilovic E, Zubrowski M, Huang A, Wong WL, Callahan MK, Merghoub T, et al. Relief of profound feedback inhibition of mitogenic signaling by RAF inhibitors attenuates their activity in BRAFV600E melanomas. Cancer Cell. 2012;**22**(5):668-682

[70] Hernandez MA, Patel B, Hey F, Giblett S, Davis H, Pritchard C. Regulation of BRAF protein stability by a negative feedback loop involving the MEK-ERK pathway but not the FBXW7 tumour suppressor. Cellular Signalling. 2016;**28**(6):561-571

[71] Wan L, Chen M, Cao J, Dai X, Yin Q, Zhang J, Song SJ, Lu Y, Liu J, Inuzuka H, et al. The APC/C E3 ligase complex activator FZR1 restricts BRAF oncogenic function. Cancer Discovery. 2017;**7**(4):424-441

[72] Chakraborty A, Diefenbacher ME, Mylona A, Kassel O, Behrens A. The E3 ubiquitin ligase Trim7 mediates c-Jun/AP-1 activation by Ras signalling. Nature Communications. 2015;**6**:6782

[73] Delmas A, Cherier J, Pohorecka M, Medale-Giamarchi C, Meyer N, Casanova A, Sordet O, Lamant L, Savina A, Pradines A, et al. The c-Jun/RHOB/AKT pathway confers resistance of BRAF-mutant melanoma cells to MAPK inhibitors. Oncotarget. 2015;**6**(17):15250-15264

[74] McClurg UL, Robson CN. Deubiquitinating enzymes as oncotargets. Oncotarget. 2015;**6**(12):9657

[75] Wilkinson KD. DUBs at a glance. Journal of Cell Science. 2009;**122**(14):2325-2329

[76] Carbone M, Yang H, Pass HI, Krausz T, Testa JR, Gaudino G. BAP1 and cancer. Nature Reviews Cancer. 2013;**13**(3):153

[77] Machida YJ, Machida Y, Vashisht AA, Wohlschlegel JA, Dutta A. The deubiquitinating enzyme BAP1 regulates cell growth via interaction with HCF-1. The Journal of Biological Chemistry. 2009;**284**(49):34179-34188

[78] Shembade N, Harhaj EW. Regulation of NF-κB signaling by the A20 deubiquitinase. Cellular & Molecular Immunology. 2012;**9**(2):123

[79] Shembade N, Ma A, Harhaj EW. Inhibition of NF-κB signaling by A20 through disruption of ubiquitin enzyme complexes. Science. 2010;**327**(5969):1135-1139

[80] Honma K, Tsuzuki S, Nakagawa M, Tagawa H, Nakamura S, Morishima Y, Seto M. TNFAIP3/A20 functions as a novel tumor suppressor gene in several subtypes of non-Hodgkin lymphomas. Blood. 2009;**114**(12):2467-2475

[81] Giordano M, Roncagalli R, Bourdely P, Chasson L, Buferne M, Yamasaki S, Beyaert R, Van Loo G, Auphan-Anezin N, Schmitt-Verhulst A-M. The tumor necrosis factor alpha-induced protein 3 (TNFAIP3, A20) imposes a brake on antitumor activity of CD8 T cells. Proceedings of the National Academy of Sciences. 2014;**111**(30):11115-11120

[82] Bignell GR, Warren W, Seal S, Takahashi M, Rapley E, Barfoot R, Green H, Brown C, Biggs PJ, Lakhani SR. Identification of the familial cylindromatosis tumour-suppressor gene. Nature Genetics. 2000;**25**(2):160-165

[83] Brummelkamp TR, Nijman SM, Dirac AM, Bernards R. Loss of the cylindromatosis tumour suppressor inhibits apoptosis by activating NF-κB. Nature. 2003;**424**(6950):797-801

[84] Ke H, Massoumi R. The role of CYLD in blocking oncogenic cell signaling in melanoma. Journal of Cancer Therapy. 2013;**4**(06):32

[85] Qiu H, Yuan S, Lu X. miR-186 suppressed CYLD expression and promoted cell proliferation in human melanoma. Oncology Letters. 2016;**12**(4):2301-2306

[86] Zhang K, Guo L. MiR-767 promoted cell proliferation in human melanoma by suppressing CYLD expression. Gene. 2018;**641**:272-278

[87] Staal J, Driege Y, Bekaert T, Demeyer A, Muyllaert D, Van Damme P, Gevaert K, Beyaert R. T-cell receptor-induced JNK activation requires proteolytic inactivation of CYLD by MALT1. The EMBO Journal. 2011;**30**(9):1742-1752

[88] Alameda J, Fernandez-Acenero M, Moreno-Maldonado R, Navarro M, Quintana R, Page A, Ramirez A, Bravo A, Casanova M. CYLD regulates keratinocyte differentiation and skin cancer progression in humans. Cell Death & Disease. 2011;**2**(9):e208

[89] Ke H, Augustine CK, Gandham VD, Jin JY, Tyler DS, Akiyama SK, Hall RP, Zhang JY. CYLD inhibits melanoma growth and progression through suppression of the JNK/AP-1 and beta1-integrin signaling pathways. The Journal of Investigative Dermatology. 2013;**133**(1):221-229

[90] Miliani de Marval P, Lutfeali S, Jin JY, Leshin B, Selim MA, Zhang JY. CYLD inhibits tumorigenesis and metastasis by blocking JNK/AP1 signaling at multiple levels. Cancer Prevention Research (Philadelphia, Pa.). 2011

[91] Reiley WW, Jin W, Lee AJ, Wright A, Wu X, Tewalt EF, Leonard TO, Norbury CC, Fitzpatrick L, Zhang M. Deubiquitinating enzyme CYLD negatively regulates the ubiquitin-dependent kinase Tak1 and prevents abnormal T cell responses. The Journal of Experimental Medicine. 2007;**204**(6):1475-1485

[92] Trompouki E, Hatzivassiliou E, Tsichritzis T, Farmer H, Ashworth A, Mosialos G. CYLD is a deubiquitinating enzyme that negatively regulates NF-κB activation by TNFR family members. Nature. 2003;**424**(6950):793

[93] Stegmeier F, Sowa ME, Nalepa G, Gygi SP, Harper JW, Elledge SJ. The tumor suppressor CYLD regulates entry into mitosis. Proceedings of the National Academy of Sciences. 2007;**104**(21):8869-8874

[94] Tsunoda K, Oikawa H, Tada H, Tatemichi Y, Muraoka S, Miura S, Shibazaki M, Maeda F, Takahashi K, Akasaka T. Nucleus accumbens-associated 1 contributes to cortactin deacetylation and augments the migration of melanoma cells. The Journal of Investigative Dermatology. 2011;**131**(8):1710-1719

[95] Wickström SA, Masoumi KC, Khochbin S, Fässler R, Massoumi R. CYLD negatively regulates cell-cycle progression by inactivating HDAC6 and increasing the levels of acetylated tubulin. The EMBO Journal. 2010;**29**(1):131-144

[96] Sanchez-Tillo E, Liu Y, de Barrios O, Siles L, Fanlo L, Cuatrecasas M, Darling DS, Dean DC, Castells A, Postigo A. EMT-activating transcription factors in cancer: Beyond EMT and tumor invasiveness. Cellular and Molecular Life Sciences: CMLS. 2012;**69**(20):3429-3456

[97] Massoumi R, Kuphal S, Hellerbrand C, Haas B, Wild P, Spruss T, Pfeifer A, Fassler R, Bosserhoff AK. Down-regulation of CYLD expression by snail promotes tumor progression in malignant melanoma. The Journal of Experimental Medicine. 2009;**206**(1):221-232

[98] Pharoah PD, Guilford P, Caldas C. Incidence of gastric cancer and breast cancer in CDH1 (E-cadherin) mutation carriers from hereditary diffuse gastric cancer families. Gastroenterology. 2001;**121**(6):1348-1353

[99] Risinger JI, Berchuck A, Kohler MF, Boyd J. Mutations of the E–cadherin gene in human gynecologic cancers. Nature Genetics. 1994;**7**(1):98

[100] Hsu M-Y, Meier FE, Nesbit M, Hsu J-Y, Van Belle P, Elder DE, Herlyn M. E-cadherin expression in melanoma cells restores keratinocyte-mediated growth control and down-regulates expression of invasion-related adhesion receptors. The American Journal of Pathology. 2000;**156**(5):1515-1525

[101] Li G, Satyamoorthy K, Herlyn M. N-cadherin-mediated intercellular interactions promote survival and migration of melanoma cells. Cancer Research. 2001;**61**(9):3819-3825

[102] Lade-Keller J, Riber-Hansen R, Guldberg P, Schmidt H, Hamilton-Dutoit SJ, Steiniche T. E-to N-cadherin switch in melanoma is associated with decreased expression of phosphatase and tensin homolog and cancer progression. The British Journal of Dermatology. 2013;**169**(3):618-628

[103] Kuphal S, Palm HG, Poser I, Bosserhoff AK. Snail-regulated genes in malignant melanoma. Melanoma Research. 2005;**15**(4):305-313

[104] Rotte A, Martinka M, Li G. MMP2 expression is a prognostic marker for primary melanoma patients. Cellular Oncology. 2012;**35**(3):207-216

[105] Mueller BM. Different Roles for Plasminogen Activators and Metalloproteinases in Melanoma Metastasis. In: Günthert U, Birchmeier W, editors. Attempts to Understand Metastasis Formation I. Current Topics in Microbiology 213/I and Immunology. Vol. 213/1. Berlin, Heidelberg: Springer; 1996. pp. 65-85

[106] Howard JD, Moriarty WF, Park J, Riedy K, Panova IP, Chung CH, Suh KY, Levchenko A, Alani RM. Notch signaling mediates melanoma-endothelial cell communication and melanoma cell migration. Pigment Cell & Melanoma Research. 2013;**26**(5):697-707

[107] Golan T, Messer AR, Amitai-Lange A, Melamed Z, Ohana R, Bell RE, Kapitansky O, Lerman G, Greenberger S, Khaled M, et al. Interactions of melanoma cells with distal keratinocytes trigger metastasis via notch signaling inhibition of MITF. Molecular Cell. 2015;**59**(4):664-676

[108] Krepler C, Xiao M, Samanta M, Vultur A, Chen HY, Brafford P, Reyes-Uribe PI, Halloran M, Chen T, He X, et al. Targeting notch enhances the efficacy of ERK inhibitors in BRAF-V600E melanoma. Oncotarget. 2016;**7**(44):71211-71222

[109] Zhang K, Wong P, Salvaggio C, Salhi A, Osman I, Bedogni B. Synchronized targeting of notch and ERBB signaling suppresses melanoma tumor growth through inhibition of Notch1 and ERBB3. The Journal of Investigative Dermatology. 2016;**136**(2):464-472

[110] Wang L, YR Dent S. Functions of SAGA in development and disease. Epigenomics. 2014;**6**(3):329-339

[111] Luise C, Capra M, Donzelli M, Mazzarol G, Jodice MG, Nuciforo P, Viale G, Di Fiore PP, Confalonieri S. An atlas of altered expression of deubiquitinating enzymes in human cancer. PLoS One. 2011;**6**(1):e15891

[112] Liu YL, Yang YM, Xu H, Dong XS. Increased expression of ubiquitin-specific protease 22 can promote cancer progression and predict therapy failure in human colorectal cancer. Journal of Gastroenterology and Hepatology. 2010;**25**(11):1800-1805

[113] Didier R, Mallavialle A, Ben Jouira R, Domdom MA, Tichet M, Auberger P, Luciano F, Ohanna M, Tartare-Deckert S, Deckert M. Targeting the proteasome-associated deubiquitinating enzyme USP14 impairs melanoma cell survival and overcomes resistance to MAPK-targeting therapies. Molecular Cancer Therapeutics. 2018

[114] Potu H, Peterson LF, Kandarpa M, Pal A, Sun H, Durham A, Harms PW, Hollenhorst PC, Eskiocak U, Talpaz M. Usp9x regulates Ets-1 ubiquitination and stability to control NRAS expression and tumorigenicity in melanoma. Nature Communications. 2017;**8**:14449

[115] Kapuria V, Peterson LF, Fang D, Bornmann WG, Talpaz M, Donato NJ. Deubiquitinase inhibition by small-molecule WP1130 triggers aggresome formation and tumor cell apoptosis. Cancer Research. 2010;**70**(22):9265-9276

10

The Landscape of Histone Modification in Cancer Metastasis

Zhaoping Qiu, Jianlin Wang and Yadi Wu

Abstract

Metastasis represents one of the most devastating aspects of cancer. Epithelial to mesenchymal transition (EMT) has been shown to play a critical role in tumorigenic metastasis. During metastatic progression, both genetic and epigenetic modifications endow cancer cells with properties that modulate the capacity for metastatic success. Histone modification is profoundly altered in cancer cells and contributes to cancer metastasis by controlling different metastatic phenotypes. Here, we first review histone modifications and discuss their roles in EMT and metastasis, with a particular focus on histone methylation and acetylation. Second, we review the major histone modification enzymes that control chromatin in cancer metastasis. Third, we discuss the transcriptional regulation concerted by these enzymes with EMT transcription factors at different molecular layers. Finally, we discuss pharmacologic manipulation of histone modification enzymes for metastasis treatment. A comprehensive understanding of histone modification in metastasis will not only provide new insights into our knowledge of cancer progression and metastasis, but also offer a novel approach for the development of innovative therapeutic strategies.

Keywords: EMT, epigenetic, histone modification, metastasis, inhibitor

1. Introduction

Approximately 90% of cancer deaths are caused by metastasis [1]. Cancer metastasis is an exceedingly complex process involving tumor cell motility, intravasation, and circulation in the blood or lymph system, extravasation, and growth in new tissues and organs [2, 3]. During invasion, tumor cells lose cell–cell adhesion, gain mobility and leave the site of the primary tumor to invade adjacent tissues. In intravasation, tumor cells penetrate through the endothelial barrier and enter the systemic circulation through blood and lymphatic vessels. In extravasation, cells that survive the anchorage-independent growth conditions in the bloodstream attach to vessels at distant sites and leave the bloodstream. Finally, in metastatic colonization, tumor cells form macrometastases in the new host environment [2, 3]. All of these steps, from initial breakdown of tissue structure, through increased invasiveness, and ultimately distribution and colonization throughout the body, are developmental characteristics of the processes, epithelial to mesenchymal transition (EMT) and mesenchymal to epithelial transition (MET). EMT is a distinctive morphogenic process that occurs during embryonic development, chronic degeneration and fibrosis of organs, and tumor invasion and metastasis [4–6]. The similarity of genetic controls and biochemical mechanisms that underlie the acquisition of an invasive phenotype and the subsequent systemic spread of cancer cells highlights the concept that tumor cells usurp this developmental pathway for metastatic dissemination. In total, EMT provides tumor cells with the proclivity for early metastasis, renders them resistance to therapeutics and endows cells with cancer stem cell (CSC)-like traits [6].

The hallmark of EMT is the loss of E-cadherin expression, an important caretaker of the epithelial phenotype. Loss of E-cadherin expression is often correlated with the tumor grade and stage because it results in the disruption of the cell–cell adhesion and an increase in the nuclear β-catenin. Several transcription factors have been implicated in the regulation of EMT, including the zinc finger proteins of the SNAIL family (SNAIL1/2/3), the basic helix–loop–helix (HLH) factor TWIST (TWIST1/2, E12/E47), and two double zinc finger and homeodomain ZEB family (ZEB1/ZEB2). These factors act as a molecular switch for the EMT program by repressing a subset of common genes that encode cadherins, claudins, integrins, mucins, plakophilin, occludin and ZO1, and thereby induce EMT.

EMT is a dynamic process that preserves plasticity [6]. In this instance, the reprogramming of gene expression provides a rapid and dynamic regulatory mechanism to switch between the epithelial and mesenchymal conditions during cancer progression. Consistent with this, these EMT-activating transcriptional factors (EMT-TFs) are liable proteins that turn over rapidly and do not have long residence times at their binding sites. Interestingly, disseminating cells orchestrate a metastatic cascade without a concomitant need for genomic mutations, which indicates that this dissemination is epigenetically templated. Both EMT and epigenetic modification (DNA methylation and histone modifications) are dynamic and efficient processes during development, differentiation and carcinogenesis. These studies indicate that the epigenetic mechanism plays an important role in modulating the induction of EMT and tumor metastasis.

2. Epigenetics and histone modification

2.1. Epigenetic and chromatin structure

The term "epigenetics" was first coined by Conrad H. Waddington in his Principles of Embryology textbook in 1942 to designate a process in which gene regulation modulated development. The final definition of epigenetics was confirmed in the Epigenetic Meeting held by the Banbury Conference Center and Cold Spring Harbor Laboratory in 2008 as "a stably heritable phenotype resulting from changes in a chromosome without alterations in the DNA sequence." In general, epigenetic regulation includes changes that impact histone modification, DNA methylation, histone variants, chromatin looping, noncoding RNAs and nucleosomal occupancy and remodeling.

Genomic DNA is tightly packaged in chromatin by both histone and nonhistone proteins in the nucleus of eukaryotic cells. The basic chromatin subunits, nucleosomes, are formed by wrapping 146 base pairs (bp) of DNA around an octamer of four core histones: H2A, H2B, H3, and H4. Whereas the nucleosomal core is compact, eight flexible lysine-rich histone tails protrude from the nucleosome that modulate internucleosomal contacts and provide binding sites for nonhistone proteins. From the perspective of gene transcription, chromatin structure can be divided into two distinct categories: euchromatin and heterochromatin. "Euchromatin" is an open chromatin structure that affords accessibility of transcription factors to DNA, resulting in gene activation. In contrast, "heterochromatin" is a closed chromatin structure with a low interaction between transcription factors and the genome, leading to gene repression.

2.2. Histone modifications and histone code hypothesis

The histone code hypothesis was first proposed by Strahl and Allis in 2000. They suggested that "multiple histone modifications, acting in a combinatorial or sequential fashion on one or multiple histone tails, specify unique downstream functions" [7]. The histone "language," based on this "histone code," is encoded in these modifications and read by chromatin-associated proteins. So far, several histone post-translational modifications (PTMs) have been identified, including acetylation, methylation, phosphorylation, ubiquitination, sumoylation, ADP ribosylation, proline isomerization, biotinylation, citrullination and their various combinations [8]. These modifications constitute a unique "code" to regulate histone interactions with other proteins and thereby allow modification (either overcoming or solidifying) of the intrinsic histone barrier to transcription. Accordingly, with these modifications, the various proteins that add, recognize and remove these PTMs, termed writers, readers and erasers, respectively, have been identified and structurally characterized. While "writer" and "eraser" enzymes modify histones by catalyzing the addition and removal of histone PTMs, respectively; "reader" proteins recognize these modified histones and 'translate' the PTMs by executing distinct cellular programs. In addition, numerous core histone chaperones also facilitate core histone deposition or removal from chromatin. Histone modifications control dynamic transitions between transcriptionally active or silent chromatin states, and regulate the transcription of genetic information encoded in DNA (the "genetic code") [9]. Analyses of genome-wide profiles of histone modifications and gene expression identified three distinct types of configurations: repressed, active and bivalent. First, the closed chromatin configuration is linked with suppression of gene transcription, the repressed state. Second, an open chromatin configuration is associated with active gene transcription, the active state. Third, bivalent chromatin consists of domains that have both repressive and active histone markers, predominately on developmental genes, which allows phenotypic plasticity before committing to a specific cell fate.

During EMT, histone modifications provide a regulatory platform to orchestrate the repression or activation between epithelial and mesenchymal genes. Here, we only focus on the well-studied histone acetylation and methylation, and discuss their diverse regulation and role in transcriptional reprogramming of tumor metastasis (**Table 1**).

Modification				Writer	Eraser
Acetylation			H3K9, H3K27	P300, PCAF, MOF, Tip60	HDAC
Methylation	Lysine	Activating	H3K4	MLL1–4, Set 1a, Set 1b, Ash1L, Set7/9, and SMYD	KDM1, KDM2, KDM5, JARID2 and NO66
			H3K36	KMT3, NSD2, NSD3 and SMYD	KDM2, KDM4/JMJD and NO66
			H3K79	KMT4	PHF8
		Repressing	H3K9	KMT1	KDM1, KDM3, KDM4, PHF8, and JHDM1D
			H3K20	KMT5, KMT7 and SET8	Unknown
			H3K27	PRC2	KDM6, UTY and JHDM1D
	Arginine		H4R3me2a, H3R8, H3R2me2a,H4R3me2s	PRMT1, PRMT2, PRMT3, CARM1/PRMT4, PRMT5, PRMT6, PRMT7, PRMT8, and PRMT9	Unknown

Table 1. Histone modifying enzymes involved in metastasis.

3. Histone acetylation

Evidence has established that histone acetylation is associated with gene activation. A genome-wide study demonstrated that all forms of histone acetylation are positively correlated with gene expression [10]. Histones contain amino acids with basic side chains that are positively charged and attracted to the negatively charged genomic DNA. Ultimately, histone acetylation reduces the positive charge on histones and decreases the interaction between nucleosomes and DNA. Generally, histone acetylation is greater in the promoters of active genes and influences both the initiation and elongation of gene transcription. Histone acetylation also stabilizes the binding of chromatin remodeling factors at promoter regions and induces nucleosomes unfolding as well as reduces nucleosome occupancy. The acetylation state of a chromatin leads to the structural modification of the nucleosome. Acetylated (or hyperacetylated) chromatin is in a relaxed confirmation and associated with active transcription. In contrast, deacetylated (or hypoacetylated) chromatin is condensed and supercoiled, and is associated with transcriptional silencing (and, in the context of cancer, the inhibition of tumor suppressor genes).

Histone acetylation is a rapid and reversible process controlled by histone acetyltransferases (HATs) and histone deacetylases (HDAC)s. The HATs transfer acetyl groups from acetyl-coenzyme A (CoA) to the ε-amino groups of lysine residues in histone tails, which results in gene activation. HATs contain a bromodomain that recognizes and binds to acetylated histones, categorized into three major families, GNAT (GCN5 and PCAF), MYST (Tip60 and MOF), and CBP/p300. The HDACs remove acetyl groups from lysine residues, leading to gene silencing. Sequence homology, subcellular location, and the features of the catalytic site have been used to classify the 18 members of the human HDAC family into 4 groups: class

I (HDACs 1, 2, 3, and 8), class II (HDACs 4, 5, 6, 7, 9, and 10), class III (SIRT1, SIRT2, SIRT3, SIRT4, SIRT5, SIRT6, and SIRT7), and class IV (HDAC11) [11]. Class I HDACs have sequence homology to class II HDACs and class IV HDACs but not class III HDACs. Class I, II, and IV HDACs are zinc-dependent, whereas class III HDACs are nicotinamide adenine dinucleotide $(NAD)^+$-dependent. Genome-wide mapping of the binding of HATs and HDACs to the human genome demonstrate that these enzymes regulate the activation and repression of transcription, respectively. The dysfunctional balance between acetylation and deacetylation is clearly associated with human disease and tumorigenesis.

p300 cooperates in an epigenetic manner with a DOT1L-c-Myc complex to induce EMT in breast metastasis [12]. The elevated level of p300-DOT1L-c-Myc is associated with the acquisition of CSC-like properties during breast carcinogenesis, which implies that p300 functions as a potential oncogene to influence the clinical outcome of breast cancer. In addition, transforming growth factor-beta (TGF-β) and WNT co-operated to mediate EMT. TGF-β induces the translocation of β-catenin to the nucleus where it binds to T- cell Factor (TCF); this complex recruits p300/CBP to assemble a transcriptional complex on target gene promoters that promotes EMT signaling. Intriguingly, over-expression of SNAIL/SLUG up-regulates TGF-β-receptor 2 (TGFBR2) expression with an increase of H3K9 acetylation on TGFBR2 promoter to increase TGF-β signaling [13]. In contrast, however, p300 was reportedly recruited by the hepatocyte nuclear factor (HNF) 3 to the E-cadherin promoter, increasing expression, and thus reducing the metastatic potential of breast cancer cells [14]. Similarly, the p300-CBP-associated factor (PCAF) has functions that can differ among cancer types. PCAF is an anti-oncogene and its expression is down-regulated and negatively correlated with tumor metastasis in hepatocellular carcinoma (HCC) [15]. This complex plays an important role in suppressing EMT and HCC metastasis and by targeting Gli1 [16]. However, it was also reported that PCAF acetylates the enhancer of zeste homolog 2 (EZH2) at K348 to augment EZH2 stability, and thus promotes lung cancer cell migration and invasion [17]. These reports indicate that the role of PCAF is context-dependent. In several breast cancer cell lines, hMOF catalyzes promoter H4K16 acetylation, which is critical to maintain expression of EMT-related tumor suppressor genes [18]. Consistent with this, MOF also acetylates the histone demethylase lysine-specific histone demethylase 1 (LSD1), to suppress EMT, indicating that MOF is a critical suppressor of EMT and tumor progression [19]. Recently, we found that Tip60 appears to be an important regulator of TWIST activity by acetylating at H3K73 and H3K76 of the GK-X-GK motif, resulting in an interaction between BRD4 and TWIST, hence promoting the aggressiveness of basal-like breast cancer (BLBC) [20].

Dysfunctional class I HDAC expression and activity is associated with cancer metastasis. HDAC1 regulates invasiveness by increasing matrix metalloproteinase (MMP) expression. Furthermore, HIF-2α is a transcriptional regulator of the *HDAC1* gene, and hypoxia increase HIF-2α and HDAC1 expression [21]. TGF-β-driven E-cadherin silencing and EMT in human pancreatic cancer cells also depend on HDAC activity [22]. HDAC1 and HDAC2 form a transcriptional repressor complex with SNAIL to downregulate the E-cadherin expression of pancreatic cancer cells during metastasis. Intriguingly, SNAIL also recruits the HDAC1/2-containing SIN3A complex to deacetylate histones on the E-cadherin promoter for gene silencing [23]. In a similar manner, SLUG recruits the HDAC1-containing CtBP complex to silence genes by binding to the E-box on the BRCA2 promoter [24]. ZEB1/2 also recruits the CtBP/HDAC1 complex to the E-cadherin promoter, while ZEB1 recruits SIRT1, a class III HDAC, to silence E-cadherin and promote EMT and metastasis in prostate cancer cells [25, 26]. Moreover, ZEB1-induced EMT is accomplished by repression of other epithelial genes, including EPCAM, ESRP1 and RAB25, and is accomplished by a reduced acetylation of H3K9 and H3K27 at their promoters. In fact, evidence suggests that H3K27 deacetylation is a key epigenetic event in ZEB1-induced transcriptional reprogramming [27]. In addition to the EMT transcriptional factors, HDAC1 co-purifies with TCF12 and promotes migration and invasion; elevated expression of TCF12 and HDAC1 correlate with a poor prognosis in gallbladder cancer. These findings suggest that this HLH transcription factor TCF12 could also target HDACs for epithelial gene silencing during EMT [28]. The expression of the HDAC1 and HDAC3 correlates with nuclear receptor (NR) (i.e., ER and PR) status. HDAC assembles a complex with ERα that binds to the SLUG promoter to repress expression [29]. Interestingly, HDAC6 and SIRT1 counteract the p300-catalyzed acetylation on Cortactin, which enhances its F-actin binding ability to facilitate EMT and tumor progression [30]. Conversely, HDAC6 and ERα are co-localized in the cytoplasm of renal cell carcinoma (RCC) cells and HDAC6 enhances cell motility by decreasing acetylated α-tubulin expression [21]. Loss of α-Tubulin acetylation by HDAC6 is also associated with TGF-β-induced EMT [31].

Recently, the clinical relevance of HDACs and the therapeutic potential of HDAC inhibitors (HDACi) have been reported. HDACi can generally be classified into hydroximates, cyclic peptides, aliphatic acids, and benzamides [32], and grouped according to their specificity. Thus far three HDACi: vorinostat (SAHA), romidepsin (Istodax) and PTCL (Belinostat or Beleodaq) are approved by the FDA for some T-cell lymphomas [33]. However, these molecules have not produced favorable and expected outcomes in solid tumors. Currently, a number of small molecules HDACi were investigated in clinical trials with variety of solid neoplasms, including breast cancer, either alone or in combination with hormonal treatments. Entinostat (MS-275), a benzamide with high specificity for the class I HDACs, is currently in a phase II/III trial for advanced ER^+ breast cancer [34, 35]. Vorinostat exerts EMT reversal effects by restoring the expression of E-cadherin. An expanded screen on 41 HDACi further identified 28 HDACi compounds, such as the class I-specific inhibitors Mocetinosat, Entinostat and CI994, that restore E-cadherin and ErbB3 expressions in ovarian, pancreatic and bladder carcinoma cells [36]. Mocetinostat, but not other HDACi, specifically interferes with ZEB1 function, restores miR-203 expression, represses stemness properties, and induces sensitivity against chemotherapy by restoring histone acetylation on the E-cadherin promoter [37]. Given that persistent genes activation may require targeting of multiple epigenetic silencing machineries, a combination of HDACi with anticancer drugs and/or radiotherapy demonstrate synergistic or additive effects in clinical trials. For example, HDACi have been utilized in combination with 5 Aza-dC as a synergistic strategy [38]. However, recent reports also found that HDACi could promote EMT in prostate and nasopharyngeal cancer cells [39, 40], indicating the application of HDACi in anti-cancer therapy is cancer-context dependent and may limit application.

4. Histone methylation

Histone methylation occurs at specific lysine or arginine residues on the histone tails. This modification is associated with either transcriptional activation or repression. Histone methylation does not change the electrostatic charge of histones or affect the chromatin structure. The functional effects of histone methylation are affected by both the position of the modified residues and number of methyl groups. Histone methyltransferases (HMTs) transfer methyl groups from S-adenosylmethionine (SAM) to either lysine or arginine residues, whereas histone demethylases (HDMs) remove methyl groups. The HMTs and HDMs specifically catalyze particular lysine or arginine residues.

4.1. Lysine methylation

Methylation of lysine residues on histones was first identified in the 1960s. Histone lysines can have four states of methylation at different lysine sites. Histones H2B lysine 5 (H2BK5), H3K4, H3K9, H4K20, H3K27, H3K36, and H3K79 are subject to unmethylated, mono-methylation (me1), di-methylation (me2), or tri-methylation (me3) on the ε-amino groups of lysine residues. These lysine methylations change the chromatin structure and regulate gene transcription. Histone lysine methylation is a reversible modification and is maintained by the balance lysine methyltransferases (KMTs) and lysine demethylases (KDMs). The KMTs recruit SAM as a cofactor and catalyze the addition of methyl groups to lysine residues through the SET domain. The KMTs are grouped into the SET domain-containing enzyme families (KMT1–3 and KMT5–7), the KMT4/DOT1 family, and others. The KDMs include the flavin adenine dinucleotide- (FAD-) dependent monoamine oxidase family (KDM1/LSD), the Jumonji C domain-containing demethylase (JMJD) families (KDM2–6), and others. Methylation of H3K4, H3K36, and H3K79 usually correlate with gene activation, whereas methylation of H3K9, H3K20, H3K27, and H3K56 are associated with transcriptional silencing.

4.1.1. Transcriptional activation and lysine methylation

H3K4: H3K4 methylation (H3K4me) is present in euchromatic regions and is usually associated with transcriptional activation. H3K4me3 occurs principally at the 5′ end of actively transcribed genes, near the transcription start site (TSS). H3K4me2 is located throughout genes, but frequently found towards the middle of the coding region of transcribed genes, and H3K4me1 is more abundant at the 3′ ends [41]. H3K4me2 marks can be present at both active and inactive euchromatic genes, whereas H3K4me3 is present exclusively at active genes. H3K4me favors transcriptional activation by facilitating H3 acetylation and the recruitment of RNA polymerase II, but it also antagonizes gene repression by preventing the binding of nucleosome remodeling and deacetylase co-repressor complexes, such as NuRD, and interfering with substrate recognition by the variegation 3–9 (SUV39H) methyltransferases [42]. The balance between KMTs and KDMs is an important dynamics for H3K4me and the regulation of gene transcription. More than ten H3K4 KMTs have been identified, including the mixed-lineage leukemia (MLL)1–4 proteins, along with Set 1a and Set 1b, Ash1L, Set7/9, and also the

SET and MYND domain-containing enzymes (SMYD) family members (SMYD1 and SMYD3). SMYD are involved in many cellular processes, including tumorigenesis and invasiveness. For example, SMYD3 is a novel histone H3K4-specific N-lysine di- and tri-methyltransferase, and highly characteristic active transcription. SMYD3 exerts its effects on initiation, invasion and metastasis of diverse tumors (e.g., esophageal squamous cell carcinoma (ESCC), gastric cancer, HCC, cholangiocarcinoma, breast cancer, prostate cancer, and leukemia). SMYD3 stimulates EZR and LOXL2 transcription to enhance proliferation, migration and invasion by directly binding to sequences of the promoter regions of these target genes [43]. SMYD3 is also capable of increasing cell migration through MMP-9 expression [44]. The MLL proteins (Trithorax homologs in Drosophila) are important for the regulation of developmental genes such as the Hox cluster, and deficiency of MLL1 or MLL2 causes embryonic lethality [45]. MLL1 coordinates with HIF1α and regulates hypoxia-induced HOTAIR expression to facilitate tumorigenesis [46]. In addition, MLL1 interacts with β-catenin to promote cervical carcinoma cell tumorigenesis and metastasis [47]. KMT2B/MLL2 is highly expressed in ESCC and promotes tumor progression by inducing EMT [48]. Another member of MLL family, MLL3 is reportedly mutated in multiple cancers. MLL3 regulates many migration-related genes and downregulation of MLL3 has a profound impact on the progression of ESCC [49]. Furthermore, Kim et al. [50] showed that KMT2D/MLL4 expression is associated with poor survival in breast cancer and regulates tumor proliferation and invasiveness.

Histone lysine methylation is a reversible process. H3K4 is demethylated by the KDM1 family (LSD1 and LSD2), the KDM2 family (FBXL10 and FBXL11), and the KDM5 family (JARID1A, JARID1B, JARID1C, and JARID1D) as well as JARID2 and NO66. The LSD subgroup of KDMs specifically targets the mono- and dimethylated lysines. This group demethylates substrates through a flavin adenine dinucleotide-dependent oxidative reaction, producing lysine and formaldehyde. KDM1A/LSD1 was the first H3K4 lysine-specific demethylase to be identified. We and others demonstrated that SNAIL recruits LSD1 to epithelial gene promoters with demethylation of H3K4me2 and subsequent silencing of target genes to enhance tumor metastasis [51]. SLUG also interacts with LSD1 to facilitate tumor metastasis [52]. In addition, both SNAIL and SLUG recruit LSD1 and bind to a series of E-boxes located within the BRCA1 promoter to repress BRCA1 expression. LSD1 overexpression promoted metastasis whereas knockdown of LSD1 inhibited tumor spread, suggesting that LSD1 is a key regulator of ESCC metastasis [53]. LSD1 and LSD2 act differently in the regulation of gene transcription and chromatin remodeling. However, both of KDM1A and KDM1B are overexpressed in invasive breast carcinoma, and depletion results in high levels of H3K4me1–2. The KDM5/JARID1 family is frequently found in the promoter region of transcriptionally active genes, and results in repressed expression of the target genes. KDM5A is highly expressed in ovarian cancer tissues and facilitates EMT and metastasis [54]. KDM5A promotes an increase in TNC expression, which augments breast cancer cell invasion and metastasis [55]. Reports indicate that, in gastric cancer cell, KDM5A is induced by TGF-β1 and recruited by p-SMAD3 to silence the *E-cadherin* promoter and promote tumor progression [56]. KDM5B plays a role in cell differentiation, stem cell self-renewal and other developmental progresses. Recent studies showed that KDM5B expression was increased in breast, bladder, lung, prostate and many other tumors and promote tumor initiation, invasion and metastasis. Mechanistically, KDM5B exerts its function through modulation of H3K4me3 at the PTEN gene promoter [57].

KDM5C/JARID1C is overexpressed in breast cancer, and its expression is significantly associated with metastasis. This demethylase modulates the status of H3K4 methylation in the breast cancer metastasis suppressor-1 (BRMS1) promoter, and thereby controls the expression of BRMS1 to inhibit tumor progression. Accordingly, the expression of KDM5C and BRMS1 are inversely correlated in human breast cancer [58].

H3K36: Because the level of H3K36me3 is high at the promoter site in active genes, H3K36me3 is involved in active transcription. In contrast, the H3K36me1 signal has a low association with active promoters. H3K36 is methylated by the KMT3 family (SETD2 and NSD1) as well as by NSD2, NSD3, SMYD1, SMYD2, SMYD3, SMYD4, and SMYD5. SETD2 plays a tumor suppressor role in tumor metastasis. Interestingly, SETD2 is frequently either deleted or mutated [59]. In contrast, H3K36 is demethylated by the KDM2 family (FBXL10 and FBXL11), the KDM4/JMJD family (JMJD2A, JMJD2B, and JMJD2C), and NO66. KDM2A expression is increased in breast cancer and associated with poor clinical outcomes [60]. KDM2A promotes lung tumorigenesis by epigenetically enhancing ERK1/2 signaling through demethylation of H3K36 [61]. In addition, KDM8/JMJD5 also demethylates H3K36me2, and overexpression of JMJD5 promotes cell invasion and is significantly correlated with clinical stage, histological grade and lymph node metastasis [62].

H3K79: H3K79me3 is associated with active transcription in yeast, whereas it is localized at both active and silent promoters in humans. H3K79me1 and H3K79me2 do not have any association with either active or silent promoters. H3K79 is methylated by the KMT4 family (DOT1L) and demethylated by PHF8 [63]. Methylation of H3K79 has been implicated in cell cycle regulation and the DNA damage response [63]. Disruption of this methylation can lead to cancers, making DOT1L a potential therapeutic target for cancers such as leukemia [64]. More recently, DOT1L has been implicated in the stimulation of proliferation, self-renewal, and metastatic potential of breast cancer cells [65]. DOTL1 cooperates with c-Myc-p300 complex to epigenetically activate EMT regulators in breast cancer progression. Clinically, DOTL1 expression is associated with poorer survival and aggressiveness of breast cancer [12]. PHF8 is highly expressed in metastatic prostate tissues and plays an important role in controlling invasion and metastasis [66]. PHF8 also interacts with β-catenin, and binds to the promoter region of vimentin, leading to the promotion of gastric cancer progression and metastasis [67].

4.1.2. Transcriptional repression and lysine methylation

H3K9: The methylation of H3K9 (H3K9me) was the first mechanism of gene repression to be linked to KMT. Studies in *Drosophila* showed that the gene *Su(var)39*, later shown to encode a H3K9 HMT, had an important role in the regulation of position-effect variegation [68] and similar enzymes were subsequently discovered in humans (SUV39H1/H2, G9a and Riz1 among others) [69]. H3K9 methylation is important for chromatin condensation and heterochromatin formation. H3K9me is recognized and bound by heterochromatin protein 1 (HP1), which recruits SUV39H, to reinforce the silencing process. H3K9 methylation plays a critical role in the formation of transcriptionally silent heterochromatin and the stable inheritance of the heterochromatin state. H3K9me1 and H3K9me2 are associated with euchromatic gene repression, whereas H3K9me3 is associated with stably silenced heterochromatin. H3K9me2 marks contribute to the maintenance of gene repression in differentiated tissues in large genomic regions known as 'large organized chromatin K9–modifications (LOCKs)', and require the activity of the methyltransferase G9a [70]. H3K9me is methylated by the KMT1 family (SUV39H1, SUV39H2, G9a, GLP, SETDB1, and SETDB2). H3K9 is demethylated by the KDM1 family (LSD1), the KDM3 family (JMJD1A, JMJD1B and JMJD1C), and the KDM4 family (JMJD2A, JMJD2B, JMJD2C, and JMJD2D) as well as PHF8 and KDM7A/JHDM1D. SUV39H1 generates H3K9me3, and is involved in breast carcinogenesis. In addition, we found that SUV39H1 cooperates with SNAIL to repress the expression of E-cadherin. Knockdown of SUV39H1 blocked the formation of H3K9me3 and DNA methylation and inhibited cell migration, invasion and metastasis of BLBC [71]. Furthermore, we demonstrated that knocking down G9a resulted in suppression of H3K9 methylation and inhibition of tumor cell migration or invasion [72]. Mechanically, we found that G9a interacted with SNAIL and is critical for SNAIL-mediated E-cadherin repression in human breast cancer. Consistent with our research, Huang et al. [73] demonstrated that knocking down G9a or pharmacological inhibition of its activity suppressed tumor cell growth, colony formation, invasion and migration in non-small-cell lung cancer cells (NSCLC). G9a is also associated with an increased expression in lung cancer [74]. SETDB1 is the most significantly up-regulated epigenetic regulator in human HCCs and prostate cancer [75, 76]. Knockdown of SETDB1 decreases cell migration and invasion and reduces EMT and CSC properties [77]. SETDB1 indirectly up-regulates STAT3 expression and induces TWIST. KDM3A catalyzes the demethylation of H3K9 associated with transcriptional repression, resulting in the derepression and activation of genes involved with invasion and metastasis [78]. Global gene expression profiling demonstrated KDM3A regulates genes and pathways that augment cell migration and metastasis. KDM3A promotes both migration *in vitro* and metastasis *in vivo* by targeting melanoma cell adhesion molecule (MCAM) [79]. Surprisingly, increased expression of KDM3B correlates with improved clinical outcomes [80]. Accordingly, JMJD1B and JMJD2B are associated with PRL-3, a gene crucial to metastasis in colorectal cancer (CRC). However, JMJD1B seems to be a candidate tumor suppressor while JMJD2B seems to be a potential oncoprotein for CRC metastasis and progression [81]. With respect to the breast cancer, KDM4A is a regulator of cancer cell growth and metastasis, which correlates with breast cancer progression, and is associated with the attenuation of the tumor suppressor ARHI [82]. KDM4B is physically associated with β-catenin and binds to the promoter of the β-catenin target gene *vimentin* to increase its transcription by inducing H3K9 demethylation [83]. Inhibition of JMJD2B attenuates migration and invasion of gastric cancer cells *in vitro* and metastasis *in vivo*. KDM4C expression correlates significantly with genes driving metabolic alterations in breast cancer; the mechanism involves an interaction between KDM4C and HIF1α, which is recruited to a subset of genes involved in metabolic remodeling and metastasis [84].

H4K20: H4K20 methylation is also associated with repressed chromatin. A recent genome-wide analysis demonstrated that H4K20me3 was associated with heterochromatin and played a pivotal role in chromatin integrity. In addition, loss of histone H4K20me3 predicts poor prognosis in breast cancer and is associated with invasive activity. On the other hand, H4K20me1 is located in the promoters or coding regions of active genes and co-localizes with H3K9me1, which suggest that H4K20me1 is associated with transcriptional activity. H4K20 is methylated by the KMT5 family (PR-Set7, SUV4-20H1, and SUV4-20H2) and the KMT7 family (SET7/9). KDMs that catalyze H4K20 demethylation have not been reported. Moreover, ectopic expression of SUV420H1 and SUV420H2 in breast cancer cells suppressed cell invasiveness, whereas knockdown of SUV420H2 activated invasion by normal mammary epithelial-cell *in vitro* [85]. Through its repressive H4K20me3 mark, SUV420H2 silences several key drivers of the epithelial state. Knockdown of SUV420H2 elicited MET on a molecular and functional level. An analysis of human pancreatic cancer biopsies suggests that high levels of SUV420H2 correlate with a loss of epithelial characteristics and progressively invasive cancer [86]. SET8 (also known as PR-Set7/9, SETD8, KMT5A), a member of the SET domain-containing methyltransferase family that specifically target H4K20 for monomethylation, physically interacts with TWIST to promote EMT and invasion by breast cancer cells [87]. Interestingly, SET8 acts as a dual epigenetic modifier on the promoters of E-cadherin and N-cadherin through its H4K20 monomethylation activity [88]. These bipolar roles of SET8 in EMT were also found in prostate cancer, which were mediated by ZEB1 [89]. A recent report indicates that the activation of the Shh pathway is required for EMT in NSCLCs [90]. SET7-mediated Gli3 methylations contribute to the tumor growth and metastasis in NSCLCs *in vitro* and *in vivo* [91].

H3K27: Another important repressive mark is H3K27 methylation which plays an essential role in embryogenesis, cell differentiation and organogenesis. H3K27me3 is associated with constitutive heterochromatin and maintenance of gene repression during early development. According to a genome-wide analysis, the levels of H3K27me2 and H3K27me3 are elevated in silent promoters and reduced in both active promoters and genic regions, whereas the level of H3K27me1 is high in promoters engaged in active transcription, especially downstream of the TSS [92, 93]. In embryonic stem cells (ESCs), H3K27 methylation usually overrides the effect of H3K4me3 in bivalent regions, maintaining them in a repressed state. Upon differentiation, these regions become exclusively marked by either of these modifications, leading to gene activation or repression [92]. H3K27 methylation is catalyzed by the polycomb repressive complex 2 (PRC2), which is composed mainly of suppressor of zeste 12 (SUZ12), embryonic ectoderm development (EED) and EZH2. H3K27 is demethylated by the KDM6 family (KDM6A/UTX and KDM6B/JMJD3), as well as UTY and JHDM1D [94, 95]. EZH2 is overexpressed in prostate and breast cancers and correlates with poor prognosis. Interestingly, EZH2 is essential for CSC self-renewal, and these CSCs provide the seeds for metastatic dispersal and differentiate into tumor-associated endothelial cells. Pre-clinical studies showed that EZH2 can silence several anti-metastatic genes (e.g., E-cadherin and tissue inhibitors of metalloproteinases), thereby favoring cell invasion and anchorage-independent growth. Accordingly, Tiwari and colleagues delineated an elegant pathway wherein TGF-β induces EZH2 expression to elicit EMT programs and metastasis of breast cancers by reprogramming the epigenome [96]. EZH2 represses TIMP2 transcription, which leads to increased activity of MMP-2 and MMP-9 and the invasive capacity of BLBC cells [97]. In pancreatic cancer cells, SNAIL recruits PRC to the E-cadherin promoter by binding to SUZ12 [98]. Increased KDM6A expression is associated with poor prognosis, along with derepression/activation of genetic programs that induce cell proliferation, luminal to basal-like transition, and metastasis. Furthermore, the function of KDM6A correlates with the activity of the MLL4, and increased expression of these epigenetic enzymes correlates with poor survival outcomes in breast cancer [50]. UTX interacts with the

MLL4 complex to activate several pro-metastatic genes including MMP9 and SIX1, leading to increased EMT and metastasis of breast cancer [50]. In colon cancer, KDM6A not only demethylates H3K27me3 at the E-cadherin promoter but also recruits CBP to the E-cadherin promoter, resulting in increased H3K27ac [99]. However, it was also reported that KDM6A inhibited EMT by epigenetic repression of EMT genes in cooperation with LSD1 and HDAC1 [100]. Therefore, the role of KDM6A an EMT suppressor or enhancer requires further investigation. KDM6B expression is also increased in invasive breast carcinomas and enforcing KDM6B overexpression induces EMT, invasive migration, stem cell-like traits, and metastatic properties. The mechanism involves demethylation associated with increased SNAIL or SLUG expression mediating the EMT [101]. Interestingly, KDM6B also modulates the tumor microenvironment and promotes melanoma progression and metastasis through upregulation several targets of NF-κB and BMP signaling, including stanniocalcin 1 (STC1) and chemokine (C-C motif) ligand 2 (CCL2) [102].

In summary, histone lysine methylation modulates chromatin accessibility, transcriptional status, and control of tumor suppressor and oncogene expression in aberrant cell metastasis. Dynamic regulation of the either permissive or repressive histone methylation at different genomic loci and through different molecular mechanisms facilitates the dynamic EMT process.

4.2. Arginine methylation

Histone arginine methylation also occurs in many arginine sites, histone H3 arginine 2 (H3R2), H3R8, H3R17, H3R26, and H4R3 undergo monomethylation (me1), symmetrical dimethylation (me2s), or asymmetrical dimethylation (me2a) on the guanidinyl groups of arginine residues. The N-arginine methyltransferases (PRMTs) are a class of enzymes that transfer a methyl group from SAM to the guanidino nitrogen of arginine. PRMTs generate three arginine methylation forms: monomethylarginine (MMA), asymmetric dimethylarginine (aDMA), and symmetric dimethylarginine (sDMA). Human PRMTs are composed of nine members that are categorized into three groups based on the type of arginine methylation reaction each member catalyzes. Type I is comprised of PRMT1, PRMT2, PRMT3, CARM1/PRMT4, PRMT6, and PRMT8; these catalyze both mono-methyl and asymmetric dimethyl arginine reactions. The type II group is made up of two members, PRMT5 and PRMT9, which catalyze both mono-methyl arginine and symmetric dimethyl arginine. Finally, PRMT7 is, at this point, considered the only bona fide type III methyltransferase and can generate only mono-methyl arginines. Many studies demonstrated that PRMTs regulate a wide range of genetic programs and cellular processes including cell cycle, RNA splicing and differentiation. Although the consequence of lysine methylation is relatively well studied, the role of PRMT action in tumorgenesis is poorly understood. Here, we provide a description of these PRMTs regarding tumor metastasis.

PRMT1: PRMT1 has been extensively studied in many fields. Its activity is responsible for a substantial percentage of methylated arginine residues and modulates a wide range of cell types. Specifically, asymmetric dimethylation on H4R3 by PRMT1 is involved in transcriptional activation, thereby driving oncogenic pathways. PRMT1 is an important regulator of EMT, cancer cell migration, and invasion. PRMT1 can generate H4R3me2a on the promoter region of ZEB1 and TWIST, which play a critical role in EMT [103, 104]. Furthermore, PRMT1 is overexpressed in melanoma; silencing PRMT1 significantly suppresses tumor growth and metastatic ability by targeting activated leukocyte cell adhesion molecule (ALCAM) [105]. Similarly, downregulation of PRMT1 inhibits cell migration and invasion in HCC and oral squamous cell carcinoma (OSCC) [106, 107]. Because of complex alternative splicing in the 5′ region of its pre-mRNA, there are seven distinct PRMT1 isoforms [108]. Each of these isoforms, named PRMT1v1-v7, has distinct characteristics in terms of expression. PRMT1v1 is the most abundantly expressed isoform and likely represents the isoform that is described as PRMT1 in most reports. The expression of alternatively spliced PRMT1 (PRMT1v2) isoform, which is generated through inclusion of alternative exon 2, is significantly altered in breast cancer and promotes invasiveness. The RNA binding protein RALY regulates the PRMT1v2 isoform and promotes metastatic potential [109].

PRMT2: PRMT2 is also reported to be overexpressed in breast cancer [110]. PRMT2 interacts with many NRs, including ERα and ERβ *in vitro* [111]. Interestingly, the activation of these receptors within cells has both distinct and in some cases opposing effects, which suggests that the functional role(s) PRMT2 are quite diverse. Recently, four alternatively spliced PRMT2 isoforms (PRMT2L2, PRMT2α, β, and γ) in addition to the original PRMT2 isoform were identified [112]. Several splice variants (*i.e.*, PRMT2-α, $-\beta$, $-\gamma$) were identified as induced in breast cancer, particularly in ER, PR-positive breast cancer [110]. PRMT2 directly binds and enhances estrogen-mediated transactivation of ERα, and enhances the promoter activity of the downstream target gene SNAIL. These findings suggest that the increased PRMT2 expression is associated with breast aggressiveness and metastasis [110].

PRMT4: PRMT4, more commonly known as coactivator-associated arginine methyltransferase 1 (CARM1), is involved in the regulation of a number of cellular processes including transcription, pre-mRNA splicing and cell cycle progression. The expression of CARM1 is dysregulated in colorectal, prostate and breast cancer. CARM1 methylates the chromatin-remodeling SWI/SNF core subunit, BAF155 in breast cancer [113]. The methylation of arginine 1064 residue of BAF155 is associated with breast cancer recurrence and metastasis, indicating that CARM1 plays an important role in tumorigenic activity through BAF155. Accordingly, CARM1-induced tumorigenic effects and its expression is increased in invasive breast cancer, and correlates with a high tumor grade [114]. Interestingly, the *CARM1* gene also transcribes four isoforms: the primary isoform CARM1 (CARM1v1) and three alternative isoforms, v2, v3 and v4 [115]. Whether these isoform are responsible for the methylation of distinct substrates and their individual functions requires further study.

PRMT5: PRMT5 is a type II enzyme that generates symmetric dimethylarginine (sDMA). The PRMT5 symmetrically methylates H3R8 site and functions in gene silencing. H3R8me2s strongly associates with H4R3me2s, because both modifications are catalyzed by PRMT5. However, acetylation of H3K9 and H3K14 prevents H3R8 methylation. PRMT5 also acts as a novel cofactor of SHARPIN (Shank-associated RH domain interacting protein), which plays a central role in controlling lung cancer cell metastasis. SHARPIN-PRMT5 is essential for the monomethylation of histones at key metastasis-related genes [116]. PRMT5 has another distinct function; PRMT5 coordinates with multiple Mediator complex subunits to dimethylate H4R3 at the promoter regions of immune response genes and C/EBPβ target genes [117]. Conversely, PRMT5 methylation of histone H3R2 recruits WDR5 and the MLL complex, stimulating H3K4 methylation and euchromatin maintenance [118]. In the context of cancer metastasis, PRMT5 is involved in TGF-β-WDR77 signaling, which induces cancer cell invasion [119]; this report indicates PRMT5 interacts with the WDR77 complex to catalyze arginine methylation. With respect to the acquisition of EMT via TGF-β signaling, epigenetic PRMT5-WDR77 activity is necessary for tumor invasion and metastasis. Furthermore, PRMT5 appears to be recruited by AJUBA to SNAIL and functions as a co-repressor. PRMT5, AJUBA and SNAIL form ternary complex to repress E-cadherin, concomitant with increase arginine methylation at the locus [120]. PRMT5 also modulates metastasis by methylating KLF4. Methylation blocks ubiquitylation of KLF4 by the von Hippel–Lindau tumor suppressor, and as a result, arginine methylation of KLF4 via PRMT5 increases the level of KLF4 protein and increases the probability of breast carcinogenesis [121].

PRMT6: PRMT6 primarily catalyzes asymmetric dimethylation of H3R2. H3R2me2a counter-correlates with the methylation of H3K4, which suggests that H3R2me2a is a repressive marker. However, PRMT6 also methylates H3K4 since both H3R2me2a and H3K4me3 markers are likely to coexist. Furthermore, genome-wide analyses indicate that both H3R2me1 and H3R2me2a are associated with active genes [93]. Thus, the data on the H3R2me2a marker are contradictory, and further studies are required to resolve this issue. There is also emerging evidence of an oncogenic role of PRMT6 in cancer. Overexpression of PRMT6 is associated with several cancer types, including breast, cervix, prostate, and lung cancers, indicating that PRMT6 might play an important role for the onset, incidence, and metastasis of cancer [122]. Furthermore, Dowhan et al. [123] demonstrated a PRMT6-dependent signature that influences long-term survival in patients with breast cancer.

PRMT7: The oncogenic role of PRMT7 has been emerging over the past few years. There are two isoforms, PRMT7α and β, which are active and have slightly different methylation profiles and locations. PRMT7α localizes to the cytoplasm and nucleus, whereas PRMT7β is exclusively cytoplasmic. R531 of PRMT7 is self-methylated and loss of PRMT7 automethylation leads to a reduced recruitment to the E-cadherin promoter by YY1, which consequently derepresses E-cadherin expression by decreasing the H4R3me2's level [124]. In terms of the functional role of PRMT7, this methytransferase is highly expressed in breast cancer and induces EMT by inhibiting E-cadherin. Baldwin et al. [125] also showed that PRMT7 promotes a well-known metastasis mediator, MMP9 and induces breast cancer cell invasion. Importantly, a gene expression analysis of independent data sets of more than 1200 breast tumors identified PRMT7 expression as significantly increased. In addition, this gene is located 16q22, where the chromosomal region was correlated with an increased metastatic potential of breast cancer [126].

PRMT9: PRMT9 and PRMT5 are the only known mammalian enzymes capable of forming sDMA residues as type II PRMTs. However, the specificity of these enzymes for their substrates is distinct and not redundant. Interestingly Yang et al. [127] showed that PRMT9 is also nonhistone methyltransferase. For example, it methylates the arginine 508 site of the alternative splicing factor SAP145. Given that alternative splicing is of paramount importance in RNA processing, PRMT9 might play a key role in many cellular programs including cancer biology. Recent reports demonstrate that overexpression of PRMT9 strongly promotes HCC invasion and metastasis through EMT by regulating SNAIL expression via activation of the PI3K/Akt/GSK-3β/SNAIL signaling pathway [128].

Many HMTs and HDMs inhibitors have been developed and evaluated in clinical trials, such as chaetocin, BIX-01294, BIX-01338, UNC0638 and DZNep. Chaetocin, a natural fungal substance, is the first inhibitor of an HMT, which targets SUV39H1 without high selectively [129]. Treatment with Chaetocin induces expression of E-cadherin while reducing H3K9me3 but does not produce a global H3K9 methylation on its promoter in multiple tumor cells [130]. By the contrast, BIX-01294 specifically reduces the dimethylation of H3K9me2 through an inhibition of the enzymatic activities of G9a and GLP [131]. Treatment of BIX-01294 activates E-cadherin expression and reverse EMT phenotypes in a variety of cancer cells, and is accompanied by reduced H3K9me2 and increased H3K9 acetylation on the E-cadherin promoter [132]. Another G9a/GLP inhibitor, UNC0638, was developed with higher potency and selectively [133]. UNC0638 treatment not only resulted in lower global H3K9me2 levels but also markedly reduced the abundance of H3K9me2 marks at promoters of known G9a-regulated endogenous genes. UNC0638 treatment activates E-cadherin expression and reverses EMT in PANC-1 pancreatic cancer cells and triple negative breast cancer (TNBC) and suppresses migration and invasion [134]. Because of the importance of H3K27 methylation in cancer, several highly specific EZH2 inhibitors have been developed, such as GSK2816126 and EPZ-6438, which are currently being evaluated in clinical trials for lymphoma and solid tumor/lymphoma respectively [135]. Another EZH2 inhibitor, 3-deazaneplanocin A (DZNep), selectively inhibits H3K27me3 and H4K20me3 [136]. DZNep dampens TGF-β-induced EMT signals and reduces tumor metastasis in pancreatic cancer and colon cancer [136, 137]. We found that Parnate, an LSD1 inhibitor, activates E-cadherin expression and suppresses motility and invasiveness in breast cancer cells [51]. Two highly specific LSD1 inhibitors, GSK2879552 and ORY-1001 are employed to clinical trials for the treatment of small cell lung cancer and acute leukemia [135]. Several inhibitors targeting HDMs also have been developed as well. For example, JIB-04, a specific inhibitor targeting the JMJC-domain, inhibits the activity of H3K4 and H4K9 and attenuates lung cancer cell proliferation [138]. The first reported small molecule PRMT inhibitors, including AMI-1 and AMI-5 were identified through virtual screening and high throughput screening [139]. AMI-1 was reported as type I PRMT and PRMT5 inhibitor [140]. AMI-1 inhibits proliferation and decreases cell migratory activity of CRC cells *in vitro* and in xenograft mouse models [141].

5. Histone modification readers

Sometimes, histone modifications can directly regulate the chromatin dynamic. However, in most cases, the modifications are recognized by proteins containing distinct recognition domains, which act as "readers" and bind to different histone modifications. For example, bromodomain acts as lysine acetylation "readers" of modified histones that mediate signaling transduction changes in gene regulatory networks. In the human genome, there are 61 bromodomains found within 46 proteins that can be divided into eight families based on structure/sequence similarity. Among them, bromodomain and the extra-terminal domain (BET) family recognize acetylated lysine residues in histones H3 and H4. BRD4 is a member of the BET family that carries two bromodomains. Recently, our studies revealed that the di-acetylated TWIST, mediated by Tip60, recruits BRD4 and related transcriptional components to the super-enhancer of its targeted genes during tumor progression in BLBC [20]. In addition, pharmacologic inhibition of BRD4 with the BET-specific bromodomain inhibitors, JQ1 and MS417, effectively reduces WNT5A expression and suppresses invasion, CSC-like properties and tumorigenicity of breast cancer cells *in vitro* and *in vivo* [20]. Given the extensive cancer-related functions of BRD4 and the proof-of-concept demonstrated by disruption of the BRD4–acetyl-lysine interactions as a therapeutic target, significant efforts have thus been made to develop BRD4 inhibitors from both pharmaceutical and academic settings. BRD4 inhibitors have several chemical classifications including azepines, 3,5-dimethylisoxazoles, pyridones, triazolopyrazines, tetrahydroquinolines (THQs), 4-acyl pyrroles and 2-thiazolidinones [142]. BET inhibitor treatment results in AMIGO2 silencing and changes in PTK7 proteolytic processing, and thus inhibit melanoma metastasis [143].

Histone methylation provides docking sites and is recognized by specific reader proteins that contain a methyllysine binding protein, which has emerged as a focus of epigenetic research due to its critical role in gene regulation and oncogenesis. This reader harbors specific motifs, including Chromodomain (CD), MBT, WD40 repeat, PHD finger, PWWP, Tudor and Ankyrin repeat. Methyllysine binding proteins distinguish methylation marks on different residues as well as different methylation states on the same residue and in turn mediate distinct downstream functions [144]. CD-containing HP1 proteins were the first identified methyl-lysine binding proteins and recognize methylated-H3K9 (methyl-H3K9) [145]. HP1α was down-regulated in metastatic cells of colon cancer and thyroid carcinomas relative to non-metastatic cells, indicating HP1α may be directly involved in the silencing of genes that potentiate cancer cell invasive potential and metastasis. Recent evidence implicate HP1α in EMT. The association of HP1α to major satellite repeat sequences located in pericentric heterochromatin decreased during the initial steps of TGF-β-induced EMT in a SNAIL/LOXL2-dependent manner [146]. In addition, HP1α post-translational modifications could participate in the heterochromatin dynamics associated with EMT. In a different set of modifications, four MBT-repeats domain of SFMBT1 recognize H3K4me2/3 and form a stable complex with LSD1. SFMBT1 is essential for SNAIL-dependent recruitment of LSD1 to chromatin, demethylation of H3K4me2, transcriptional repression of epithelial markers, and induction of EMT by TGF-β [147]. H3K4me2/3 is also recognized by the WD40 repeat domain of WDR5, which is also important for the assembly and activity of the SET1 protein complex catalyzing H3K4me3 [148]. Under hypoxic conditions, WDR5 is induced, interacts with HDAC3 and further recruits SET1 complex to activate mesenchymal gene expression to promote EMT [149]. Furthermore, the PRC2 component, EED, also contains a WD40 repeat that recognizes H3K27me3. EED recruits PRC2 to chromatin with pre-existing H3K27me3 to spread the same methylation into adjacent regions [150]. Intriguingly, G9a and GLP itself contain a methyl-lysine binding module (the ankyrin repeat domains), which generates and reads the same epigenetic mark [151]. Several small molecule compounds targeting the lysine methylation reader domain have been developed, including UNC1215 and UNC3866 that block the methyl-lysine binding mediated by the MBT domain-containing protein L3MBTL3, and the CD-containing protein CBX4/7 respectively [152, 153]. However, whether these inhibitors reverse EMT and tumor progression remains unknown.

6. Coordinated histone modification regulation

Because different chromatin modifying enzymes coexist in the same protein complex, and because diverse catalyzed modifications have been implicated in regulating the same set of genes, it is likely that these processes act in concert to orchestrate transcriptional regulation during EMT. For example, HDAC1/2, G9a/GLP, LSD1, HP1 and ZEB1/2 were co-purified in the CtBP1 co-repressor complex [154, 155]. ZEB1/2 could first target the complex to E-cadherin promoter to initiate repression. Next, HADC1/2 would deacetylate histones while the primed H3K9 was methylated by G9a/GLP. Meanwhile, LSD1, which removes H3K4me1/2, whereby the un-methylated H3K4 could also prevent H3K9 from re-acetylation [156, 157]. An affinity purification of Flag-TWIST identified several components of the NuRD chromatin remodeling complex. Among them, TWIST directly interacts with Mi2β, MTA2 and RbAp46 and likely targets the NuRD complex for histone deacetylation and chromatin remodeling on E-cadherin promoter. Together, these epigenetic events lead to gene silencing and promote EMT and breast cancer metastasis [158]. In addition, TWIST was also co-purified with SET8, BRCA1-associated protein (BRAP), NF-kB subunit RelA, PPP2CA and HES6 in MCF7 breast cancer cells [88]. SET8 interacts with TWIST. However, SET8 and TWIST are functionally interdependent in promoting EMT. SET8 mediates E-cadherin repression and N-cadherin activation simultaneously via its H4K20 monomethylation to promote cell invasion and EMT. However, the molecular mechanism that underlies the same repressive protein complex that contributes to opposite functions on different genomic loci remains an open question. Our recent study found that TWIST is diacetylated by Tip60, which was further recognized by BRD4, thereby constructing an activated TWIST/BRD4/P-TEFβ/RNA-Pol II complex at the WNT5A promoter and enhancer to promote EMT and breast cancer cell metastasis [20]. In breast cancer cells, the UTX-MLL4 forms a complex with LSD1/HDAC1/DNMT1 on the promoter of several EMT-TFs and decreases H3K4mes and H3 acetylation. UTX facilitates epigenetic silencing of EMT-TFs by inducing competition between MLL4 and the H3K4 demethylase LSD1, which results in inhibition of EMT and CSC-like properties [100].

MPP8, another methy-H3K9 binding protein, bridges DNMT3A and G9a/GLP to assemble a repressive trimeric protein complex on chromatin by binding to different methyl-lysines. MPP8 also couples H3K9 methylation and DNA methylation to silence epithelial genes and EMT [159, 160]. Interestingly, MPP8 also cooperates with the SIRT1 in this process through a physical interaction [161]. SIRT1 and MPP8 reciprocally promote each other's function and coordinate epithelial gene silencing and EMT. SIRT1 antagonizes PCAF-catalyzed MPP8-K439 acetylation to protect MPP8 from ubiquitin-proteasome-mediated proteolysis. Conversely, MPP8 recruits SIRT1 for H4K16 deacetylation after binding to methyl-H3K9 on target promoters. Therefore, MPP8 not only promote DNA-methylation but also H4K16 deacetylation to fine-tune the transcriptional regulation of EMT.

7. Conclusions and perspectives

Increasing evidences show that aberrant profiles of histone modifications contribute to a dysregulation those results in the metastatic cascade. The biochemically reversible nature of histone modifications provides a platform for rapid changes in a variety of epithelia and mesenchymal genes during EMT and MET. In concert with different ETM-TFs and oncogenic signaling, pleiotropic histone modifications form a sophisticated and regulated network to coordinate the plasticity and dynamic change required for EMT.

Recent research identifies the critical role of histone modifications in metastasis, but leaves many important, open questions. First, do tumor microenvironmental signals trigger the formation of histone modification enzyme complexes present on different EMT-TFs? Whether these extrinsic signals affect enzyme activity indirectly through intracellular signaling pathways or directly through the EMT-TFs remains to be determined. Second, how do these EMT-TFs form distinct complexes that coordinate the epigenetic regulation of gene expression programs during EMT? Third, EMT is usually activated only transiently and partially. Therefore, which and how do different histone modifying enzymes and the catalyzed modifications contribute to these dynamic changes? Finally, what consequences do epigenetic instabilities have on cancer cell fitness? Do these activities increase plasticity and/or lead to vulnerabilities that it could influence the metastasis?

We know that histone modification enzymes are highly correlated with tumor progression and a poor clinical outcome. Therefore, these enzymes can serve not only as effective biomarkers for earlier diagnosis, but also present multiple therapeutic opportunities. Over the last decade, considerable progress has been made in the discovery and development of potent and selective small molecule inhibitors targeting specific histone modifiers. Many of these molecules are currently under extensive preclinical testing or being evaluated in clinical trials. These inhibitors show great potential as clinically useful drugs. Additionally, inhibitors to specific histone modifying enzymes could serve as useful chemical probes to characterize the function of different epigenetic pathways in EMT *in vivo* as well as many other important pathological diseases.

In all, advances in our understanding of the landscape of histone modifications in metastasis will provide a better sense of the molecular mechanisms associated with metastasis and thus help speed the development of new therapeutic strategies and biomarkers for metastasis.

Acknowledgements

We thank Dr. Cathy Anthony for the critical editing of this manuscript. Our research was supported by the Shared Resources of the University of Kentucky Markey Cancer Center (P30CA177558). Our research was also supported by grants from American Cancer Society Research Scholar Award (RSG13187) and NIH (P20GM121327 and CA230758) (to Y Wu).

Conflict of interest

The authors have declared that no conflict of interests exists.

Author details

Zhaoping Qiu[1,2], Jianlin Wang[1,2] and Yadi Wu[1,2*]

*Address all correspondence to: yadi.wu@uky.edu

1 Department of Pharmacology and Nutritional Sciences, University of Kentucky School of Medicine, Lexington, KY, USA

2 Department of Markey Cancer Center, University of Kentucky School of Medicine, Lexington, KY, USA

References

[1] Van't Veer LJ, Weigelt B. Road map to metastasis. Nature Medicine. 2003;**9**:999-1000

[2] Chambers AF, Groom AC, MacDonald IC. Dissemination and growth of cancer cells in metastatic sites. Nature Reviews. Cancer. 2002;**2**:563-572. DOI: 10.1038/nrc865

[3] Pantel K, Brakenhoff RH. Dissecting the metastatic cascade. Nature Reviews. Cancer. 2004;**4**:448-456. DOI: 10.1038/nrc1370

[4] Thiery JP. Epithelial-mesenchymal transitions in tumor progression. Nature Reviews. Cancer. 2002;**2**:442-454

[5] Thiery JP, Acloque H, Huang RY, Nieto MA. Epithelial-mesenchymal transitions in development and disease. Cell. 2009;**139**:871-890. DOI: S0092-8674(09)01419-6 [pii] 10.1016/j.cell.2009.11.007

[6] Brabletz T, Kalluri R, Nieto MA, Weinberg RA. EMT in cancer. Nature Reviews. Cancer. 2018;**18**:128-134. DOI: 10.1038/nrc.2017.118

[7] Strahl BD, Allis CD. The language of covalent histone modifications. Nature. 2000;**403**: 41-45. DOI: 10.1038/47412

[8] Tessarz P, Kouzarides T. Histone core modifications regulating nucleosome structure and dynamics. Nature Reviews. Molecular Cell Biology. 2014;**15**:703-708. DOI: 10.1038/nrm3890

[9] Jenuwein T, Allis CD. Translating the histone code. Science. 2001;**293**:1074-1080. DOI: 10.1126/science.1063127

[10] Wang Z, Zang C, Rosenfeld JA, Schones DE, Barski A, Cuddapah S, et al. Combinatorial patterns of histone acetylations and methylations in the human genome. Nature Genetics. 2008;**40**:897-903. DOI: 10.1038/ng.154

[11] de Ruijter AJ, van Gennip AH, Caron HN, Kemp S, van Kuilenburg AB. Histone deacetylases (HDACs): Characterization of the classical HDAC family. The Biochemical Journal. 2003;**370**:737-749. DOI: 10.1042/BJ20021321

[12] Cho MH, Park JH, Choi HJ, Park MK, Won HY, Park YJ, et al. DOT1L cooperates with the c-Myc-p300 complex to epigenetically derepress CDH1 transcription factors in breast cancer progression. Nature Communications. 2015;**6**:7821. DOI: 10.1038/ncomms8821

[13] Dhasarathy A, Phadke D, Mav D, Shah RR, Wade PA. The transcription factors Snail and Slug activate the transforming growth factor-beta signaling pathway in breast cancer. PLoS One. 2011;**6**:e26514. DOI: 10.1371/journal.pone.0026514

[14] Liu YN, Lee WW, Wang CY, Chao TH, Chen Y, Chen JH. Regulatory mechanisms controlling human E-cadherin gene expression. Oncogene. 2005;**24**:8277-8290. DOI: 10.1038/sj.onc.1208991

[15] Tuo H, Zheng X, Tu K, Zhou Z, Yao Y, Liu Q. Expression of PCAF in hepatocellular carcinoma and its clinical significance. Xi Bao Yu Fen Zi Mian Yi Xue Za Zhi. 2013;**29**:297-300

[16] Li Q, Liu Z, Xu M, Xue Y, Yao B, Dou C, et al. PCAF inhibits hepatocellular carcinoma metastasis by inhibition of epithelial-mesenchymal transition by targeting Gli-1. Cancer Letters. 2016;**375**:190-198. DOI: 10.1016/j.canlet.2016.02.053

[17] Wan J, Zhan J, Li S, Ma J, Xu W, Liu C, et al. PCAF-primed EZH2 acetylation regulates its stability and promotes lung adenocarcinoma progression. Nucleic Acids Research. 2015;**43**:3591-3604. DOI: 10.1093/nar/gkv238

[18] Taipale M, Rea S, Richter K, Vilar A, Lichter P, Imhof A, et al. hMOF histone acetyltransferase is required for histone H4 lysine 16 acetylation in mammalian cells. Molecular and Cellular Biology. 2005;**25**:6798-6810. DOI: 10.1128/mcb.25.15.6798-6810.2005

[19] Luo H, Shenoy AK, Li X, Jin Y, Jin L, Cai Q, et al. MOF acetylates the histone demethylase LSD1 to suppress epithelial-to-mesenchymal transition. Cell Reports. 2016;**15**:2665-2678. DOI: 10.1016/j.celrep.2016.05.050

[20] Shi J, Wang Y, Zeng L, Wu Y, Deng J, Zhang Q, et al. Disrupting the interaction of BRD4 with diacetylated Twist suppresses tumorigenesis in basal-like breast cancer. Cancer Cell. 2014;**25**:210-225. DOI: 10.1016/j.ccr.2014.01.028

[21] Ramakrishnan S, Ku S, Ciamporcero E, Miles KM, Attwood K, Chintala S, et al. HDAC 1 and 6 modulate cell invasion and migration in clear cell renal cell carcinoma. BMC Cancer. 2016;**16**:617. DOI: 10.1186/s12885-016-2604-7

[22] von Burstin J, Eser S, Paul MC, Seidler B, Brandl M, Messer M, et al. E-cadherin regulates metastasis of pancreatic cancer in vivo and is suppressed by a SNAIL/HDAC1/HDAC2 repressor complex. Gastroenterology. 2009;**137**:361-71, 371.e1-5. DOI: 10.1053/j.gastro.2009.04.004

[23] Peinado H, Ballestar E, Esteller M, Cano A. Snail mediates E-cadherin repression by the recruitment of the Sin3A/histone deacetylase 1 (HDAC1)/HDAC2 complex. Molecular and Cellular Biology. 2004;**24**:306-319

[24] Tripathi MK, Misra S, Khedkar SV, Hamilton N, Irvin-Wilson C, Sharan C, et al. Regulation of BRCA2 gene expression by the SLUG repressor protein in human breast cells. The Journal of Biological Chemistry. 2005;**280**:17163-17171. DOI: 10.1074/jbc.M501375200

[25] Aghdassi A, Sendler M, Guenther A, Mayerle J, Behn CO, Heidecke CD, et al. Recruitment of histone deacetylases HDAC1 and HDAC2 by the transcriptional repressor ZEB1 downregulates E-cadherin expression in pancreatic cancer. Gut. 2012;**61**:439-448. DOI: 10.1136/gutjnl-2011-300,060

[26] Byles V, Zhu L, Lovaas JD, Chmilewski LK, Wang J, Faller DV, et al. SIRT1 induces EMT by cooperating with EMT transcription factors and enhances prostate cancer cell migration and metastasis. Oncogene. 2012;**31**:4619-4629. DOI: 10.1038/onc.2011.612

[27] Roche J, Nasarre P, Gemmill R, Baldys A, Pontis J, Korch C, et al. Global decrease of histone H3K27 acetylation in ZEB1-induced epithelial to mesenchymal transition in lung cancer cells. Cancers (Basel). 2013;**5**:334-356. DOI: 10.3390/cancers5020334

[28] He J, Shen S, Lu W, Zhou Y, Hou Y, Zhang Y, et al. HDAC1 promoted migration and invasion binding with TCF12 by promoting EMT progress in gallbladder cancer. Oncotarget. 2016;**7**:32754-32764. DOI: 10.18632/oncotarget.8740

[29] Ye Y, Xiao Y, Wang W, Yearsley K, Gao JX, Barsky SH. ERalpha suppresses slug expression directly by transcriptional repression. The Biochemical Journal. 2008;**416**:179-187. DOI: 10.1042/bj20080328

[30] Zhang X, Yuan Z, Zhang Y, Yong S, Salas-Burgos A, Koomen J, et al. HDAC6 modulates cell motility by altering the acetylation level of cortactin. Molecular Cell. 2007;**27**: 197-213. DOI: 10.1016/j.molcel.2007.05.033

[31] Gu S, Liu Y, Zhu B, Ding K, Yao TP, Chen F, et al. Loss of alpha-tubulin acetylation is associated with TGF-beta-induced epithelial-mesenchymal transition. The Journal of Biological Chemistry. 2016;**291**:5396-5405. DOI: 10.1074/jbc.M115.713123

[32] Dokmanovic M, Marks PA. Prospects: histone deacetylase inhibitors. Journal of Cellular Biochemistry. 2005;**96**:293-304. DOI: 10.1002/jcb.20532

[33] Eckschlager T, Plch J, Stiborova M, Hrabeta J. Histone deacetylase inhibitors as anticancer drugs. International Journal of Molecular Sciences. 2017;**18**. DOI: 10.3390/ijms18071414

[34] Trapani D, Esposito A, Criscitiello C, Mazzarella L, Locatelli M, Minchella I, et al. Entinostat for the treatment of breast cancer. Expert Opinion on Investigational Drugs. 2017;**26**:965-971. DOI: 10.1080/13543784.2017.1353077

[35] Damaskos C, Garmpis N, Valsami S, Kontos M, Spartalis E, Kalampokas T, et al. Histone deacetylase inhibitors: An attractive therapeutic strategy against breast cancer. Anticancer Research. 2017;**37**:35-46. DOI: 10.21873/anticanres.11286

[36] Tang HM, Kuay KT, Koh PF, Asad M, Tan TZ, Chung VY, et al. An epithelial marker promoter induction screen identifies histone deacetylase inhibitors to restore epithelial differentiation and abolishes anchorage independence growth in cancers. Cell Death Discovery. 2016;**2**:16041. DOI: 10.1038/cddiscovery.2016.41

[37] Meidhof S, Brabletz S, Lehmann W, Preca BT, Mock K, Ruh M, et al. ZEB1-associated drug resistance in cancer cells is reversed by the class I HDAC inhibitor mocetinostat. EMBO Molecular Medicine. 2015;**7**:831-847. DOI: 10.15252/emmm.201404396

[38] Kristensen LS, Nielsen HM, Hansen LL. Epigenetics and cancer treatment. European Journal of Pharmacology. 2009;**625**:131-142. DOI: 10.1016/j.ejphar.2009.10.011

[39] Jiang GM, Wang HS, Zhang F, Zhang KS, Liu ZC, Fang R, et al. Histone deacetylase inhibitor induction of epithelial-mesenchymal transitions via up-regulation of Snail facilitates cancer progression. Biochimica et Biophysica Acta. 2013;**1833**:663-671. DOI: 10.1016/j.bbamcr.2012.12.002

[40] Kong D, Ahmad A, Bao B, Li Y, Banerjee S, Sarkar FH. Histone deacetylase inhibitors induce epithelial-to-mesenchymal transition in prostate cancer cells. PLoS One. 2012;**7**:e45045. DOI: 10.1371/journal.pone.0045045

[41] Pokholok DK, Harbison CT, Levine S, Cole M, Hannett NM, Lee TI, et al. Genome-wide map of nucleosome acetylation and methylation in yeast. Cell. 2005;**122**:517-527. DOI: 10.1016/j.cell.2005.06.026

[42] Lachner M, Jenuwein T. The many faces of histone lysine methylation. Current Opinion in Cell Biology. 2002;**14**:286-298

[43] Zhu Y, Zhu MX, Zhang XD, Xu XE, Wu ZY, Liao LD, et al. SMYD3 stimulates EZR and LOXL2 transcription to enhance proliferation, migration, and invasion in esophageal squamous cell carcinoma. Human Pathology. 2016;**52**:153-163. DOI: 10.1016/j.humpath.2016.01.012.

[44] Liu Y, Liu H, Luo X, Deng J, Pan Y, Liang H. Overexpression of SMYD3 and matrix metalloproteinase-9 are associated with poor prognosis of patients with gastric cancer. Tumor Biology. 2015;**36**:4377-4386. DOI: 10.1007/s13277-015-3077-z

[45] Yu BD, Hess JL, Horning SE, Brown GA, Korsmeyer SJ. Altered Hox expression and segmental identity in Mll-mutant mice. Nature. 1995;**378**:505-508. DOI: 10.1038/378505a0

[46] Bhan A, Deb P, Shihabeddin N, Ansari KI, Brotto M, Mandal SS. Histone methylase MLL1 coordinates with HIF and regulate lncRNA HOTAIR expression under hypoxia. Gene. 2017;**629**:16-28. DOI: 10.1016/j.gene.2017.07.069

[47] Qiang R, Cai N, Wang X, Wang L, Cui K, Wang X, et al. MLL1 promotes cervical carcinoma cell tumorigenesis and metastasis through interaction with beta-catenin. Onco Targets and Therapy. 2016;**9**:6631-6640. DOI: 10.2147/ott.s114370

[48] Abudureheman A, Ainiwaer J, Hou Z, Niyaz M, Turghun A, Hasim A, et al. High MLL2 expression predicts poor prognosis and promotes tumor progression by inducing EMT in esophageal squamous cell carcinoma. Journal of Cancer Research and Clinical Oncology. 2018. DOI: 10.1007/s00432-018-2625-5

[49] Xia M, Xu L, Leng Y, Gao F, Xia H, Zhang D, et al. Downregulation of MLL3 in esophageal squamous cell carcinoma is required for the growth and metastasis of cancer cells. Tumor Biology. 2015;**36**:605-613. DOI: 10.1007/s13277-014-2616-3

[50] Kim JH, Sharma A, Dhar SS, Lee SH, Gu B, Chan CH, et al. UTX and MLL4 coordinately regulate transcriptional programs for cell proliferation and invasiveness in breast cancer cells. Cancer Research. 2014;**74**:1705-1717. DOI: 10.1158/0008-5472.can-13-1896

[51] Lin Y, Wu Y, Li J, Dong C, Ye X, Chi YI, et al. The SNAG domain of Snail1 functions as a molecular hook for recruiting lysine-specific demethylase 1. The EMBO Journal. 2010;**29**:1803-1816. DOI: 10.1038/emboj.2010.63

[52] Wu ZQ, Li XY, Hu CY, Ford M, Kleer CG, Weiss SJ. Canonical Wnt signaling regulates Slug activity and links epithelial-mesenchymal transition with epigenetic Breast Cancer 1, Early Onset (BRCA1) repression. Proceedings of the National Academy of Sciences of the United States of America. 2012;**109**:16654-16659. DOI: 10.1073/pnas.1205822109

[53] Alsaqer SF, Tashkandi MM, Kartha VK, Yang YT, Alkheriji Y, Salama A, et al. Inhibition of LSD1 epigenetically attenuates oral cancer growth and metastasis. Oncotarget. 2017; **8**:73372-73,386. DOI: 10.18632/oncotarget.19637

[54] Feng T, Wang Y, Lang Y, Zhang Y. KDM5A promotes proliferation and EMT in ovarian cancer and closely correlates with PTX resistance. Molecular Medicine Reports. 2017;**16**:3573-3580. DOI: 10.3892/mmr.2017.6960

[55] Cao J, Liu Z, Cheung WK, Zhao M, Chen SY, Chan SW, et al. Histone demethylase RBP2 is critical for breast cancer progression and metastasis. Cell Reports. 2014;**6**:868-877. DOI: 10.1016/j.celrep.2014.02.004

[56] Liang X, Zeng J, Wang L, Shen L, Ma X, Li S, et al. Histone demethylase RBP2 promotes malignant progression of gastric cancer through TGF-beta1-(p-Smad3)-RBP2-E-cadherin-Smad3 feedback circuit. Oncotarget. 2015;**6**:17661-17674. DOI: 10.18632/oncotarget.3756

[57] Tang B, Qi G, Tang F, Yuan S, Wang Z, Liang X, et al. JARID1B promotes metastasis and epithelial-mesenchymal transition via PTEN/AKT signaling in hepatocellular carcinoma cells. Oncotarget. 2015;**6**:12723-12739. DOI: 10.18632/oncotarget.3713

[58] Wang Q, Wei J, Su P, Gao P. Histone demethylase JARID1C promotes breast cancer metastasis cells via down regulating BRMS1 expression. Biochemical and Biophysical Research Communications. 2015;**464**:659-666. DOI: 10.1016/j.bbrc.2015.07.049

[59] Wang L, Zehir A, Nafa K, Zhou N, Berger MF, Casanova J, et al. Genomic aberrations frequently alter chromatin regulatory genes in chordoma. Genes, Chromosomes and Cancer. 2016;**55**:591-600. DOI: 10.1002/gcc.22362

[60] Chen JY, Li CF, Chu PY, Lai YS, Chen CH, Jiang SS, et al. Lysine demethylase 2A promotes stemness and angiogenesis of breast cancer by upregulating Jagged1. Oncotarget. 2016;**7**:27689-27710. DOI: 10.18632/oncotarget.8381

[61] Wagner KW, Alam H, Dhar SS, Giri U, Li N, Wei Y, et al. KDM2A promotes lung tumorigenesis by epigenetically enhancing ERK1/2 signaling. The Journal of Clinical Investigation. 2013;**123**:5231-5246. DOI: 10.1172/jci68642

[62] Zhao Z, Sun C, Li F, Han J, Li X, Song Z. Overexpression of histone demethylase JMJD5 promotes metastasis and indicates a poor prognosis in breast cancer. International Journal of Clinical and Experimental Pathology. 2015;**8**:10325-10334

[63] Nguyen AT, Zhang Y. The diverse functions of Dot1 and H3K79 methylation. Genes and Development. 2011;**25**:1345-1358. DOI: 10.1101/gad.2057811

[64] Daigle SR, Olhava EJ, Therkelsen CA, Majer CR, Sneeringer CJ, Song J, et al. Selective killing of mixed lineage leukemia cells by a potent small-molecule DOT1L inhibitor. Cancer Cell. 2011;**20**:53-65. DOI: 10.1016/j.ccr.2011.06.009

[65] Zhang L, Deng L, Chen F, Yao Y, Wu B, Wei L, et al. Inhibition of histone H3K79 methylation selectively inhibits proliferation, self-renewal and metastatic potential of breast cancer. Oncotarget. 2014;**5**:10665-10677. DOI: 10.18632/oncotarget.2496

[66] Bjorkman M, Ostling P, Harma V, Virtanen J, Mpindi JP, Rantala J, et al. Systematic knockdown of epigenetic enzymes identifies a novel histone demethylase PHF8 overexpressed in prostate cancer with an impact on cell proliferation, migration and invasion. Oncogene. 2012;**31**:3444-3456. DOI: 10.1038/onc.2011.512

[67] Li S, Sun A, Liang X, Ma L, Shen L, Li T, et al. Histone demethylase PHF8 promotes progression and metastasis of gastric cancer. American Journal of Cancer Research. 2017; **7**:448-461

[68] Tschiersch B, Hofmann A, Krauss V, Dorn R, Korge G, Reuter G. The protein encoded by the Drosophila position-effect variegation suppressor gene Su(var)3-9 combines domains of antagonistic regulators of homeotic gene complexes. The EMBO Journal. 1994;**13**:3822-3831

[69] Shilatifard A. Molecular implementation and physiological roles for histone H3 lysine 4 (H3K4) methylation. Current Opinion in Cell Biology. 2008;**20**:341-348. DOI: 10.1016/j.ceb.2008.03.019

[70] Wen B, Wu H, Shinkai Y, Irizarry RA, Feinberg AP. Large histone H3 lysine 9 dimethylated chromatin blocks distinguish differentiated from embryonic stem cells. Nature Genetics. 2009;**41**:246-250. DOI: 10.1038/ng.297

[71] Dong C, Wu Y, Wang Y, Wang C, Kang T, Rychahou PG, et al. Interaction with Suv39H1 is critical for Snail-mediated E-cadherin repression in breast cancer. Oncogene. 2013; **32**:1351-1362. DOI: 10.1038/onc.2012.169

[72] Dong C, Wu Y, Yao J, Wang Y, Yu Y, Rychahou PG, et al. G9a interacts with Snail and is critical for Snail-mediated E-cadherin repression in human breast cancer. The Journal of Clinical Investigation. 2012;**122**:1469-1486. DOI: 10.1172/jci57349

[73] Huang T, Zhang P, Li W, Zhao T, Zhang Z, Chen S, et al. G9A promotes tumor cell growth and invasion by silencing CASP1 in non-small-cell lung cancer cells. Cell Death and Disease. 2017;**8**:e2726. DOI: 10.1038/cddis.2017.65

[74] Chen MW, Hua KT, Kao HJ, Chi CC, Wei LH, Johansson G, et al. H3K9 histone methyltransferase G9a promotes lung cancer invasion and metastasis by silencing the cell adhesion molecule Ep-CAM. Cancer Research. 2010;**70**:7830-7840. DOI: 10.1158/0008-5472.can-10-0833

[75] Sun Y, Wei M, Ren SC, Chen R, Xu WD, Wang FB, et al. Histone methyltransferase SETDB1 is required for prostate cancer cell proliferation, migration and invasion. Asian Journal of Andrology. 2014;**16**:319-324. DOI: 10.4103/1008-682x.122812

[76] Wong CM, Wei L, Law CT, Ho DW, Tsang FH, Au SL, et al. Up-regulation of histone methyltransferase SETDB1 by multiple mechanisms in hepatocellular carcinoma promotes cancer metastasis. Hepatology. 2016;**63**:474-487. DOI: 10.1002/hep.28304

[77] Zhang H, Cai K, Wang J, Wang X, Cheng K, Shi F, et al. MiR-7, inhibited indirectly by lincRNA HOTAIR, directly inhibits SETDB1 and reverses the EMT of breast cancer stem cells by downregulating the STAT3 pathway. Stem Cells. 2014;**32**:2858-2868. DOI: 10.1002/stem.1795

[78] Ramadoss S, Guo G, Wang CY. Lysine demethylase KDM3A regulates breast cancer cell invasion and apoptosis by targeting histone and the non-histone protein p53. Oncogene. 2017;**36**:47-59. DOI: 10.1038/onc.2016.174

[79] Sechler M, Parrish JK, Birks DK, Jedlicka P. The histone demethylase KDM3A, and its downstream target MCAM, promote Ewing Sarcoma cell migration and metastasis. Oncogene. 2017;**36**:4150-4160. DOI: 10.1038/onc.2017.44

[80] Paolicchi E, Crea F, Farrar WL, Green JE, Danesi R. Histone lysine demethylases in breast cancer. Critical Reviews in Oncology/Hematology. 2013;**86**:97-103. DOI: 10.1016/j.critrevonc.2012.11.008

[81] Liu Y, Zheng P, Liu Y, Ji T, Liu X, Yao S, et al. An epigenetic role for PRL-3 as a regulator of H3K9 methylation in colorectal cancer. Gut. 2013;**62**:571-581. DOI: 10.1136/gutjnl-2011-301,059

[82] Li LL, Xue AM, Li BX, Shen YW, Li YH, Luo CL, et al. Erratum to: JMJD2A contributes to breast cancer progression through transcriptional repression of the tumor suppressor ARHI. Breast Cancer Research. 2016;**18**:114. DOI: 10.1186/s13058-016-0776-3

[83] Zhao L, Li W, Zang W, Liu Z, Xu X, Yu H, et al. JMJD2B promotes epithelial-mesenchymal transition by cooperating with beta-catenin and enhances gastric cancer metastasis. Clinical Cancer Research. 2013;**19**:6419-6429. DOI: 10.1158/1078-0432.ccr-13-0254

[84] Luo W, Chang R, Zhong J, Pandey A, Semenza GL. Histone demethylase JMJD2C is a coactivator for hypoxia-inducible factor 1 that is required for breast cancer progression. Proceedings of the National Academy of Sciences of the United States of America. 2012;**109**:E3367-E3376. DOI: 10.1073/pnas.1217394109

[85] Yokoyama Y, Matsumoto A, Hieda M, Shinchi Y, Ogihara E, Hamada M, et al. Loss of histone H4K20 trimethylation predicts poor prognosis in breast cancer and is associated with invasive activity. Breast Cancer Research. 2014;**16**:R66. DOI: 10.1186/bcr3681

[86] Viotti M, Wilson C, McCleland M, Koeppen H, Haley B, Jhunjhunwala S, et al. SUV420H2 is an epigenetic regulator of epithelial/mesenchymal states in pancreatic cancer. The Journal of Cell Biology. 2018;**217**:763-777. DOI: 10.1083/jcb.201705031

[87] Fang J, Feng Q, Ketel CS, Wang H, Cao R, Xia L, et al. Purification and functional characterization of SET8, a nucleosomal histone H4-lysine 20-specific methyltransferase. Current Biology. 2002;**12**:1086-1099

[88] Yang F, Sun L, Li Q, Han X, Lei L, Zhang H, et al. SET8 promotes epithelial-mesenchymal transition and confers TWIST dual transcriptional activities. The EMBO Journal. 2012;**31**:110-123. DOI: 10.1038/emboj.2011.364

[89] Hou L, Li Q, Yu Y, Li M, Zhang D. SET8 induces epithelialmesenchymal transition and enhances prostate cancer cell metastasis by cooperating with ZEB1. Molecular Medicine Reports. 2016;**13**:1681-1688. DOI: 10.3892/mmr.2015.4733

[90] Della Corte CM, Bellevicine C, Vicidomini G, Vitagliano D, Malapelle U, Accardo M, et al. SMO gene amplification and activation of the Hedgehog pathway as novel mechanisms of resistance to anti-epidermal growth factor receptor drugs in human lung cancer. Clinical Cancer Research. 2015;**21**:4686-4697. DOI: 10.1158/1078-0432.ccr-14-3319

[91] Fu L, Wu H, Cheng SY, Gao D, Zhang L, Zhao Y. Set7 mediated Gli3 methylation plays a positive role in the activation of Sonic Hedgehog pathway in mammals. eLife. 2016;**5**. DOI: 10.7554/eLife.15690

[92] Bernstein BE, Meissner A, Lander ES. The mammalian epigenome. Cell. 2007;**128**:669-681. DOI: 10.1016/j.cell.2007.01.033

[93] Barski A, Cuddapah S, Cui K, Roh TY, Schones DE, Wang Z, et al. High-resolution profiling of histone methylations in the human genome. Cell. 2007;**129**:823-837. DOI: 10.1016/j.cell.2007.05.009

[94] Hublitz P, Albert M, Peters AH. Mechanisms of transcriptional repression by histone lysine methylation. The International Journal of Developmental Biology. 2009;**53**:335-354. DOI: 10.1387/ijdb.082717 ph

[95] Xiang Y, Zhu Z, Han G, Lin H, Xu L, Chen CD. JMJD3 is a histone H3K27 demethylase. Cell Research. 2007;**17**:850-857. DOI: 10.1038/cr.2007.83

[96] Tiwari N, Tiwari VK, Waldmeier L, Balwierz PJ, Arnold P, Pachkov M, et al. Sox4 is a master regulator of epithelial-mesenchymal transition by controlling Ezh2 expression and epigenetic reprogramming. Cancer Cell. 2013;**23**:768-783. DOI: 10.1016/j.ccr.2013.04.020

[97] Chien YC, Liu LC, Ye HY, Wu JY, Yu YL. EZH2 promotes migration and invasion of triple-negative breast cancer cells via regulating TIMP2-MMP-2/−9 pathway. American Journal of Cancer Research. 2018;**8**:422-434

[98] Herranz N, Pasini D, Diaz VM, Franci C, Gutierrez A, Dave N, et al. Polycomb complex 2 is required for E-cadherin repression by the Snail1 transcription factor. Molecular and Cellular Biology. 2008;**28**:4772-4781. DOI: 10.1128/MCB.00323-08

[99] Zha L, Cao Q, Cui X, Li F, Liang H, Xue B, et al. Epigenetic regulation of E-cadherin expression by the histone demethylase UTX in colon cancer cells. Medical Oncology. 2016;**33**:21. DOI: 10.1007/s12032-016-0734-z

[100] Choi HJ, Park JH, Park M, Won HY, Joo HS, Lee CH, et al. UTX inhibits EMT-induced breast CSC properties by epigenetic repression of EMT genes in cooperation with LSD1 and HDAC1. EMBO Reports. 2015;**16**:1288-1298. DOI: 10.15252/embr.201540244

[101] Tang B, Qi G, Tang F, Yuan S, Wang Z, Liang X, et al. Aberrant JMJD3 expression upregulates slug to promote migration, invasion, and stem cell-like behaviors in hepatocellular carcinoma. Cancer Research. 2016;**76**:6520-6532. DOI: 10.1158/0008-5472.can-15-3029

[102] Park WY, Hong BJ, Lee J, Choi C, Kim MY. H3K27 demethylase JMJD3 employs the NF-kappaB and BMP signaling pathways to modulate the tumor microenvironment and promote melanoma progression and metastasis. Cancer Research. 2016;**76**:161-170. DOI: 10.1158/0008-5472.can-15-0536

[103] Gao Y, Zhao Y, Zhang J, Lu Y, Liu X, Geng P, et al. The dual function of PRMT1 in modulating epithelial-mesenchymal transition and cellular senescence in breast cancer cells through regulation of ZEB1. Scientific Reports. 2016;**6**:19874. DOI: 10.1038/srep19874

[104] Avasarala S, Van Scoyk M, Karuppusamy Rathinam MK, Zerayesus S, Zhao X, Zhang W, et al. PRMT1 is a novel regulator of epithelial-mesenchymal-transition in non-small cell lung cancer. The Journal of Biological Chemistry. 2015;**290**:13479-13489. DOI: 10.1074/jbc.M114.636050

[105] Li L, Zhang Z, Ma T, Huo R. PRMT1 regulates tumor growth and metastasis of human melanoma via targeting ALCAM. Molecular Medicine Reports. 2016;**14**:521-528. DOI: 10.3892/mmr.2016.5273

[106] Gou Q, He S, Zhou Z. Protein arginine N-methyltransferase 1 promotes the proliferation and metastasis of hepatocellular carcinoma cells. Tumor Biology. 2017;**39**. DOI: 10.1177/1010428317691419

[107] Zhou W, Yue H, Li C, Chen H, Yuan Y. Protein arginine methyltransferase 1 promoted the growth and migration of cancer cells in esophageal squamous cell carcinoma. Tumor Biology. 2016;**37**:2613-2619. DOI: 10.1007/s13277-015-4098-3

[108] Goulet I, Gauvin G, Boisvenue S, Cote J. Alternative splicing yields protein arginine methyltransferase 1 isoforms with distinct activity, substrate specificity, and subcellular localization. The Journal of Biological Chemistry. 2007;**282**:33009-33021. DOI: 10.1074/jbc.M704349200

[109] Bondy-Chorney E, Baldwin RM, Didillon A, Chabot B, Jasmin BJ, Cote J. RNA binding protein RALY promotes protein arginine methyltransferase 1 alternatively spliced isoform v2 relative expression and metastatic potential in breast cancer cells. The International Journal of Biochemistry and Cell Biology. 2017;**91**:124-135. DOI: 10.1016/j.biocel.2017.07.008

[110] Zhong J, Cao RX, Hong T, Yang J, Zu XY, Xiao XH, et al. Identification and expression analysis of a novel transcript of the human PRMT2 gene resulted from alternative polyadenylation in breast cancer. Gene. 2011;**487**:1-9. DOI: 10.1016/j.gene.2011.06.022

[111] Qi C, Chang J, Zhu Y, Yeldandi AV, Rao SM, Zhu YJ. Identification of protein arginine methyltransferase 2 as a coactivator for estrogen receptor alpha. The Journal of Biological Chemistry. 2002;**277**. DOI: 28624-30. DOI: 10.1074/jbc.M201053200

[112] Zhong J, Cao RX, Zu XY, Hong T, Yang J, Liu L, et al. Identification and characterization of novel spliced variants of PRMT2 in breast carcinoma. The FEBS Journal. 2012;**279**:316-335. DOI: 10.1111/j.1742-4658.2011.08426.x

[113] Wang L, Zhao Z, Meyer MB, Saha S, Yu M, Guo A, et al. CARM1 methylates chromatin remodeling factor BAF155 to enhance tumor progression and metastasis. Cancer Cell. 2014;**25**:21-36. DOI: 10.1016/j.ccr.2013.12.007

[114] Habashy HO, Rakha EA, Ellis IO, Powe DG. The estrogen receptor coactivator CARM1 has an oncogenic effect and is associated with poor prognosis in breast cancer. Breast Cancer Research and Treatment. 2013;**140**:307-316. DOI: 10.1007/s10549-013-2614-y

[115] Ohkura N, Takahashi M, Yaguchi H, Nagamura Y, Tsukada T. Coactivator-associated arginine methyltransferase 1, CARM1, affects pre-mRNA splicing in an isoform-specific manner. The Journal of Biological Chemistry. 2005;**280**:28927-28935. DOI: 10.1074/jbc.M502173200

[116] Fu T, Lv X, Kong Q, Yuan C. A novel SHARPIN-PRMT5-H3R2me1 axis is essential for lung cancer cell invasion. Oncotarget. 2017;**8**:54809-54820. DOI: 10.18632/oncotarget.18957

[117] Tsutsui T, Fukasawa R, Shinmyouzu K, Nakagawa R, Tobe K, Tanaka A, et al. Mediator complex recruits epigenetic regulators via its two cyclin-dependent kinase subunits to repress transcription of immune response genes. The Journal of Biological Chemistry. 2013;**288**:20955-20965. DOI: 10.1074/jbc.M113.486746

[118] Migliori V, Muller J, Phalke S, Low D, Bezzi M, Mok WC, et al. Symmetric dimethylation of H3R2 is a newly identified histone mark that supports euchromatin maintenance. Nature Structural and Molecular Biology. 2012;**19**:136-144. DOI: 10.1038/nsmb.2209

[119] Chen H, Lorton B, Gupta V, Shechter D. A TGFbeta-PRMT5-MEP50 axis regulates cancer cell invasion through histone H3 and H4 arginine methylation coupled transcriptional activation and repression. Oncogene. 2017;**36**:373-386. DOI: 10.1038/onc.2016.205

[120] Hou Z, Peng H, Ayyanathan K, Yan KP, Langer EM, Longmore GD, et al. The LIM protein AJUBA recruits protein arginine methyltransferase 5 to mediate SNAIL-dependent transcriptional repression. Molecular and Cellular Biology. 2008;**28**:3198-3207. DOI: 10.1128/mcb.01435-07

[121] Hu D, Gur M, Zhou Z, Gamper A, Hung MC, Fujita N, et al. Interplay between arginine methylation and ubiquitylation regulates KLF4-mediated genome stability and carcinogenesis. Nature Communications. 2015;**6**:8419. DOI: 10.1038/ncomms9419

[122] Yoshimatsu M, Toyokawa G, Hayami S, Unoki M, Tsunoda T, Field HI, et al. Dysregulation of PRMT1 and PRMT6, Type I arginine methyltransferases, is involved in various types of human cancers. International Journal of Cancer. 2011;**128**:562-573. DOI: 10.1002/ijc.25366

[123] Dowhan DH, Harrison MJ, Eriksson NA, Bailey P, Pearen MA, Fuller PJ, et al. Protein arginine methyltransferase 6-dependent gene expression and splicing: association with

breast cancer outcomes. Endocrine-Related Cancer. 2012;**19**:509-526. DOI: 10.1530/erc-12-0100

[124] Geng P, Zhang Y, Liu X, Zhang N, Liu Y, Liu X, et al. Automethylation of protein arginine methyltransferase 7 and its impact on breast cancer progression. The FASEB Journal. 2017;**31**:2287-2300. DOI: 10.1096/fj.201601196R

[125] Baldwin RM, Haghandish N, Daneshmand M, Amin S, Paris G, Falls TJ, et al. Protein arginine methyltransferase 7 promotes breast cancer cell invasion through the induction of MMP9 expression. Oncotarget. 2015;**6**:3013-3032. DOI: 10.18632/oncotarget.3072

[126] Thomassen M, Tan Q, Kruse TA. Gene expression meta-analysis identifies chromosomal regions and candidate genes involved in breast cancer metastasis. Breast Cancer Research and Treatment. 2009;**113**:239-249. DOI: 10.1007/s10549-008-9927-2

[127] Yang Y, Hadjikyriacou A, Xia Z, Gayatri S, Kim D, Zurita-Lopez C, et al. PRMT9 is a type II methyltransferase that methylates the splicing factor SAP145. Nature Communications. 2015;**6**:6428. DOI: 10.1038/ncomms7428

[128] Jiang H, Zhou Z, Jin S, Xu K, Zhang H, Xu J, et al. PRMT9 promotes hepatocellular carcinoma invasion and metastasis via activating PI3K/Akt/GSK-3beta/Snail signaling. Cancer Science. 2018. DOI: 10.1111/cas.13598

[129] Greiner D, Bonaldi T, Eskeland R, Roemer E, Imhof A. Identification of a specific inhibitor of the histone methyltransferase SU(VAR)3-9. Nature Chemical Biology. 2005;**1**:143-145. DOI: 10.1038/nchembio721

[130] Lakshmikuttyamma A, Scott SA, DeCoteau JF, Geyer CR. Reexpression of epigenetically silenced AML tumor suppressor genes by SUV39H1 inhibition. Oncogene. 2010;**29**:576-588. DOI: 10.1038/onc.2009.361

[131] Kubicek S, O'Sullivan RJ, August EM, Hickey ER, Zhang Q, Teodoro ML, et al. Reversal of H3K9me2 by a small-molecule inhibitor for the G9a histone methyltransferase. Molecular Cell. 2007;**25**:473-481. DOI: 10.1016/j.molcel.2007.01.017

[132] Liu S, Ye D, Guo W, Yu W, He Y, Hu J, et al. G9a is essential for EMT-mediated metastasis and maintenance of cancer stem cell-like characters in head and neck squamous cell carcinoma. Oncotarget. 2015;**6**:6887-6901. DOI: 10.18632/oncotarget.3159

[133] Vedadi M, Barsyte-Lovejoy D, Liu F, Rival-Gervier S, Allali-Hassani A, Labrie V, et al. A chemical probe selectively inhibits G9a and GLP methyltransferase activity in cells. Nature Chemical Biology. 2011;**7**:566-574. DOI: 10.1038/nchembio.599

[134] Liu XR, Zhou LH, Hu JX, Liu LM, Wan HP, Zhang XQ. UNC0638, a G9a inhibitor, suppresses epithelialmesenchymal transitionmediated cellular migration and invasion in triple negative breast cancer. Molecular Medicine Reports. 2018;**17**:2239-2244. DOI: 10.3892/mmr.2017.8190

[135] Finley A, Copeland RA. Small molecule control of chromatin remodeling. Chemistry and Biology. 2014;**21**:1196-1210. DOI: 10.1016/j.chembiol.2014.07.024

[136] Tan J, Yang X, Zhuang L, Jiang X, Chen W, Lee PL, et al. Pharmacologic disruption of Polycomb-repressive complex 2-mediated gene repression selectively induces apoptosis in cancer cells. Genes and Development. 2007;**21**:1050-1063. DOI: 10.1101/gad.1524107

[137] Mody HR, Hung SW, AlSaggar M, Griffin J, Govindarajan R. Inhibition of S-adenosylmethionine-dependent methyltransferase attenuates TGFbeta1-induced EMT and metastasis in pancreatic cancer: Putative roles of miR-663a and miR-4787-5p. Molecular Cancer Research. 2016;**14**:1124-1135. DOI: 10.1158/1541-7786.mcr-16-0083

[138] Wang L, Chang J, Varghese D, Dellinger M, Kumar S, Best AM, et al. A small molecule modulates Jumonji histone demethylase activity and selectively inhibits cancer growth. Nature Communications. 2013;**4**:2035. DOI: 10.1038/ncomms3035

[139] Cheng D, Yadav N, King RW, Swanson MS, Weinstein EJ, Bedford MT. Small molecule regulators of protein arginine methyltransferases. The Journal of Biological Chemistry. 2004;**279**:23892-23899. DOI: 10.1074/jbc.M401853200

[140] Castellano S, Milite C, Ragno R, Simeoni S, Mai A, Limongelli V, et al. Design, synthesis and biological evaluation of carboxy analogues of arginine methyltransferase inhibitor 1 (AMI-1). ChemMedChem. 2010;**5**:398-414. DOI: 10.1002/cmdc.200900459

[141] Zhang B, Dong S, Zhu R, Hu C, Hou J, Li Y, et al. Targeting protein arginine methyltransferase 5 inhibits colorectal cancer growth by decreasing arginine methylation of eIF4E and FGFR3. Oncotarget. 2015;**6**:22799-22811. DOI: 10.18632/oncotarget.4332

[142] Liu Z, Wang P, Chen H, Wold EA, Tian B, Brasier AR, et al. Drug discovery targeting bromodomain-containing protein 4. Journal of Medicinal Chemistry. 2017;**60**:4533-4558. DOI: 10.1021/acs.jmedchem.6b01761

[143] Fontanals-Cirera B, Hasson D, Vardabasso C, Di Micco R, Agrawal P, Chowdhury A, et al. Harnessing BET inhibitor sensitivity reveals AMIGO2 as a melanoma survival gene. Molecular Cell. 2017;**68**:731-744.e9. DOI: 10.1016/j.molcel.2017.11.004

[144] Wagner T, Robaa D, Sippl W, Jung M. Mind the methyl: methyllysine binding proteins in epigenetic regulation. ChemMedChem. 2014;**9**:466-483. DOI: 10.1002/cmdc.201300422

[145] Maison C, Almouzni G. HP1 and the dynamics of heterochromatin maintenance. Nature Reviews. Molecular Cell Biology. 2004;**5**:296-304. DOI: 10.1038/nrm1355

[146] Millanes-Romero A, Herranz N, Perrera V, Iturbide A, Loubat-Casanovas J, Gil J, et al. Regulation of heterochromatin transcription by Snail1/LOXL2 during epithelial-to-mesenchymal transition. Molecular Cell. 2013;**52**:746-757. DOI: 10.1016/j.molcel.2013.10.015

[147] Tang M, Shen H, Jin Y, Lin T, Cai Q, Pinard MA, et al. The malignant brain tumor (MBT) domain protein SFMBT1 is an integral histone reader subunit of the LSD1 demethylase complex for chromatin association and epithelial-to-mesenchymal transition. The Journal of Biological Chemistry. 2013;**288**:27680-27691. DOI: 10.1074/jbc.M113.482349

[148] Wysocka J, Swigut T, Milne TA, Dou Y, Zhang X, Burlingame AL, et al. WDR5 associates with histone H3 methylated at K4 and is essential for H3 K4 methylation and vertebrate development. Cell. 2005;**121**:859-872. DOI: 10.1016/j.cell.2005.03.036

[149] Wu MZ, Tsai YP, Yang MH, Huang CH, Chang SY, Chang CC, et al. Interplay between HDAC3 and WDR5 is essential for hypoxia-induced epithelial-mesenchymal transition. Molecular Cell. 2011;**43**:811-822. DOI: 10.1016/j.molcel.2011.07.012

[150] Margueron R, Justin N, Ohno K, Sharpe ML, Son J, Drury WJ 3rd, et al. Role of the polycomb protein EED in the propagation of repressive histone marks. Nature. 2009; **461**:762-767. DOI: 10.1038/nature08398

[151] Collins RE, Northrop JP, Horton JR, Lee DY, Zhang X, Stallcup MR, et al. The ankyrin repeats of G9a and GLP histone methyltransferases are mono- and dimethyllysine binding modules. Nature Structural and Molecular Biology. 2008;**15**:245-250. DOI: 10.1038/nsmb.1384

[152] James LI, Barsyte-Lovejoy D, Zhong N, Krichevsky L, Korboukh VK, Herold JM, et al. Discovery of a chemical probe for the L3MBTL3 methyllysine reader domain. Nature Chemical Biology. 2013;**9**:184-191. DOI: 10.1038/nchembio.1157

[153] Stuckey JI, Dickson BM, Cheng N, Liu Y, Norris JL, Cholensky SH, et al. A cellular chemical probe targeting the chromodomains of Polycomb repressive complex 1. Nature Chemical Biology. 2016;**12**:180-187. DOI: 10.1038/nchembio.2007

[154] Shi Y, Sawada J, Sui G, Affar el B, Whetstine JR, Lan F, et al. Coordinated histone modifications mediated by a CtBP co-repressor complex. Nature. 2003;**422**:735-738. DOI: 10.1038/nature01550

[155] Shi Y, Lan F, Matson C, Mulligan P, Whetstine JR, Cole PA, et al. Histone demethylation mediated by the nuclear amine oxidase homolog LSD1. Cell. 2004;**119**:941-953. DOI: 10.1016/j.cell.2004.12.012

[156] Nishioka K, Chuikov S, Sarma K, Erdjument-Bromage H, Allis CD, Tempst P, et al. Set9, a novel histone H3 methyltransferase that facilitates transcription by precluding histone tail modifications required for heterochromatin formation. Genes and Development. 2002;**16**:479-489. DOI: 10.1101/gad.967202

[157] Wang H, Cao R, Xia L, Erdjument-Bromage H, Borchers C, Tempst P, et al. Purification and functional characterization of a histone H3-lysine 4-specific methyltransferase. Molecular Cell. 2001;**8**:1207-1217

[158] Fu J, Qin L, He T, Qin J, Hong J, Wong J, et al. The TWIST/Mi2/NuRD protein complex and its essential role in cancer metastasis. Cell Research. 2011;**21**:275-289. DOI: 10.1038/cr.2010.118

[159] Chang Y, Sun L, Kokura K, Horton JR, Fukuda M, Espejo A, et al. MPP8 mediates the interactions between DNA methyltransferase Dnmt3a and H3K9 methyltransferase GLP/G9a. Nature Communications. 2011;**2**:533. DOI: 10.1038/ncomms1549

[160] Kokura K, Sun L, Bedford MT, Fang J. Methyl-H3K9-binding protein MPP8 mediates E-cadherin gene silencing and promotes tumor cell motility and invasion. The EMBO Journal. 2010;**29**:3673-3687. DOI: 10.1038/emboj.2010.239

[161] Sun L, Kokura K, Izumi V, Koomen JM, Seto E, Chen J, et al. MPP8 and SIRT1 crosstalk in E-cadherin gene silencing and epithelial-mesenchymal transition. EMBO Reports. 2015;**16**:689-699. DOI: 10.15252/embr.201439792

11

Prognostic Biomarkers for Breast Cancer Metastasis

Kwok Kin Lee, Wee Joo Chng and Sudhakar Jha

Abstract

Breast cancer treatment has improved rapidly through the years, starting from surgery, to hormonal therapy, to targeted therapy. Despite this, tumor metastasis remains the highest cause of breast cancer–related death. The current regime to deter metastasis is through adjuvant therapy, but such therapy frequently yields undesirable side effects. As such, prognostic markers for metastasis are important to stratify patients for adjuvant therapy so as to ameliorate the standard of living of patients with low metastatic potential. So far, only a few well-characterized prognostic biomarkers for metastasis are used in clinics. This chapter will cover both established and novel prognostic biomarkers for breast cancer metastasis and metastatic breast cancer prognosis. The potential of using these biomarkers as predictive biomarkers or new targeted therapy will also be discussed.

Keywords: metastasis, prognostic biomarker, metastatic breast cancer, relapse, recurrence, distant-free metastasis survival, overall survival

1. Introduction

Breast cancer remains the most frequently diagnosed cancer in women worldwide. In the United States (US), the American Cancer Society estimates that in 2018, the highest frequency of cancer diagnosed and the second highest cancer-related death in women will be breast cancer, at 30 and 14%, respectively [1]. Breast cancer survival statistics have improved tremendously over the years with a decrease of 39% mortality from 1989 to 2015 [1, 2]. This is mainly due to mammogram screening resulting in early detection and intervention [3, 4]. When diagnosed at a localized stage, the 5-year survival rate is 99% [5]. However, metastasis remains the major cause of mortality in breast cancer patients. Five-year survival rate decreases dramatically according to spread of cancer, with regional and distant metastasis spreads at 85 and 27%, respectively [1]. Ten-year survival rate for stage IV metastatic breast cancer female patients is only approximately 13% [6]. These statistics indicate that metastasis is the major barrier against breast cancer eradication.

Breast cancer can be categorized largely into two types, *in situ* and invasive breast cancer [2]. *In situ* represents the subset in which the cancer is still confined within the transformed origin. Ductal carcinoma *in situ* (DCIS) and lobular carcinoma *in situ* (LCIS) are the two main types of frequently diagnosed *in situ* breast cancer at 83 and 13%, respectively [2]. DCIS, as its name suggests, refers to cancer originating from the epithelial cells of the breast ducts, whereas LCIS arises from the lobules of the breast. On the other hand, majority (80%) of breast cancer will become invasive, i.e., that they will outgrow into surrounding breast tissue [2].

The primary treatment for *in situ* breast cancer is surgery. This includes lumpectomy where only the tumor and surrounding tissues are removed or mastectomy in which the entire breast is removed [2]. Very often, radiation and adjuvant therapy are recommended after surgery to prevent recurrence and to eliminate breast tumor cells which might have spread [2]. Examples of adjuvant therapy are cytotoxic chemotherapy, hormone therapy, and targeted therapy [2, 3]. These will be discussed in more detail in the later sections.

Although adjuvant therapy has been shown to be beneficial in preventing metastatic recurrence, the patient's quality of life is severely affected in many cases. Side effects include fatigue, osteoporosis, increased thromboembolic events, premature menopause, weight gain, and mild memory loss [7, 8]. Although as many as 80% of patients receive adjuvant treatment, only 40% of them relapse and die from metastatic breast cancer indicating that majority of patients are over-treated and suffer unnecessary side effects [3]. In addition, only 15% of patients treated with tamoxifen after surgery will have distant recurrence, indicating that 85% of patients will be overtreated if chemotherapy is mandatory [9].

One solution to overcome unnecessary treatment is through identifying patients with high and low risk of metastasis using prognostic biomarkers. Current established metastasis biomarkers are available but have poor predictive power [10]. With new concepts such as gene expression profiling and circulating tumor cells, new prognostic markers with greater accuracy could be identified. The following sections will describe established markers as well as new upcoming markers for the prediction of survival, metastasis risk, and recurrence risk for metastatic breast cancer. Current and potential use of these markers in the clinic as predictive biomarkers for treatment and as potential targets is also discussed.

2. Established biomarkers

2.1. Tumor size and lymph node status

The tumor-node-metastasis (TNM) staging system is commonly used to stage breast cancer progression during initial diagnosis [11]. It constitutes a manner to measure the aggressiveness of the cancer. The abbreviations represent different characteristics of the cancer. "T" represents tumor size, "N" indicates the number of lymph nodes that the cancer has spread to, and "M" conveys the presence of distant metastasis [11]. In the absence of distant metastasis ("M"), tumor size and lymph node status are established prognostic markers for likelihood of metastasis. Specifically, primary tumors that are less than 2 cm have low prognosis for developing into metastatic breast cancer. Tumor sizes of 2–5 cm and more than 5 cm have a high and very high likelihood of progressing into metastatic cancer respectively [12–15]. Likewise, breast cancer patients with no detectable lymph node metastases are at low risk of distant metastasis. Patients with presence of lymph node metastasis have high risk of metastasis, and more than four lymph node metastases represent a high probability progressing to distant metastasis [12–15].

2.2. Histological grade

Histological grade is the determination of how differentiated a tumor is. As the histological grade increases, the tumor appears more poorly differentiated [16]. The determination of histological grade is performed by a trained pathologist using certain characteristics of the cancer tissue section such as mitotic count, extent of tubule or gland formation, and nuclear pleomorphism [16]. Histological grade 1 tumors have low risk of metastasis, while grade 2 and 3 tumors have intermediate- and high-risk tumors [12, 14, 17]. Integrating histological grade with the aforementioned tumor size and lymph node status, several prognostic indices such as the Nottingham Prognostic Index, the Kalmar Prognostic Index, and the St. Gallen guidelines have been established and used in clinics to aid in adjuvant treatment decision [16].

2.3. Angioinvasion

Angioinvasion is the presence of blood vessel invasion by cancer cells. In lymph node negative patients, angioinvasion has some prognostic value in predicting metastasis [18, 19]. In particular, tumor emboli in more than three blood vessels suggest a high risk of metastasis [18, 19]. Although these tumor characteristics (tumor size, lymph node status, histological grade, and angioinvasion) represent a simple and cheap method to predict metastasis, statistics show that these prognostic factors only accurately predict metastatic outcome in 30% of patients [3, 16]. As such, better prognostic markers are required for the remaining 70%.

2.4. Molecular subtype

Invasive breast cancer can be divided into four main molecular subtypes based on the presence of hormone receptors (estrogen or progesterone) (HR) and human epidermal growth factor receptor 2 (HER2) [2]. The four subtypes are luminal A (HR+/HER2−), luminal B (HR+/HER2+), HER2 enriched (HR−/HER2+), and triple negative (HR−/HER2−) at frequencies of 71, 12, 5, and 12% of all invasive breast cancer, respectively [2].

In general, luminal A and B subtypes are associated with the most favorable prognosis and least aggressive, followed by HER2 enriched and triple negative sequentially [2, 20–23]. In a 6.9-year follow-up study on patients who were initially diagnosed with localized breast cancer, the frequency of distant metastasis increases progressively in the following order, luminal A (6.4%), luminal B (12.1%), HER2-enriched (19.2%), and triple negative (27.4%) [24]. Another study involving metastatic breast cancer found that luminal A exhibited the longest survival rate (34.4 months), followed by luminal B (24.8 months), HER2 enriched (19.8 months), and triple negative (8.8 months) [25]. Similarly, follow-up on patients with early stage breast cancer found that survival with distant metastasis showed similar patterns [26]. Luminal A survived the longest duration (2.2 years), followed by luminal B (1.6 years), HER2 enriched (0.7 years), and triple negative (0.5 years) [26]. These findings strongly suggest that molecular subtype correlates with metastasis rate and survival and can be used as a prognostic marker for metastasis.

In fact, molecular subtypes are already routinely used in clinics as prognostic and predictive biomarkers for overall survival and stratification of patients to targeted therapy [2]. As a predictive biomarker, patients who are either HR+ or HER2+ benefit majorly due to targeted therapy options. The estrogen receptor (ER) in breast cancer plays an important tumor promoting role by activating downstream intracellular signals for proliferation and survival [27]. As such, patients with ER+ breast cancer are routinely treated with selective estrogen receptor modulators (SERMs) [8]. Tamoxifen is the first approved SERM to be used for the treatment of ER+ metastatic breast cancer [8]. Five-year use of tamoxifen as an adjuvant significantly reduced local and distant recurrences by 40–50% making ER status both a prognostic and predictive biomarker [28].

Apart from using SERMs, aromatase inhibitors (AIs) are an alternative targeted treatment for ER+ breast cancer patients. These inhibitors function to block estrogen production by inhibiting the aromatase enzyme [8]. Studies have found that there is no difference in efficacy and time to distant recurrence when compared to tamoxifen treatment [29]. In addition, both tamoxifen and AI treatment are associated with increased overall survival and distant metastasis-free survival [30]. Since ovaries are the main source of estrogen, ovarian surgery, ovarian irradiation, or ovarian suppression by drugs have been shown to improve therapeutic outcomes [2, 31]. Particularly, in a clinical study, 5-year disease free survival was as high as 91.1%, when ER+ premenopausal women were treated with adjuvant ovarian suppression combined with AI treatment [31]. Additionally, use of AI with ovarian suppression significantly decreased recurrence as compared to tamoxifen with ovarian suppression [31]. These evidences strongly illustrate the use of ER status for metastatic survival prognosis and for tamoxifen or AI adjuvant therapy decision.

Historically, HER2-enriched metastatic breast cancer is associated with high aggressiveness and has a poor prognosis [2, 32–34]. That is until the first anti-HER2 targeted therapy Trastuzumab clinical trial emerged, which showed improved clinical outcomes by including Trastuzumab into adjuvant treatment with chemotherapy for HER2-enriched metastatic breast cancer [35]. Trastuzumab is a monoclonal antibody which binds and targets the extracellular portion of the HER2 receptor protein [8]. Specifically, combining Trastuzumab with standard chemotherapy for HER2-enriched metastatic breast cancer resulted in increased time to progression, overall survival, and duration of response [35, 36].

In recent years, many new biologics targeting HER2 have been approved for advanced metastatic HER2-enriched breast cancer [37]. Pertuzumab, another monoclonal antibody which inhibits HER2 dimerization, is approved for use in combination with trastuzumab in metastatic HER2+ breast cancer [38]. Treatment of HER2-enriched metastatic breast cancer patients using a combination of Pertuzumab, Trastuzumab, and Docetaxel resulted in a significant increase in median overall survival of 15.7 months as compared to just treating with Trastuzumab and Docetaxel [38]. Increase in progression free survival and duration of response by 6.3 months and 7.7 months, respectively, were also noted when Pertuzumab was used in combination [38].

Another recently approved biologic for HER2+ advanced breast cancer is the antibody-drug conjugate T-DM1 [39, 40]. It involves the ingenious exploitation of Trastuzumab's specificity to HER2+ breast cancer cells to deliver the linked cytotoxic microtubule-inhibitory drug DM1 directly to HER2+ cancer cells [39, 40]. It is particularly effective in slowing disease progression for HER2+ advanced breast cancer patients who were initially treated with first line Trastuzumab/Taxane combination [39]. Progression free survival when treated with T-DM1 was significantly longer (9.6 months) as compared to the standard second line treatment (6.4 months) [39]. Overall survival improved significantly from 25.1 to 30.9 months [39]. Additionally, patients treated with T-DM1 experienced less toxicity as compared to the standard second line treatment [39]. Taken together, it is recommended that the Docetaxel/Trastuzumab/Pertuzumab combination be used as a first line choice and T-DM1 as a second line therapy [37].

The importance of HER2-targeted therapy for metastatic breast cancer is further emphasized by the finding that as many as 16% of initially HER2 negative breast cancer exhibits HER2 expression upon metastasis [37]. This indicates that HER2-targeted therapies could be extended to treat metastasis in this select group of patients, and it is recommended in clinics that HER2 status in metastatic cells be tested by fluorescence in situ hybridization or immunohistochemistry staining to evaluate eligibility for HER2-targeted therapy regardless of initial subtype of the primary tumor [37]. Overall, these findings highlight the importance of using HER2 status as both a prognostic and predictive biomarker in clinics for metastatic breast cancer.

As for triple negative cancers which do not currently have their own targeted therapy, neoadjuvant anthracycline-based chemotherapy has been found to benefit this group [41]. Clinical response in triple negative was 85% as compared to luminal (47%) or HER2 positive (70%), and all subtypes had equally good prognosis after treatment [41]. However, this only applies to triple negative patients who exhibited pathologic complete response from treatment, which constitutes only 27% [41]. As such, for majority of triple negative patients who do not display complete pathologic response after chemotherapy, more studies need to be done to discover targets specific against triple negative breast cancer.

In addition to metastasis frequency and survival, molecular subtypes could potentially predict distant metastasis tumor sites and distant relapse sites. With the exception of triple negative basal subtype, bone metastasis is the most common metastasized site among all subtypes, with the luminal subtypes displaying the highest frequency [26, 42]. Correspondingly, bone is the most frequent metastatic relapse site, with luminal subtypes exhibiting the highest frequency [43, 44]. The subtypes with the highest brain and lung metastasis rates are HER2 enriched and triple negative [26]. Among all subtypes, metastatic lung and brain relapse are highest for triple negative [43, 44]. HER2-enriched subtype has the highest liver metastasis rate, whereas triple negative has more distant lymph node metastasis as compared to other subtypes [26, 42]. The importance of determining site of metastasis is covered in the next section.

2.5. Site of distant metastasis

The significance of predicting site of metastasis for metastatic breast cancer patients is highlighted by the intrinsic correlation with overall survival and survival after distant recurrence. In the following order, breast cancer patients with single site brain, lung or liver, and bone metastasis have the worst to best prognosis [42, 45]. Median overall survival rates for patients with brain, lung, liver, and bone metastasis are 11 months, 30 months, 31 months, and 41 months, respectively [42]. In addition, the survival trend holds true when patients are stratified based on HR indicating that it is independent of HR status [45].

Postmetastasis distant recurrence is also associated with the site of recurrence. In particular, first visceral (including brain) site recurrence is associated with a poorer prognosis as compared to first bone recurrence with 3-year breast cancer specific survival (BCSS) rate at 13 (visceral) and 23% (bone), respectively [46]. When compared to recurrences closer to the primary tumor, first local and first lymph node recurrences 3-year BCSS are significantly higher at 83 and 33%, respectively, indicating that metastatic site proximity to primary tumor origin site is also strongly linked to prognosis [46].

Apart from the site of distant metastasis, the number of initial metastatic sites is also prognostic of survival. Patients with multiple metastatic sites have significantly poorer overall survival than patients with single metastatic site in both HR+ (9 months) and HR– (5 months) patients [45]. Multiple metastatic sites are also more prone to occur in HR– patients, which are in line with the poorer prognosis of HR– patients [45].

2.6. Age of diagnosis

Indubitably, as with many diseases, age is a major determinant of prognosis in metastatic breast cancer. Survival rate in stage IV invasive breast cancer patients significantly decreases with age [6]. Ten-year breast cancer specific survival rates for three groups of stage IV patients namely, below the age of 40 years, between 41 and 50 years, and between 51 and 70 years, drops from 15.7 to 14.9% to 11.7%, respectively [6]. Likewise, another study found similar trends in metastatic breast cancer patients, where overall survival decreases significantly with age, from 32 months (age < 50 years) to 25 months (50–69 years) to 16 months (>69 years) [47]. One plausible explanation is that younger patients are more physically fit to endure treatment than elder patients, and this is supported by a significantly higher rate of surgery and radiation therapy underwent by patients below 69 years [47].

Age is also a determinant in the prediction of distant metastasis site. In accordance with the age-related survival trend, frequency of the deadlier lung metastasis increases significantly with age from 5.9% (age < 50 years) to 7.6% (50–69 years) to 14.2% (> 69 years), respectively [47]. Correspondingly, a significantly lower rate of the less lethal distant lymphatic metastasis is observed as age increases with rates at 7.3, 5.4, and 4.0% for patient age of less than 50 years, 50–69 years, and more than 69 years, respectively [47]. Metastasis to the brain, liver or bone is not dependent on age [47]. Interestingly, multiple metastatic sites, which are associated with poorer prognoses, occurred more frequently in younger patients (<69 years) than in older patients (>69 years) at approximately 34.9 (age < 50 years) and 36.2% (50–69 years), and 28.3% (>69 years), respectively [47]. This discrepancy could be explained by the higher rate of treatment in younger patients, suggesting that patients with multiple metastatic sites could benefit from surgery and radiation therapy [47]. Overall, age at diagnosis is a strong independent prognostic factor for metastatic breast cancer patient survival and for predicting the site of metastasis [47].

2.7. Urokinase-type plasminogen activator (uPA) and plasminogen activator type 1 inhibitor (PAI-1)

The urokinase-type plasminogen activator (uPA), which is a serine protease, and its inhibitor plasminogen activator type 1 inhibitor (PAI-1) are involved in the degradation of extracellular matrix, which is a crucial process in the initial stages of metastasis [48]. Although PAI-1 inhibits uPA activity, it has been found to promote tumor invasion and angiogenesis through other means [49]. As such, both uPA and PAI-1 could potentially be used as metastasis prognostic markers. Supporting this, high uPA and PAI-1 levels are correlated with lower metastasis-free survival and overall survival in breast cancer patients [50–54]. In addition to being a prognostic marker, both uPA and PAI-1 could be used as predictive biomarkers for adjuvant therapy. In a study, patients with high uPA and PAI-1 levels benefited significantly from adjuvant chemotherapy compared to patients with low uPA and PAI-1 levels [55]. This indicates that patients with high uPA and PAI-1 levels could be treated with chemotherapy after surgery.

Furthermore, since uPA functions by binding to its receptor, urokinase plasminogen activator receptor (uPAR), the interaction could be exploited for metastasis targeted therapy. Indeed, one of the developments in this area is the use of an antibody to target uPAR [56, 57]. Remarkably, the antibody is shown to inhibit invasion of cancer cells and induce apoptosis, indicating its potential use for metastatic breast cancer [57].

2.8. Gene expression profiling

With the advent of gene expression profiling, treatment options are expected to shift toward a more personalized approach [58]. Although the idea of sequencing every cancer patient for individualized prognosis and treatment remains elusive, using multigene signatures to stratify patients into groups with different prognosis and therapeutic options has been very well established and routinely used in clinics. The first report of using high throughput methods for stratification of patients started in diffuse large B-cell lymphoma (DLBCL) patients [59, 60]. Based on their gene signatures from microarray, two subtypes of DLBCL, namely germinal center B-like DLBCL and activated B-like DLBCL, were characterized and were prognostic of overall survival [59]. In fact, molecular subtypes of breast cancer (mentioned in previous sections) were also identified using microarray-based gene expression profiling and are routinely used in clinical settings for prognosis [20–23].

Following the clinical success of using multigene signatures to identify and stratify patients with different clinical outcomes, two different gene expression profiling panels have emerged and are currently used in clinical settings. Each platform relies on different gene panel and is routinely used for predicting metastasis risk, local and distant metastasis recurrence, and for treatment decisions [61]. These are Oncotype DX and MammaPrint. Other gene expression profiling panels such as the PAM50 [62], two-gene expression ratio [63], and MapQuant DX [64] are not covered here [65].

Oncotype DX is the most widely used multigene panel tool for the prediction of distant recurrence risk in the United States [2]. It is a reverse-transcription-polymerase-chain-reaction (RT-PCR) based assay which measures the expression of 16 cancer-related genes and 5 reference genes in tumor tissue [9]. Based on the expression level of the 21 genes, an algorithm computes a recurrence score which quantifies the probability of distant recurrence [9]. Using the recurrence score, a patient with higher score is considered high risk and would likely benefit from chemotherapy as compared to a patient with lower score who could avoid chemotherapy altogether [2, 9].

Oncotype DX is currently utilized in clinics to predict distant recurrence for ER+, lymph node negative breast cancer patients who had prior tamoxifen treatment [9]. In the original paper, 51% of ER+, lymph node negative, tamoxifen-treated patients were classified under low-risk, and indeed, only 6.8% of this group had distant recurrence within 10 years [9]. This is in comparison with the high-risk group consisting of 27% of patients who had a 30.5% distant recurrence rate within 10 years [9]. In addition, recurrence score could also predict overall survival and relapse-free survival [9]. In support, a recent prospective validation study showed that Oncotype DX could potentially select low recurrence patients with high probability to forgo chemotherapy [66]. Five-year recurrence free rate from all sites and distant site, for patients with low recurrence score and only underwent tamoxifen treatment, were a high 98.7 and 99.3%, respectively [66]. Overall survival and invasive disease-free rates were up to 98 and 93.8%, respectively [66]. These findings show the clinical applicability of Oncotype DX to select for patients who could forgo chemotherapy and its unnecessary side effects.

The second most commonly used multigene panel for prognosis and treatment decision is MammaPrint [65, 67]. It utilizes an oligonucleotide microarray to measure the expression of 70 genes to identify gene signatures that stratify patients into a "good" or "poor" prognosis that predicts metastasis risk in lymph node negative early breast cancer patients [68–72]. Sensitivity and specificity of MammaPrint are 91 and 73%, respectively [3]. Genes involved in "poor" prognosis signature include angiogenesis, cell cycle, invasion, and metastasis [69].

In one of the earlier studies depicting the prognostic value of MammaPrint patient stratification, 10-year distant metastasis free probabilities were lower for "poor" prognosis group at 50.0% than in "good" prognosis group at 85.2% [68]. Overall survival rates were also significantly different between groups at 50.6 and 85.2% for "poor" and "good" prognosis groups correspondingly [68].

In a follow-up study with longer term survival statistics, 25-year distant metastasis free survival was significantly lower for "poor" prognosis group (41.6%) as compared to "good" prognosis group (60.4%) [72]. Overall survival at 25 years also showed the same trend at 44.5 and 57.3% for "poor" and "good" prognosis groups, respectively [72]. These statistics show the relevance of using MammaPrint in clinical settings as a prognostic biomarker for metastasis risk and overall survival. It could also be applied as a predictive biomarker for selecting patients with "poor" prognosis for adjuvant treatment.

Overall, the importance of multigene expression profiling tools for prognosis and treatment decision in the clinic is apparent when compared to classical clinicopathological parameters which are determined by a trained pathologist. It is found that low agreement exists among pathologists in breast cancer grading as tumor grading includes a degree of subjectivity [9]. A study comparing the different gene expression profiling tools found that although different gene sets were used among different panels, 4 out of 5 (including Oncotype DX and MammaPrint) achieved high concordance in relation to predicting outcomes [73]. As such, tools like Oncotype DX and MammaPrint stand out in this aspect.

3. New biomarkers

3.1. Improved gene expression profiling

Although the first generation gene expression profiling tools, Oncotype DX, and MammaPrint have greatly advanced the prognosis of breast cancer patients for metastasis risk and distant recurrence, a major drawback is that they are unable to accurately predict late distant recurrence of more than 5 years [74]. Two newer gene expression profiling tools, EndoPredict and The Breast Cancer Index, have emerged successful in this aspect [74].

EndoPredict is a RT-PCR-based assay, which measures the expression of eight cancer genes and three housekeeping genes to stratify patients into high- and low-risk distant recurrence groups [75–77]. A newer version of it combines the 11 gene expression with tumor size and nodal status to calculate a risk score termed the EPclin [76]. Patients with an EPclin score of less than 3.3 are classified as low-distant recurrence risk, while more than or equals to 3.3 are classified as high-distant recurrence risk [76]. The EPclin score is the best predictor of late relapse (>5 years), when compared to the earlier version of EndoPredict or to nodal status and tumor size alone [76]. Metastasis free survival for short term (less than 5) and long term (5–12 years) are also significantly different between the EPclin-stratified high- and low-risk groups, validating its applicability to predict metastasis [76]. In addition, distant recurrence free rates at 10 years in EPclin low-risk group is higher than in EPclin high-risk group, at 98.20 and 87.69%, respectively, depicting its ability to predict distant recurrence for longer time frames [76].

The breast cancer index (BCI) is another RT-PCR-based assay, which combines two independent biomarkers namely a set of five cell cycle genes and the HOXB13 and IL17BR gene ratio to determine the recurrence probability of early stage ER+, lymph node negative breast cancer patients [63, 78, 79]. Independently, both the five gene panel and the two gene ratio are associated with distant metastasis free survival rates [78]. However, when combined, three groups could be formed, low-, intermediate-, and high-risk groups, which are significantly predictive of metastasis occurrence [78]. Ten-year distant metastasis free survival for low-, intermediate-, and high-risk groups are 98, 87, and 60%, respectively [78]. Additionally, in a study comparing the prognostic ability of BCI with Oncotype DX and another gene panel, BCI emerged as the only test capable of significantly predicting both early and late distant metastasis recurrence, whereas the other two were only able to predict early recurrence [80].

In general, both EndoPredict and BCI seem to be superior as compared to the first-generation counterparts. This is particularly in terms of predicting longer term distant recurrence while also predictive of early recurrence [74].

3.2. Circulating tumor cells

An essential part of distant metastasis requires cells from the primary tumor to migrate into the bloodstream to spread throughout the body till it finds a secondary site to establish a secondary tumor [3]. As such, it is not surprising that circulating tumor cells (CTCs) in peripheral blood could be utilized as a prognostic indicator. The peripheral blood also represents an easily accessible region, which is an added advantage of using CTCs for prognosis [81].

The history of CTCs dates back as far as the nineteenth century when researchers have just begun to study the concept of tumor cells shedding from primary tumor [82, 83]. Today, there are multiple platforms for the isolation and detection of CTCs in the peripheral blood in clinical use [84]. Termed the "golden standard", the CellSearch system is the only FDA-approved platform for such purpose in breast, prostate, and colorectal cancer [84]. The problems associated with detection of CTCs are its rare amount in the peripheral blood and the absence of a universal surface marker for different cancer cell types [84]. The CellSearch system overcomes these sensitivity and specificity issues through the use of an antibody to capture CTCs and poststaining the captured CTCs for identification [84]. Specifically, an avidin-biotin anti-EpCAM antibody complex is used to bind CTCs followed by a magnetic capture to isolate CTCs [84–86]. Following which, the captured pool of cells is stained with DAPI and cytokeratins CK8, CK18, and CK19 to select for nucleated and epithelial cells, respectively [84–86]. Additionally, to differentiate from circulating white blood cells, anti-CD45 is used to further isolate CTCs [84–86]. Other systems using size [87–89], density [90], and microfluidic [91] characteristics of CTCs for isolation exist but are not covered in this chapter [81].

Enumerating CTCs in peripheral blood holds immense potential in clinics. The early paper using the CellSearch system to study progression of metastatic breast cancer provided many useful information [86]. The first thing noted was that CTCs were only present in metastatic breast cancer patients. Two or more CTCs per 7.5 mL of blood were present in metastatic breast cancer patients, while CTCs were rare (less than or equal to 1) in both healthy and benign breast cancer women [86]. Next, CTCs were independent prognostic marker of overall survival and progression-free survival [86]. After new treatment, patients with high level of CTCs (CTCs $\geq$5) had a significantly lower median progression-free survival and overall survival than patients with low level of CTCs (CTCs <5), at 2.1 months versus 7.0 months for progression-free survival and 8.2 months versus >18 months for overall survival, respectively [86]. Additionally, the prognostic value of CTCs for overall survival and progression-free survival is also validated in two other studies, wherein one of it is a prospective study with metastatic breast cancer patients who were not treated previously [92, 93].

In terms of treatment, median progression-free and overall survival differed significantly between patients with CTCs ≥5 before treatment and CTCs <5 after treatment (1st group) and patients with decrease in CTCs after treatment but still ≥5 after treatment (2nd group) [86]. Median overall survival and progression free survival for 1st group are 7.6 months and 14.6 months, and for the 2nd group, 2.1 months and 9.2 months, respectively [86]. This suggests that CTCs could potentially be used to measure treatment efficiency, although the authors cautioned against this interpretation [86]. Following this, two other studies have also observed CTCs as a predictor of therapy efficiency for metastatic breast cancer [94, 95].

3.3. TIP60

Tat-interactive protein 60 kDa (TIP60) is a haploinsufficient tumor suppressor involved in both early and late stage breast cancer [96–99]. In particular for late stage progression, TIP60 is known to regulate epithelial to mesenchymal transition, an important pathway for cellular metastasis [96, 97]. Both *in vitro* and mouse models have shown that loss of TIP60 results in increased metastatic breast cancer cell migration and invasion, indicating that therapies to increase TIP60 in breast cancer could be a potential therapeutic approach for metastatic breast cancer [96, 97]. Additionally, the microRNA miR-22 inhibits the expression of TIP60, thereby making it a promoter of metastasis and a potential therapeutic target for metastatic breast cancer [97]. More importantly, both miR-22 and TIP60 are prognostic of overall survival and metastasis free survival [96, 97]. As such, both miR-22 and TIP60 expression levels would be invaluable tools in clinics to predict metastatic probability and prognosis of overall survival.

4. Future directions/conclusions

Using only clinicopathological characteristics for assessing metastasis risk, the St Gallen criteria and National Institutes of Health criteria each classified a low 15 and 7% of lymph node negative breast cancer as low metastasis risk, respectively [3, 68]. However, after 10 years, up to 25% of the low-risk group developed distant recurrence [3, 68]. In addition, only slightly less than half (45%) of high-risk patients developed metastasis, indicating that the remaining 55% of "high-risk" patients had adjuvant treatment and tolerated its unnecessary effects [3, 68]. In contrast, using MammaPrint in the same cohort, a high 60% of total patients were categorized as low risk, out of which only 13% of these low-risk patients developed metastasis after 10 years, showing that as many as 52.2% of overall patients were safely spared from adjuvant therapy, as compared to 5.25 to 11.25% of overall patients stratified using clinicopathological characteristics [3, 68]. These findings clearly delineate the superiority of gene expression panels for prognosis as compared to just clinicopathological characteristics.

A more beneficial solution would be to combine both clinicopathological markers and multigene expression profiling to have an additive or synergistic effect in prediction for the betterment of patient prognosis and prediction of treatment outcomes. An example is the multigene expression EPclin risk score which combines its predecessor, the EndoPredict with tumor size, and nodal status to better predict distant metastatic recurrence as compared to if the markers were used individually [76].

However, a significant problem still exists in the field of prognosis for metastatic breast cancer. Many of the gene expression profiling tools, such as Oncotype DX and BCI, are suitable only for prediction of distant metastasis recurrence in ER+, lymph node negative metastatic breast cancers [74, 100]. As such, it represents a gap in the identification of prognostic markers for other subtypes. For this, newer markers like the detection of CTCs which does not discriminate between subtypes may be used. TIP60 which also does not discriminate between subtypes in risk-free survival rates [98] may be explored and could potential be used as a prognostic biomarker for breast cancer metastasis. Other upcoming biomarkers which are not discussed here such as blood-based biomarkers [101] and long noncoding RNA [102] also holds immense potential as prognostic markers in breast cancer metastasis.

Overall, the field of metastatic breast cancer prognosis has come a long way, beginning with clinicopathological markers to molecular subtypes to multigene expression profiling and eventually CTCs. Continuing on, it is likely that future direction for this field will entail combining existing biomarkers together or with newly identified biomarkers, leading to tremendous improvements in metastatic breast cancer prognosis and in predicting metastasis.

Author details

Kwok Kin Lee[1], Wee Joo Chng[1,2,3] and Sudhakar Jha[1,4*]

*Address all correspondence to: csisjha@nus.edu.sg

1 Cancer Science Institute of Singapore, National University of Singapore, Singapore

2 Department of Medicine, Yong Loo Lin School of Medicine, National University of Singapore, Singapore

3 Department of Haematology-Oncology, National University Cancer Institute of Singapore, National University Health System, Singapore

4 Department of Biochemistry, Yong Loo Lin School of Medicine, National University of Singapore, Singapore

References

[1] Siegel RL, Miller KD, Jemal A. Cancer statistics, 2018. CA: A Cancer Journal for Clinicians. 2018;**68**(1):7-30

[2] Breast Cancer Facts & Figures 2017-2018. Atlanta: American Cancer Society, Inc.; 2017

[3] Weigelt B, Peterse JL, van 't Veer LJ. Breast cancer metastasis: Markers and models. Nature Reviews. Cancer. 2005;**5**(8):591-602

[4] Berry DA et al. Effect of screening and adjuvant therapy on mortality from breast cancer. The New England Journal of Medicine. 2005;**353**(17):1784-1792

[5] Cancer Facts & Figures 2018. Atlanta: American Cancer Society; 2018

[6] Eng LG et al. Ten-year survival in women with primary stage IV breast cancer. Breast Cancer Research and Treatment. 2016;**160**(1):145-152

[7] Eifel P et al. National Institutes of Health consensus development conference statement: Adjuvant therapy for breast cancer, November 1-3, 2000. Journal of the National Cancer Institute. 2001;**93**(13):979-989

[8] den Hollander P, Savage MI, Brown PH. Targeted therapy for breast cancer prevention. Frontiers in Oncology. 2013;**3**:250

[9] Paik S et al. A multigene assay to predict recurrence of tamoxifen-treated, node-negative breast cancer. New England Journal of Medicine. 2004;**351**(27):2817-2826

[10] Li J et al. Identification of high-quality cancer prognostic markers and metastasis network modules. Nature Communications. 2010;**1**:34

[11] Cserni G et al. The new TNM-based staging of breast cancer. Virchows Archiv. 2018;**472**(5): 697-703

[12] Page DL. Prognosis and breast cancer. Recognition of lethal and favorable prognostic types. The American Journal of Surgical Pathology. 1991;**15**(4):334-349

[13] Koscielny S et al. Breast cancer: Relationship between the size of the primary tumour and the probability of metastatic dissemination. British Journal of Cancer. 1984;**49**(6):709-715

[14] Rosen PP et al. Pathological prognostic factors in stage I (T1N0M0) and stage II (T1N1M0) breast carcinoma: A study of 644 patients with median follow-up of 18 years. Journal of Clinical Oncology. 1989;**7**(9):1239-1251

[15] Carter CL, Allen C, Henson DE. Relation of tumor size, lymph node status, and survival in 24,740 breast cancer cases. Cancer. 1989;**63**(1):181-187

[16] Rakha EA et al. Breast cancer prognostic classification in the molecular era: The role of histological grade. Breast Cancer Research. 2010;**12**(4):207

[17] Elston CW, Ellis IO. Pathological prognostic factors in breast cancer. I. The value of histological grade in breast cancer: Experience from a large study with long-term follow-up. Histopathology. 1991;**19**(5):403-410

[18] de Mascarel I et al. Obvious peritumoral emboli: An elusive prognostic factor reappraised. Multivariate analysis of 1320 node-negative breast cancers. European Journal of Cancer. 1998;**34**(1):58-65

[19] Pinder SE et al. Pathological prognostic factors in breast cancer. III. Vascular invasion: Relationship with recurrence and survival in a large study with long-term follow-up. Histopathology. 1994;**24**(1):41-47

[20] Sotiriou C et al. Breast cancer classification and prognosis based on gene expression profiles from a population-based study. Proceedings of the National Academy of Sciences. 2003;**100**(18):10393

[21] Perou CM et al. Molecular portraits of human breast tumours. Nature. 2000;**406**(6797): 747-752

[22] Sørlie T et al. Repeated observation of breast tumor subtypes in independent gene expression data sets. Proceedings of the National Academy of Sciences. 2003;**100**(14):8418

[23] Sørlie T et al. Gene expression patterns of breast carcinomas distinguish tumor subclasses with clinical implications. Proceedings of the National Academy of Sciences. 2001;**98**(19): 10869

[24] Wu X et al. Pattern of local recurrence and distant metastasis in breast cancer by molecular subtype. Cureus. 2016;**8**(12):e924

[25] Lobbezoo DJ et al. Prognosis of metastatic breast cancer subtypes: The hormone receptor/HER2-positive subtype is associated with the most favorable outcome. Breast Cancer Research and Treatment. 2013;**141**(3):507-514

[26] Kennecke H et al. Metastatic behavior of breast cancer subtypes. Journal of Clinical Oncology. 2010;**28**(20):3271-3277

[27] Renoir JM, Marsaud V, Lazennec G. Estrogen receptor signaling as a target for novel breast cancer therapeutics. Biochemical Pharmacology. 2013;**85**(4):449-465

[28] Early Breast Cancer Trialists' Collaborative Group. Relevance of breast cancer hormone receptors and other factors to the efficacy of adjuvant tamoxifen: Patient-level meta-analysis of randomised trials. Lancet. 2011;**378**(9793):771-784

[29] Dowsett M et al. Meta-analysis of breast cancer outcomes in adjuvant trials of aromatase inhibitors versus tamoxifen. Journal of Clinical Oncology. 2010;**28**(3):509-518

[30] Burstein HJ et al. Adjuvant endocrine therapy for women with hormone receptor–positive breast cancer: American Society of clinical oncology clinical practice guideline focused update. Journal of Clinical Oncology. 2014;**32**(21):2255-2269

[31] Pagani O et al. Adjuvant exemestane with ovarian suppression in premenopausal breast cancer. The New England Journal of Medicine. 2014;**371**(2):107-118

[32] Zhu X, Verma S. Targeted therapy in HER2-positive metastatic breast cancer: A review of the literature. Current Oncology. 2015;**22**(Suppl 1):S19-S28

[33] Seshadri R et al. Clinical significance of HER-2/neu oncogene amplification in primary breast cancer. The South Australian Breast Cancer Study Group. Journal of Clinical Oncology. 1993;**11**(10):1936-1942

[34] Slamon DJ et al. Human breast cancer: Correlation of relapse and survival with amplification of the HER-2/neu oncogene. Science. 1987;**235**(4785):177-182

[35] Slamon DJ et al. Use of chemotherapy plus a monoclonal antibody against HER2 for metastatic breast cancer that overexpresses HER2. The New England Journal of Medicine. 2001;**344**(11):783-792

[36] Marty M et al. Randomized phase II trial of the efficacy and safety of trastuzumab combined with docetaxel in patients with human epidermal growth factor receptor 2-positive

metastatic breast cancer administered as first-line treatment: The M77001 study group. Journal of Clinical Oncology. 2005;**23**(19):4265-4274

[37] Royce M, Herold K. New agents for the management of advanced HER2-positive breast cancer. Journal of the Advanced Practitioner in Oncology. 2016;**7**(3):295-298

[38] Swain SM et al. Pertuzumab, trastuzumab, and docetaxel in HER2-positive metastatic breast cancer. The New England Journal of Medicine. 2015;**372**(8):724-734

[39] Verma S et al. Trastuzumab emtansine for HER2-positive advanced breast cancer. The New England Journal of Medicine. 2012;**367**(19):1783-1791

[40] Lewis Phillips GD et al. Targeting HER2-positive breast cancer with trastuzumab-DM1, an antibody-cytotoxic drug conjugate. Cancer Research. 2008;**68**(22):9280-9290

[41] Carey LA et al. The triple negative paradox: Primary tumor chemosensitivity of breast cancer subtypes. Clinical Cancer Research. 2007;**13**(8):2329-2334

[42] Gong Y et al. Impact of molecular subtypes on metastatic breast cancer patients: A SEER population-based study. Scientific Reports. 2017;**7**:45411

[43] Smid M et al. Subtypes of breast cancer show preferential site of relapse. Cancer Research. 2008;**68**(9):3108-3114

[44] Soni A et al. Breast cancer subtypes predispose the site of distant metastases. American Journal of Clinical Pathology. 2015;**143**(4):471-478

[45] Largillier R et al. Prognostic factors in 1,038 women with metastatic breast cancer. Annals of Oncology. 2008;**19**(12):2012-2019

[46] Imkampe A, Bendall S, Bates T. The significance of the site of recurrence to subsequent breast cancer survival. European Journal of Surgical Oncology. 2007;**33**(4):420-423

[47] Chen M-T et al. Comparison of patterns and prognosis among distant metastatic breast cancer patients by age groups: A SEER population-based analysis. Scientific Reports. 2017;**7**:9254

[48] Duffy MJ. Urokinase plasminogen activator and its inhibitor, PAI-1, as prognostic markers in breast cancer: From pilot to level 1 evidence studies. Clinical Chemistry. 2002; **48**(8):1194-1197

[49] Andreasen PA et al. The urokinase-type plasminogen activator system in cancer metastasis: A review. International Journal of Cancer. 1997;**72**(1):1-22

[50] Janicke F, Schmitt M, Graeff H. Clinical relevance of the urokinase-type and tissue-type plasminogen activators and of their type 1 inhibitor in breast cancer. Seminars in Thrombosis and Hemostasis. 1991;**17**(3):303-312

[51] Foekens JA et al. The urokinase system of plasminogen activation and prognosis in 2780 breast cancer patients. Cancer Research. 2000;**60**(3):636-643

[52] Konecny G et al. Her-2/neu and urokinase-type plasminogen activator and its inhibitor in breast cancer. Clinical Cancer Research. 2001;**7**(8):2448-2457

[53] Janicke F et al. Randomized adjuvant chemotherapy trial in high-risk, lymph node-negative breast cancer patients identified by urokinase-type plasminogen activator and plasminogen activator inhibitor type 1. Journal of the National Cancer Institute. 2001;**93**(12):913-920

[54] Harbeck N et al. Ten-year analysis of the prospective multicentre Chemo-N0 trial validates American Society of Clinical Oncology (ASCO)-recommended biomarkers uPA and PAI-1 for therapy decision making in node-negative breast cancer patients. European Journal of Cancer. 2013;**49**(8):1825-1835

[55] Harbeck N et al. Enhanced benefit from adjuvant chemotherapy in breast cancer patients classified high-risk according to urokinase-type plasminogen activator (uPA) and plasminogen activator inhibitor type 1 (n = 3424). Cancer Research. 2002;**62**(16):4617-4622

[56] Mazar AP, Ahn RW, O'Halloran TV. Development of novel therapeutics targeting the urokinase plasminogen activator receptor (uPAR) and their translation toward the clinic. Current Pharmaceutical Design. 2011;**17**(19):1970-1978

[57] Rabbani SA, Gladu J. Urokinase receptor antibody can reduce tumor volume and detect the presence of occult tumor metastases in vivo. Cancer Research. 2002;**62**(8):2390-2397

[58] Anderson MW, Schrijver I. Next generation DNA sequencing and the future of genomic medicine. Genes. 2010;**1**(1):38-69

[59] Alizadeh AA et al. Distinct types of diffuse large B-cell lymphoma identified by gene expression profiling. Nature. 2000;**403**(6769):503-511

[60] Bertucci F et al. Gene expression profiling identifies molecular subtypes of inflammatory breast cancer. Cancer Research. 2005;**65**(6):2170

[61] Kimbung S, Loman N, Hedenfalk I. Clinical and molecular complexity of breast cancer metastases. Seminars in Cancer Biology. 2015;**35**:85-95

[62] Parker JS et al. Supervised risk predictor of breast cancer based on intrinsic subtypes. Journal of Clinical Oncology. 2009;**27**(8):1160-1167

[63] Ma X-J et al. A two-gene expression ratio predicts clinical outcome in breast cancer patients treated with tamoxifen. Cancer Cell;**5**(6):607-616

[64] Loi S et al. Definition of clinically distinct molecular subtypes in estrogen receptor-positive breast carcinomas through genomic grade. Journal of Clinical Oncology. 2007;**25**(10):1239-1246

[65] Marchionni L et al. A simple and reproducible breast cancer prognostic test. BMC Genomics. 2013;**14**:336-336

[66] Sparano JA et al. Prospective validation of a 21-gene expression assay in breast cancer. New England Journal of Medicine. 2015;**373**(21):2005-2014

[67] Committee on the Review of Omics-Based Tests for Predicting Patient Outcomes in Clinical, Trials et al. In: Micheel CM, Nass SJ, Omenn GS, editors. Evolution of Translational

Omics: Lessons Learned and the Path Forward. Washington (DC), US: National Academies Press; 2012. Copyright 2012 by the National Academy of Sciences. All rights reserved

[68] van de Vijver MJ et al. A gene-expression signature as a predictor of survival in breast cancer. The New England Journal of Medicine. 2002;**347**(25):1999-2009

[69] van 't Veer LJ et al. Gene expression profiling predicts clinical outcome of breast cancer. Nature. 2002;**415**(6871):530-536

[70] Glas AM et al. Converting a breast cancer microarray signature into a high-throughput diagnostic test. BMC Genomics. 2006;**7**:278-278

[71] Buyse M et al. Validation and clinical utility of a 70-gene prognostic signature for women with node-negative breast cancer. Journal of the National Cancer Institute. 2006;**98**(17):1183-1192

[72] Drukker CA et al. Long-term impact of the 70-gene signature on breast cancer outcome. Breast Cancer Research and Treatment. 2014;**143**(3):587-592

[73] Fan C et al. Concordance among gene-expression–based predictors for breast cancer. New England Journal of Medicine. 2006;**355**(6):560-569

[74] Győrffy B et al. Multigene prognostic tests in breast cancer: Past, present, future. Breast Cancer Research : BCR. 2015;**17**(1):11

[75] Filipits M et al. A new molecular predictor of distant recurrence in ER-positive, HER2-negative breast cancer adds independent information to conventional clinical risk factors. Clinical Cancer Research. 2011;**17**(18):6012-6020

[76] Dubsky P et al. The EndoPredict score provides prognostic information on late distant metastases in ER+/HER2– breast cancer patients. British Journal of Cancer. 2013; **109**(12):2959-2964

[77] Muller BM et al. The EndoPredict gene-expression assay in clinical practice: Performance and impact on clinical decisions. PLoS One. 2013;**8**(6):e68252

[78] Ma XJ et al. A five-gene molecular grade index and HOXB13:IL17BR are complementary prognostic factors in early stage breast cancer. Clinical Cancer Research. 2008; **14**(9):2601-2608

[79] Jankowitz RC et al. Prognostic utility of the breast cancer index and comparison to adjuvant! Online in a clinical case series of early breast cancer. Breast Cancer Research. 2011;**13**(5):R98

[80] Sgroi DC et al. Prediction of late distant recurrence in patients with oestrogen-receptor-positive breast cancer: A prospective comparison of the breast-cancer index (BCI) assay, 21-gene recurrence score, and IHC4 in the TransATAC study population. The Lancet Oncology. 2013;**14**(11):1067-1076

[81] Banys-Paluchowski M et al. Circulating tumor cells in breast cancer--current status and perspectives. Critical Reviews in Oncology/Hematology. 2016;**97**:22-29

[82] Paget S. The distribution of secondary growths in cancer of the breast. The Lancet. 1889;**133**(3421):571-573

[83] Ashworth T. A case of cancer in which cells similar to those in the tumours were seen in the blood after death. The Australasian Medical Journal. 1869;**14**:146-149

[84] Zhou L et al. Circulating tumor cells: Silent predictors of metastasis. F1000Research. 2017;**6**: pii. F1000 Faculty Rev-1445

[85] Kagan M et al. A sample preparation and analysis system for identification of circulating tumor cells. Journal of Clinical Ligand Assay. 2002;**25**(1):104-110

[86] Cristofanilli M et al. Circulating tumor cells, disease progression, and survival in metastatic breast cancer. New England Journal of Medicine. 2004;**351**(8):781-791

[87] Kulemann B et al. Circulating tumor cells found in patients with localized and advanced pancreatic cancer. Pancreas. 2015;**44**(4):547-550

[88] Freidin MB et al. An assessment of diagnostic performance of a filter-based antibody-independent peripheral blood circulating tumour cell capture paired with cytomorphologic criteria for the diagnosis of cancer. Lung Cancer. 2014;**85**(2):182-185

[89] Lin HK et al. Portable filter-based microdevice for detection and characterization of circulating tumor cells. Clinical Cancer Research. 2010;**16**(20):5011-5018

[90] Muller V et al. Circulating tumor cells in breast cancer: Correlation to bone marrow micrometastases, heterogeneous response to systemic therapy and low proliferative activity. Clinical Cancer Research. 2005;**11**(10):3678-3685

[91] Riahi R et al. A novel microchannel-based device to capture and analyze circulating tumor cells (CTCs) of breast cancer. International Journal of Oncology. 2014;**44**(6):1870-1878

[92] Cristofanilli M et al. Circulating tumor cells: A novel prognostic factor for newly diagnosed metastatic breast cancer. Journal of Clinical Oncology. 2005;**23**(7):1420-1430

[93] Bidard FC et al. Clinical validity of circulating tumour cells in patients with metastatic breast cancer: A pooled analysis of individual patient data. The Lancet Oncology. 2014;**15**(4):406-414

[94] Hayes DF et al. Circulating tumor cells at each follow-up time point during therapy of metastatic breast cancer patients predict progression-free and overall survival. Clinical Cancer Research. 2006;**12**(14 Pt 1):4218-4224

[95] Budd GT et al. Circulating tumor cells versus imaging–predicting overall survival in metastatic breast cancer. Clinical Cancer Research. 2006;**12**(21):6403-6409

[96] Gorrini C et al. Tip60 is a haplo-insufficient tumour suppressor required for an oncogene-induced DNA damage response. Nature. 2007;**448**(7157):1063-1067

[97] Pandey AK et al. TIP60-miR-22 axis as a prognostic marker of breast cancer progression. Oncotarget. 2015;**6**(38):41290-41306

[98] Bassi C et al. The acetyltransferase Tip60 contributes to mammary tumorigenesis by modulating DNA repair. Cell Death and Differentiation. 2016;**23**(7):1198-1208

[99] Zhang Y et al. TIP60 inhibits metastasis by ablating DNMT1-SNAIL2-driven epithelial-mesenchymal transition program. Journal of Molecular Cell Biology. 2016;**8**(5):384-399

[100] Gong G et al. A new molecular prognostic score for predicting the risk of distant metastasis in patients with HR+/HER2− early breast cancer. Scientific Reports. 2017;**7**:45554

[101] Berghuis AM et al. Detecting blood-based biomarkers in metastatic breast cancer: A systematic review of their current status and clinical utility. International Journal of Molecular Sciences. 2017;**18**(2):363

[102] Zhang K et al. Long non-coding RNAs as novel biomarkers for breast cancer invasion and metastasis. Oncology Letters. 2017;**14**(2):1895-1904

12

Cancer, Carcinogens and Screening in the Kidney

Michael Higgins, Ismael Obaidi and Tara McMorrow

Abstract

This chapter examines a number of different aspects of renal cancer. Firstly, an introduction into the numerous forms of renal cancers is provided, focusing on renal cell carcinomas their causes and the different treatment options currently available. This chapter also takes a look at renal cancer from a toxicological point of view. Due to the crucial role of the kidneys in blood filtration, this allows them to become susceptible to the exposure and accumulation of potentially carcinogenic chemicals. For this reason, renal carcinogens are looked at in detail focusing on the varying mechanisms of genotoxic renal carcinogens such as aristolochic acid and potassium bromate, and their non-genotoxic renal carcinogens counterparts including ochratoxin A and chlorothalonil. This chapter also examines the different methods currently used to detect a compound's carcinogenic potential, including the *in vitro* Ames test and animal based carcinogenicity screening methods.

Keywords: cancer, renal cancer, renal carcinogens, carcinogen screening, genotoxic/non-genotoxic carcinogens

1. Renal cancer

In 2016 alone there was a reported 62,700 cases of cancer involving the kidney and the renal pelvis worldwide [1]. Renal cell carcinoma (RCC) is the most common form of kidney cancer and makes up approximately 90–95% of all kidney cancers [2]. The incidence of RCC has been found to be higher in developed countries and is also more common amongst men, the exact reasons for this are currently unknown [3]. Five year survival rates for stage I RCC is 80–90%, for stage II it is 80%, for stage III it is approximately 60% and stage IV survival is estimated at just 10%. RCCs can be categorised into a number of subgroups; clear cell RCC (ccRCC), papillary RCC and chromophobe RCC [4].

Clear cell RCC (ccRCC) aptly named due to its clear cytoplasm. This clear cytoplasm is caused by its high glycogen and lipid content in the cytosol. ccRCC is the most common form of RCC, making up 70% of all kidney cancer cases [5]. ccRCC are thought to arise from proximal tubular epithelial cells and have a worse prognosis than papillary or chromophobe carcinoma [6, 7]. Approximately 95% of ccRCC are sporadic with the remaining 5% having a familial link [7]. Von Hippel–Lindau (VHL) disease is a hereditary condition that is heavily implicated in the development of familial ccRCC [8]. Mutations in the VHL are implicated in virtually all cases of familial ccRCC and approximately 57% of sporadic ccRCC [9]. Mutations in VHL also lead to the activation of hypoxia-inducible factor-1α (HIF1A) and hypoxia inducible factor-2α (HIF2A). Activation of these HIF related pathways leads to the activation of genes involved in angiogenesis and vascular endothelial growth [6]. The second most commonly mutated gene in ccRCC is polybromo 1 (PBRM1). Mutations in this gene are found in 45% of all ccRCC, its exact role in the development of tumour growth is not well understood, however it is thought that PBRM1s role is in controlling cell proliferation [10]. Components of the PI3K/AKT pathway are also believed to be implicated in ccRCC. In a study of a ccRCC database of 20 PI3K/AKT pathway panel components were assessed, 27% of the components were found to have genetic alterations related to PI3K/AKT pathway [11].

2. Other renal carcinomas

Similar to ccRCC papillary renal carcinomas are thought to arise from the epithelial cells in the proximal tubule [6]. Two hereditary conditions are linked with the development of papillary renal carcinomas, these conditions involve mutations in the MET proto-oncogene and fumarate hydrate genes, respectively [4]. However, this form of renal carcinomas is not well understood.

Chromophobe RCC (chRCC) makes up about 5% of all renal cancers [7]. chRCC is usually found in stage I or II and the tumour usually presents itself as a highly lobulated large mass, with a median tumour size of 6 cm [12]. The exact genetic alterations in chRCC are not well understood, however loss of entire chromosome 2, 10, 13, 17 and 21 occurs in almost all cases of chRCC. It is the least aggressive of all RCCs and for this reason has a low malignancy potential with a 10 year survival rate estimated at 80–90% [13]. Tumour development can also occur in the collecting duct of the kidney. This is a rare form of renal cancer that usually presents itself at an advanced stage and is believed to arise from the epithelial cells in the collecting duct [14].

3. Treatment

Fifty percent of all renal cancers are diagnosed when an ultrasound is carried out for symptoms including abdominal pain, hypertension, weight loss and elevated CRP, due to this difficulty in diagnosing renal cancer about 25% of patients present with cancer that has metastasized [15]. Surgery is commonly used in the treatment of renal cancer, depending on the severity of the disease the nephrectomy can be partial or radical. Radical nephrectomy involves the removal of the entire kidney, the adrenal gland and possibly the regionally located lymph nodes [16]. Although it is seen as an effective treatment of renal cancer, its use is associated with development of chronic kidney disease (CKD) and other cardiovascular related diseases [17]. Partial nephrectomy (also called nephron-sparing surgery) is also used, however this technique is underused due to the technical difficulties involved in removing only a part of the kidney where the tumour is localised. Partial nephrectomy has a 5 year survival rate of 87–90% [2]. Renal cell carcinomas are highly resistant to chemotherapeutic agents, for this reason the currently available drugs involve targeted therapies, including cytokines, mTOR inhibitors and targeting the vascular endothelial growth factor (VEGF) pathway [4]. A number of different cytokine related therapies are available such as interleukin 2 (IL-2) and interferon alpha (IFN-alpha), although these options have anti-cancer ability they are found not to be effective in cases where the tumour has metastasized [18]. The development of RCC is closely linked to a number of different components involved in angiogenesis, for this reason anti-angiogenic therapies have been developed targeting in particular the VEGF pathway, these include bevacizumab, sorafenib and sunitinib. These treatments have replaced interleukin related immunotherapies as a first line treatment following the partial or radical nephrectomy [19]. The mTOR pathway is involved in cell survival and its dysregulation has been shown to be heavily implicated in a number of forms of cancer [20]. Temsirolimus and everolimus, both mTOR inhibitors have been approved by the FDA for treatment of RCC, temsirolimus is considered the first line of treatment for metastatic RCC where the prognosis is poor, everolimus is used where the disease has progressed during treatment with VEGF targeted treatment [21].

4. Carcinogens

In the international agency for research on cancer (IARC) review of human carcinogens, they describe 'the term carcinogenic risk…is taken to mean that an agent is capable of causing cancer' [22]. Carcinogens are capable of inducing the process of carcinogenesis by variety of different mechanisms, these include by genotoxic (directly interacting with DNA) and non-genotoxic (indirectly lead to DNA instability) mechanisms. Carcinogenic factors have been grouped into these different categories; primary and secondary determining factor and favouring factors. Primary determining factors can be defined as a compound or chemical which is capable of inducing cancer by acting on a molecular level. Secondary determining factors are caused by hereditary factors where there is a genetic mutation with a familial link that ultimately results in cancer formation. Lastly, favouring factors are ones that may increase the possibility of tumorigenesis, these include diet, gender, age and possibly geographical location [23]. As well as carcinogens, there are also compounds called co-carcinogens that do not cause cancer by themselves but may increase the carcinogenic ability of other carcinogens [24].

5. Genotoxic vs. non-genotoxic carcinogens

Carcinogens can be classified by their mechanism of carcinogenicity. These categories include genotoxic and non-genotoxic carcinogens (**Figure 1**). In general, genotoxic carcinogens function

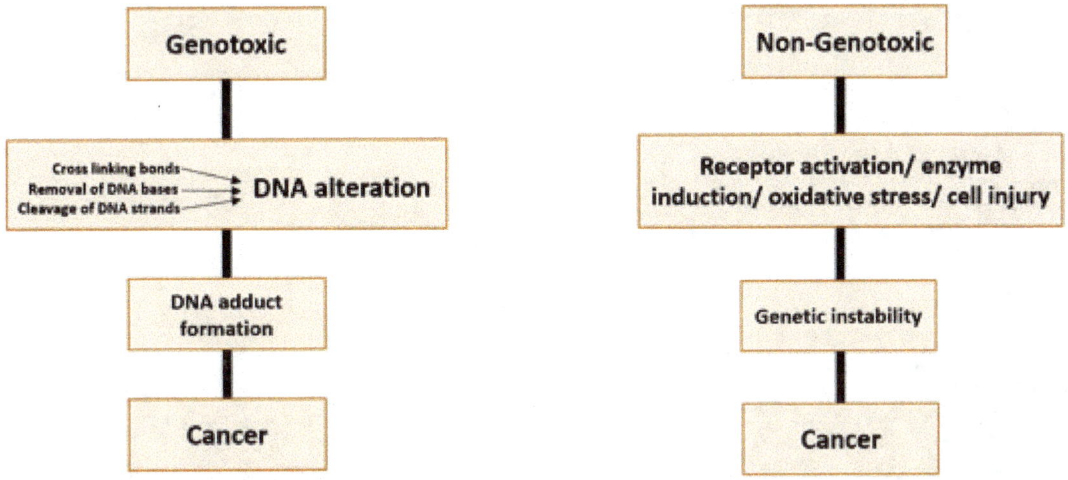

Figure 1. Mechanisms of genotoxicity and non-genotoxicity carcinogenicity. Carcinogens can be categorised as either genotoxic or non-genotoxic carcinogens. Genotoxic carcinogens induce the carcinogenesis process by directly interfering with DNA leading to genetic instability, if DNA replication occurs prior to the repair of the damage. Non-genotoxic carcinogens on the other hand indirectly interfere with DNA, this can occur by a number of mechanisms including ROS production.

by directly interfering with the patients DNA, this causes the formation of covalent bonds and eventually leads to the development of DNA adducts, while non-genotoxic carcinogens do not directly interact with DNA but act in a carcinogenic fashion through other mechanisms. Genotoxic carcinogens are believed to induce DNA damage by the formation of a cross-linking bond between two helices, the removal of DNA bases and the cleavage of DNA strands, all contributing to the alteration of DNA [25]. In general, this DNA damage would be repaired, however if DNA replication occurs before the damage is fixed the mutation may result in cancer development. As all cancers have alterations in DNA expression, non-genotoxic carcinogens are capable of inducing this genetic instability by an indirect manipulation of the natural regulation of DNA expression. In general non-genotoxic carcinogens appear to be more specific than genotoxic carcinogens in their carcinogenic ability, where they are often only capable of inducing cancer in one species, in one organ and sometimes in one sex [26]. Although the mechanisms of non-genotoxic carcinogenicity are less well understood than their genotoxic counterparts, attempts have been made to classify the main mechanisms of non-genotoxic carcinogenicity, these have included receptor activation, CYP450 induction, stimulation of oxidative stress, chronic cell injury, immunosuppression and interference with intercellular communication [26, 27].

6. Genotoxic carcinogens

Examples of genotoxic renal carcinogens are potassium bromate, 2-nitroflourene, benzo-A-pyrene, aristolochic acid and streptozotocin (**Figure 2**). Potassium bromate is a white crystal powder that is listed by the IARC as a group 2B carcinogen. Before its toxicity was established potassium bromate was widely utilised in the food industry, typically used to strengthen

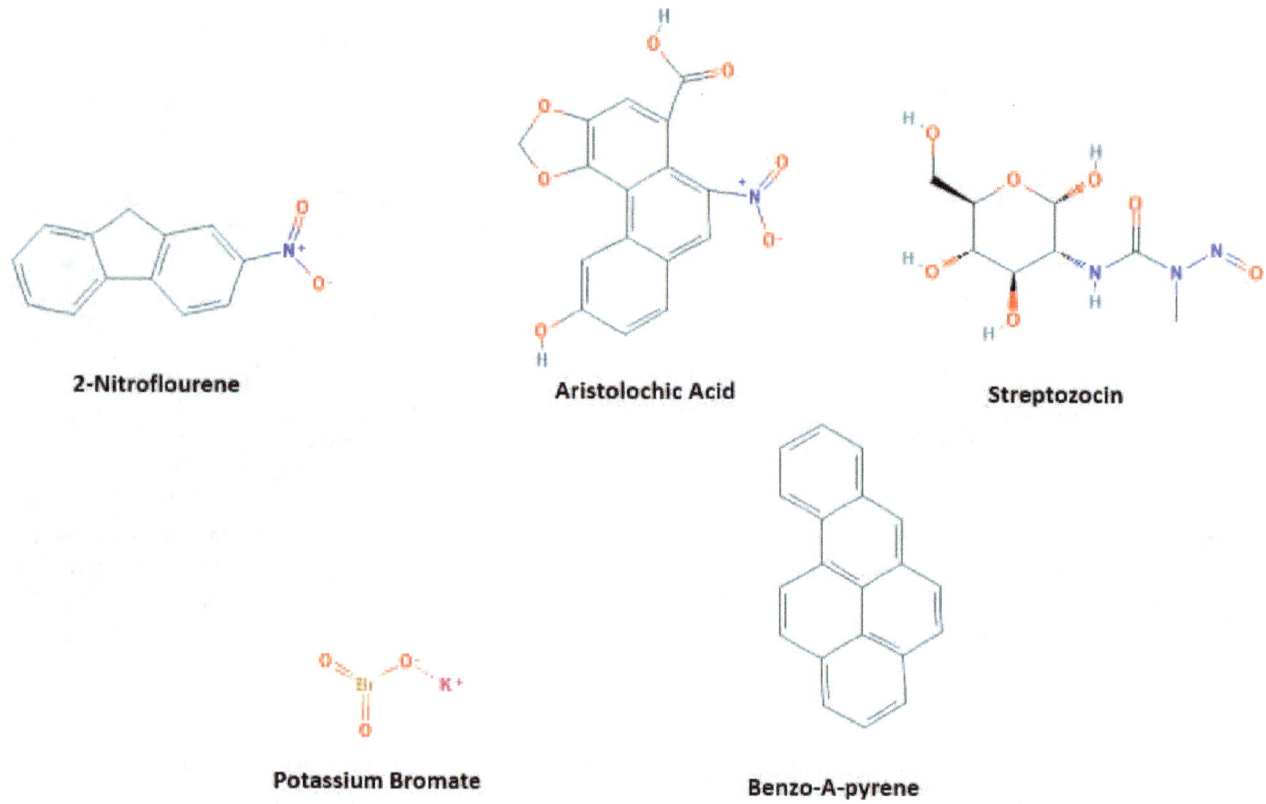

Figure 2. Chemical structure of a number genotoxic renal carcinogens (All chemical structures are adapted from https://www.ncbi.nlm.nih.gov/pccompound).

dough. Potassium bromate is a highly toxic compound that can cause oxidative DNA damage by inducing the formation of 8-hydroxyguanine (oh8Gua) [28]. 2-nitroflourene is found in the emissions from diesel fumes and kerosene heaters. This by-product of combustion is listed as a group 2B carcinogen. It has been shown to be capable of causing DNA adduct formation in rats, thus proving its genotoxicity [29]. Benzo-A-pyrene is another genotoxic carcinogen, listed as a group 1 human carcinogen. It causes a missense mutation in the tumour suppressor p53 [30]. Aristolochic acids are an extract from a plant commonly found in Asia. Plants containing aristolochic acids are classified as group 1 human carcinogens. Aristolochic acids are capable of producing DNA adducts found in tumour tissue of patients with urinary tract cancer in an area of Taiwan where the use of herbal medicine containing aristolochic acids is the most prevalent [31]. Lastly, streptozotocin is a 2B carcinogen with possible carcinogenic ability in humans and has been shown to cause tumour formation in rat kidneys and neoplastic transformation in human primary renal cells [32, 33].

7. Non-genotoxic carcinogens

Non-genotoxic renal carcinogens include ochratoxin A (OTA), monuron, bromodichloromethane and chlorothalonil (**Figure 3**). Ochratoxin A (OTA) is classified by the IARC as a group 2B carcinogen with possible human carcinogenic ability. OTA is a naturally occurring

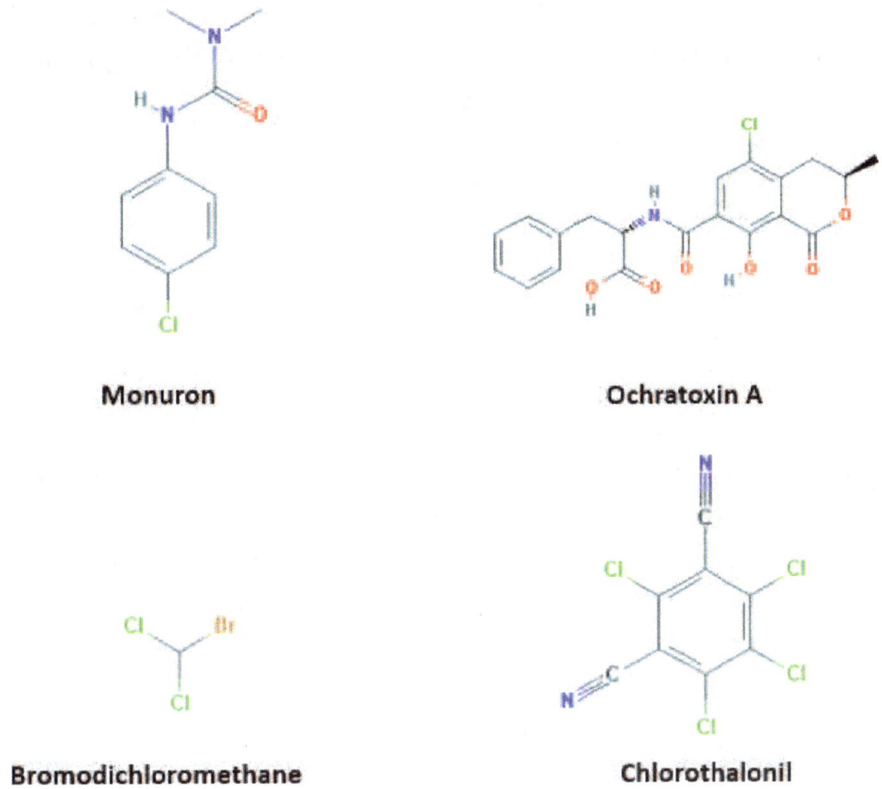

Figure 3. Chemical structure of a number of non-genotoxic renal carcinogens (All chemical structures are adapted from https://www.ncbi.nlm.nih.gov/pccompound).

mycotoxin, OTA causes contamination of food and drink products [34, 35]. OTA exposure is associated with Balkan endemic nephropathy that causes tumour formation in the urinary tract and the kidney [36]. Much work has been carried out to establish whether OTA is a genotoxic or non-genotoxic carcinogen. The formation of DNA adducts following OTA treatment would point to a possible genotoxic mechanism [37]. However, a review by Mally et al. refuted these findings where they claimed that OTA induced DNA adduct formation was not an important mechanism in OTAs overall carcinogenicity [38]. A study by Mantle et al. discussed that the reclassification of a carcinogen from a non-genotoxic to genotoxic has far reaching ramifications in terms of legislation, particularly with a contaminant found in the food and drinks industry, as a non-genotoxic carcinogen is said to have a 10-fold reduced risk to humans compared to genotoxic carcinogens [39]. This being said OTA's ability to induce the formation of reactive oxygen species is the strongest piece of evidence to suggest its non-genotoxicity [40].

Monuron is a phenylurea herbicide and a known renal carcinogen in rats as it has been shown to cause adenomas of the kidney and carcinomas of the liver [41]. In a study by Block et al. they showed that monuron induced an upregulation of genes involved in cell cycle and cell proliferation in the renal cortex [42]. Due to its unclear mechanism of carcinogenicity a number of studies have classified it as a non-genotoxic renal carcinogen [43]. Bromodichloromethane is a trihalomethane and according to the IARC is a proven carcinogen in rats and a suspected human carcinogen (Group 2B). It is also thought to cause some chromosomal aberrations

[44]. Chlorothalonil is a fungicide used in fungal control in a number of different crops. It is classified as a group 2B carcinogen to humans. A report by the *Environmental Protection Agency* in the United States declared that although an exact mechanism of carcinogenicity for chlorothalonil was unestablished it was agreed that the probable mechanism of carcinogenicity was through a non-genotoxic route as it behaved very similarly to other well established non-genotoxic carcinogens [45].

8. Bioactivation of carcinogens

In general cytochrome p450 monooxygenases play the role of detoxifying certain chemicals in the body, the opposite can also occur where these enzymes can bioactivate a particular compound where oxidation causes the conversion into a toxic by-product [46]. 2-acetylaminofluorene, a carcinogen capable of inducing tumour formation in the liver and kidney, is converted by a CYP450 mediated N-hydroxylation to produce a hydroxylamine which undergoes further transformation to become the deadly activated carcinogenic form [47]. Another example of CYP450 induced bioactivation, is the conversion of genotoxic benzo-A-pyrene to the carcinogenic benzo-a-pyrene-diol-epoxides by the enzymatic action of CYP1A1 and CYP1B1 [48]. Other families of enzymes can also carry out a similar function in converting carcinogens to their active form, including sulfotransferase. Sulfotransferase family cytosolic 1B member 1 (SULT1B1) converts the genotoxic carcinogen aristolochic acid to its active form by the action of sulfotransferase enzymes specifically SULT1B1 [49].

9. *In vitro* carcinogenicity screening

The Ames test is a bacterial mutagenicity assay, which is designed to be able to detect a chemical's ability to induce DNA damage that leads to gene mutations. The Ames test was first developed by the work of Bruce Ames, where he attempted to detect chemical mutagens with the use of bacteria [50]. This now well established assay works with the use of different strains of Salmonella that have mutations in genes involved in histidine synthesis, this causes the bacteria to be unable to grow [51]. The principle of the Ames test is based on whether a chemical can induce mutations that can cause the bacteria to again produce histidine which would then allow bacterial growth. To allow for the detection of various mutagens that function by different mechanisms different strains of salmonella are used that have varying mutations in the histidine operon [51]. Over the years the Ames test has undergone a number of modifications from the original method [52]. The most significant improvement was the incorporation of rat liver microsomes, which allowed for the screening of the original compound undergoing testing and any potentially carcinogenic metabolites that could be produced [53]. In more recent years human liver S9 microsomal fractions have been utilised to try and improve the ability to detect carcinogens in humans. The main limitation of the Ames test still remains, which is *Salmonella typhimurium* being a prokaryote, however it is still useful as an initial carcinogenic screen.

Other *in vitro* screens for identifying carcinogens are collectively called cell transformation assays (CTAs). CTAs were first developed in the 1960s, in a study by Berwald et al. they showed that a carcinogenic hydrocarbon (Benzo-A-pyrene) was able to cause a transformation from normal cells to tumour cells [54]. The three main assays used nowadays are the BALB/c 3 t3 assay (mouse embryo cells), the Syrian hamster embryo cells (SHE) assay and C3H10T1/2 assay (pluripotent stem cells) [55]. The Organisation for Economic Co-operation and Development (OECD) carried out a very comprehensive review of the BALB/c 3T3, SHE and C3H10T1/2 assays. Each of the assays were assessed based on a number of criteria including sensitivity, specificity and predictivity. The C3H10T1/2 assay had the highest predictivity percentage of human carcinogens at 95%, this was followed by SHE and BALB/c 3T3 assays that had predictivity of 88 and 77% respectively [56]. Being able to predict the carcinogenicity of non-genotoxic carcinogens has been a major problem in carcinogenic screening, this has been somewhat overcome with the use of CTAs as the transformation of cells occurs with both genotoxic and non-genotoxic carcinogens [57]. As well as being used as screens for carcinogens CTAs are also used in investigating tumour initiation, evaluating classes of chemicals and establishing mechanism of action of compounds [55].

In 2006, the EU introduced the registration, evaluation, authorisation and restriction of chemicals (REACH) initiative. The implementation of these policies highlights the needs for an improved protection of human and environmental health and safety by the identification of potentially dangerous chemicals and their exact mechanisms of hazardness. These regulations have been phased in gradually over an 11 year period since their inception [58]. This has led to much stricter rules and regulation being put in place for the chemical industry and the need for improved carcinogenicity screening methods. Although very useful in predicting carcinogenic potential, the limitations of *in vitro* testing methods must also be recognised. In a study by Walmsley et al. they highlight the challenges involved in *in vitro* screens where non-carcinogens can sometimes be determined as carcinogens and the difficulties this can cause [59].

10. Animal models based carcinogenicity screening

A 2 year rodent bioassay is widely used in carcinogenicity risk assessment. The goal of this screening method is to be able to predict potential carcinogenicity, while also characterising any potential tumour development. Before the 2-year study commences either or both 14 or 90 day pre-chronic study must be completed to establish maximum tolerated doses [60]. *The National Toxicology Programme* set out a protocol in 1976 that is still used today. This protocol involves the use of 50 animals per sex per group [61]. The testing system is categorised into acute, sub-chronic and chronic exposure and in some cases *in utero* exposure. The study concludes with a histological assessment to identify any potential carcinogenic related changes. Attempts have been made to improve on the traditional 2-year rodent method, one such suggestion by Cohen et al. proposed that the 2 year study should be replaced by an enhanced 13 week screen [62]. This study suggests a shorter more robust study is sufficient to predict carcinogenicity, thus reducing the number of animals used, as well as time and costs.

The proposed screening process involves a tiered approach where the first step is to establish genotoxicity, estrogenic/immunosuppressive activity, this would then be followed by a multi dose response screen of the compounds effects on cell proliferation and overall toxicity. However, this shortened screen could fail to predict the carcinogenicity of a chemical where the effects take longer than 13-weeks to emerge. The main arguments against the use of the well-established 2-year rodent bioassay will always be whether this particular animal is suitable for predicting disease in humans and the issue of the unnecessary use of animal models. These limitations have been further highlighted with the EU's commitment to 'reduce, refine and replace animal models' [63].

Due to the kidneys function as a blood filtration system, it allows for the exposure and accumulation of potentially carcinogenic substances, leaving the kidneys to be susceptible to the development of various forms of renal carcinomas. For this reason there is an ever increasing need to improve screening methods that are capable of detecting carcinogens particularly those known to induce the development of kidney cancers.

Acknowledgements

This work was supported by Science Foundation Ireland.

Author details

Michael Higgins, Ismael Obaidi and Tara McMorrow*

*Address all correspondence to: tara.mcmorrow@ucd.ie

School of Biomolecular and Biomedical Sciences, Conway Institute, University College Dublin, Dublin, Ireland

References

[1] Siegel RL, Miller KD, Jemal A. Cancer statistics, 2016. CA: A Cancer Journal for Clinicians. 2016;**66**(1):7-30

[2] Koul H et al. Molecular aspects of renal cell carcinoma: A review. American Journal of Cancer Research. 2011;**1**(2):240-254

[3] Znaor A, Lortet-Tieulent J, Laversanne M, Jemal A, Bray F. International variations and trends in renal cell carcinoma incidence and mortality. European Urology. March 2015;**67**(3):519-530

[4] Jonasch E, Gao JJ, Rathmell WK. Renal cell carcinoma. BMJ (British Medical Journal). 2014;**349**:g4797

[5] Cancer Facts & Figures 2013. American Cancer Society; 2013

[6] Cairns P. Renal cell carcinoma. Cancer Biomarkers. 2011;**9**(1-6):461-473

[7] Muglia VF, Prando A. Renal cell carcinoma: Histological classification and correlation with imaging findings. Radiologia Brasileira; **48**(3):166-174

[8] Su D et al. Renal cell carcinoma: molecular biology and targeted therapy. Current Opinion in Oncology; **26**(3):321-327

[9] Gnarra JR et al. Mutations of the VHL tumour suppressor gene in renal carcinoma. Nature Genetics. 1994;**7**(1):85-90

[10] Brugarolas J. Molecular genetics of clear-cell renal cell carcinoma. Journal of Clinical Oncology; **32**(18):1968-1976

[11] Guo HF et al. The PI3K/AKT pathway and renal cell carcinoma. Journal of Genetics and Genomics. 2015;**42**(7):343-353

[12] Vera-Badillo FE, Conde E, Duran I. Chromophobe renal cell carcinoma: A review of an uncommon entity. International Journal of Urology; **19**(10):894-900

[13] Amin MB et al. Chromophobe renal cell carcinoma: Histomorphologic characteristics and evaluation of conventional pathologic prognostic parameters in 145 cases. The American Journal of Surgical Pathology. 2008;**32**(12):1822-1834

[14] Dason S et al. Management of renal collecting duct carcinoma: A systematic review and the McMaster experience. Current Oncology; **20**(3):e223-e232

[15] Kell S. Renal cell carcinoma: Treatment options. British Journal of Nursing. 2011;**20**(9): 536-539

[16] Krabbe LM et al. Surgical management of metastatic renal cell carcinoma in the era of targeted therapies. World Journal of Urology; **32**(3):615-622

[17] Huang WC et al. Chronic kidney disease after nephrectomy in patients with renal cortical tumours: A retrospective cohort study. The Lancet Oncology. 2006;**7**(9):735-740

[18] Hutson TE. Renal cell carcinoma: Diagnosis and treatment, 1994-2003. Proceedings (Baylor University Medical Center). 2005;**18**(4):337-340

[19] Klatte T et al. Understanding the natural biology of kidney cancer: Implications for targeted cancer therapy. Revista de Urología. 2007;**9**(2):47-56

[20] Zarogoulidis P et al. mTOR pathway: A current, up-to-date mini-review (review). Oncology Letters; **8**(6):2367-2370

[21] Battelli C, Cho DC. mTOR inhibitors in renal cell carcinoma. Therapy; **8**(4):359-367

[22] IARC. IARC monographs of the evaluation of carcinogenic risks to humans. IARC Monograph. 25 June 2012;**100A**:1

[23] Baba AI, Câtoi C. Comparative Oncology. 2007

[24] Paolini M et al. Beta-carotene: A cancer chemopreventive agent or a co-carcinogen? Mutation Research. 2003;**543**(3):195-200

[25] Lee SJ et al. Distinguishing between genotoxic and non-genotoxic hepatocarcinogens by gene expression profiling and bioinformatic pathway analysis. Scientific Reports. 2013;**3**:2783

[26] Lima BS, Van der Laan JW. Mechanisms of nongenotoxic carcinogenesis and assessment of the human hazard. Regulatory Toxicology and Pharmacology. 2000;**32**(2):135-143

[27] van Delft JHM et al. Discrimination of genotoxic from non-genotoxic carcinogens by gene expression profiling (vol 25, pg 1265, 2004). Carcinogenesis. 2005;**26**(2):511-511

[28] Lee YS et al. Induction of oh8Gua glycosylase in rat kidneys by potassium bromate (KBrO3), a renal oxidative carcinogen. Mutation Research. 1996;**364**(3):227-233

[29] Moller L, Zeisig M. DNA adduct formation after oral administration of 2-nitrofluorene and N-acetyl-2-aminofluorene, analyzed by 32P-TLC and 32P-HPLC. Carcinogenesis. 1993;**14**(1):53-59

[30] Ruggeri B et al. Benzo[a]pyrene-induced murine skin tumors exhibit frequent and characteristic G to T mutations in the p53 gene. Proceedings of the National Academy of Sciences of the United States of America. 1993;**90**(3):1013-1017

[31] Grollman AP. Aristolochic acid nephropathy: Harbinger of a global iatrogenic disease. Environmental and Molecular Mutagenesis. 2013;**54**(1):1-7

[32] Arison RN, Feudale EL. Induction of renal tumour by streptozotocin in rats. Nature. 1967;**214**(5094):1254-1255

[33] Robbiano L et al. DNA damage induced by seven N-nitroso compounds in primary cultures of human and rat kidney cells. Mutation Research. 1996;**368**(1):41-47

[34] Majeed S et al. Aflatoxins and ochratoxin A contamination in rice, corn and corn products from Punjab, Pakistan. Journal of Cereal Science. 2013;**58**(3):446-450

[35] Duris D et al. Ochratoxin A contamination of coffee batches from Kenya in relation to cultivation methods and post-harvest processing treatments. Food Additives and Contaminants. Part A, Chemistry Analysis Control Exposure & Risk Assessment. 2010;**27**(6):836-841

[36] Clark HA, Snedeker SM. Ochratoxin A: Its cancer risk and potential for exposure. Journal of Toxicology and Environmental Health. Part B, Critical Reviews. 2006;**9**(3):265-296

[37] Grosse Y et al. Formation of Ochratoxin-A metabolites and DNA-adducts in monkey kidney-cells. Chemico-Biological Interactions. 1995;**95**(1-2):175-187

[38] Mally A, Dekant W. DNA adduct formation by ochratoxin A: Review of the available evidence. Food Additives and Contaminants. Part A, Chemistry Analysis Control Exposure & Risk Assessment. 2005;**22**:65-74

[39] Mantle PG et al. Structures of covalent adducts between DNA and ochratoxin A: A new factor in debate about genotoxicity and human risk assessment. Chemical Research in Toxicology. 2010;**23**(1):89-98

[40] Schaaf GJ et al. The role of oxidative stress in the ochratoxin A-mediated toxicity in proximal tubular cells. Biochimica et Biophysica Acta-Molecular Basis of Disease. 2002; **1588**(2):149-158

[41] NTP toxicology and carcinogenesis studies of monuron (CAS No. 150-68-5) in F344/N rats and B6C3F1 mice (feed studies). National Toxicology Program Technical Report Series. 1988;**266**:1-166

[42] Bloch KM et al. Transcriptomic alterations induced by monuron in rat and human renal proximal tubule cells in vitro and comparison to rat renal-cortex in vivo. Toxicology Research. 2015;**4**(2):423-431

[43] Elcombe CR et al. Prediction of rodent nongenotoxic carcinogenesis: Evaluation of biochemical and tissue changes in rodents following exposure to nine nongenotoxic NTP carcinogens. Environmental Health Perspectives. 2002;**110**(4):363-375

[44] Ishidate M. Data Book of Chromosomal Aberration Test In vitro. New York: Elsevier; 1987. pp. 49-50

[45] EPA. Chlorothalonil Reregistration Eligibility Decision Team. EPA 738-R-99-004. 1999

[46] Radford R et al. Mechanisms of chemical carcinogenesis in the kidneys. International Journal of Molecular Sciences. 2013;**14**(10):19416-19433

[47] Ioannides C, Lewis DFV. Cytochromes P450 in the bioactivation of chemicals. Current Topics in Medicinal Chemistry. 2004;**4**(16):1767-1788

[48] Uppstad H et al. Importance of CYP1A1 and CYP1B1 in bioactivation of benzo[a]pyrene in human lung cell lines. Toxicology Letters. 2010;**192**(2):221-228

[49] Sidorenko VS et al. Bioactivation of the human carcinogen aristolochic acid. Carcinogenesis. 2014;**35**(8):1814-1822

[50] McCann J, Ames BN. Discussion paper: The detection of mutagenic metabolites of carcinogens in urine with the salmonella/microsome test. Annals of the New York Academy of Sciences. 1975;**269**:21-25

[51] Mortelmans K, Zeiger E. The Ames Salmonella/microsome mutagenicity assay. Mutation Research, Fundamental and Molecular Mechanisms of Mutagenesis. 2000;**455**(1-2):29-60

[52] Maron DM, Ames BN. Revised methods for the Salmonella mutagenicity test. Mutation Research. 1983;**113**(3-4):173-215

[53] Malling HV. Mutagenic activation of dimethylnitrosamine and diethyl-nitrosamine in the host-mediated assay and the microsomal system. Mutation Research. 1974;**26**(6):465-472

[54] Berwald Y, Sachs L. In vitro transformation of normal cells to tumor cells by carcinogenic hydrocarbons. Journal of the National Cancer Institute. 1965;**35**(4):641-661

[55] Creton S et al. Cell transformation assays for prediction of carcinogenic potential: State of the science and future research needs. Mutagenesis; **27**(1):93-101

[56] Vasseur P, Lasne C. OECD Detailed Review Paper (DRP) number 31 on "Cell Transformation Assays for Detection of Chemical Carcinogens": Main results and conclusions. Mutation Research; **744**(1):8-11

[57] Ohmori K et al. An assay method for the prediction of tumor promoting potential of chemicals by the use of Bhas 42 cells. Mutation Research. 2004;**557**(2):191-202

[58] C1 Regulation (EC) No 1907/2006 of The European Parliament and of Council Regulation 2006. 1907/2006

[59] Walmsley RM, Billinton N. How accurate is in vitro prediction of carcinogenicity? British Journal of Pharmacology. 2011;**162**(6):1250-1258

[60] Marone PA, Hall WC, Hayes AW. Reassessing the two-year rodent carcinogenicity bioassay: A review of the applicability to human risk and current perspectives. Regulatory Toxicology and Pharmacology. 2014;**68**(1):108-118

[61] NTP. Guidelines for Carcinogen Bioassay in Small Rodents. National Cancer Institute: Carcinogenesis 1976. Technical Report Series No. 1

[62] Cohen SM. An enhanced 13-week bioassay: An alternative to the 2-year bioassay to screen for human carcinogenesis. Experimental and Toxicologic Pathology. 2010;**62**(5):497-502

[63] Parliament E. Directive 2010/63/EU of The European Parliament and of The Council of 22 September 2010 on the Protection of Animals used for Scientific Purposes. L 276/33, 2010

13

Tumour Microenvironment and Metastasis

Ke Wang

Abstract

In recent years, cancer is more and more severe harm to the health of people in the world. Although tumour diagnosis and therapy have made some progresses, there is little improvement in overall. One of the main reasons is that the pathogenesis of cancer metastasis is still enigmatic. Cancer development and metastasis are a complicated process that depends on the antigenic properties of cancer cells and a favoured environment in organs. Cancer cells metastasis causes more than 90% cancer death in the lungs, liver, brain, and bone, and a primary tumour causes less than 10% death. Therefore, understanding the process of cancer metastasis is essential, and it is convenient to deal with the problem of cancer metastasis and reduce cancer-related thrombosis. It has shown that tumour microenvironment plays a significant role in cancer progression. A variety of carcinoma-associated fibroblasts, and tumour-related macrophages play expanding and critical functions in sustaining cell proliferation, evading growth suppressors, promoting survival, activating invasion and metastasis, and reprogramming energy metabolism, but the purpose of each constituent remains unknown. This chapter will focus on discussing the role of the microenvironment on tumour invasion and metastasis to improve molecular diagnostics and therapeutics.

Keywords: cancer, metastasis, tumorigenesis, migration, invasion, tumour microenvironment, exosomes, autophagy, BMPs

1. Introduction

Cancer cells can be distant metastasis at the late stage, and they can cause damage and injury to the body of the patients. Breast cancer is a common clinical malignancy; it can metastasis to liver, bone, brain, lung and pleural metastasis, as follows. 1. Metastasis to the liver: Experts point out that the rate of breast cancer liver metastasis is 10%, the metastatic pathway has directly reached the liver through blood and lymphatic channel. There was no damage to the liver in the early stage. The liver function was normal. Liver volume could be enlarged. The condition of the patients deteriorated rapidly and died within a few months in the latter period. 2. Metastasis to bone: Bone metastases account for secondary blood metastasis of breast cancer. Common metastases places are vertebrae, ribs and pelvis. Bone metastases mainly encroach on the red bone marrow; the X-ray examination shows that it leads to irregular bone destruction, similar to the alteration of the insect specimen; some show double changes in osteoclast and osteogenesis. 3. Metastasis to brain: Brain metastases are rare, accounting for 5% of the metastatic cases of breast cancer, which can be divided into two types: meningeal metastasis and brain parenchymal metastasis. Brain metastases can cause brain oedema or brain swelling, the symptoms of increased intracranial pressure appear such as a headache, vomiting, visual impairment, convulsions and even coma. 4. Metastasis to lung and pleural: Lung and pleura are the most common metastatic sites of breast cancer. Lung metastases are often nodular and tend to be distributed in the peripheral lung field. The principal factors affecting the metastasis of breast cancer are the following factors.

2. Carcinoma-associated fibroblasts (CAFs) in the tumour microenvironment

Breast cancer mammary matrix fibroblasts can be regulated by the heat shock protein 1 [heat shock factor 1 (HSF1)] and promote the malignancy of a tumour, it indicates that CAFs may be activated before epithelial transformation [1]. CAFs are linked to the size of primary breast cancer. CAFs are triggered by the paracrine effect of various growth factors, cytokines and hormones, which can promote the proliferation of cancer cells. A large number of studies have reported that growth factors and their downstream signalling pathways produced by CAFs have a role in tumour cell survival, proliferation and cell cycle progression. At the same time, tumour cells can induce CAFs to synthesise growth factors and cytokines, and then form a positive feedback pathway to encourage tumour development. Studies have confirmed that CAFs secreted CXCL12 is linked to breast cancer cell surface homologous receptor CXCR4, promoting breast cancer cell growth [2]. HGF derived from CAFs can be bind to the C Met receptor and activate downstream signal proteins, such as tyrosine kinase, RAS/RAF/ERK, PI3K/AKT, and promote the proliferation of breast cancer cells [3]. In the co-culture of bone marrow stomatal cells and breast cancer cells, CAFs phenotype can be obtained, and the growth and aggregation of tumour cells are promoted by increasing the ratio of RANKL/OPG in breast cancer cells [4]. Besides, CAFs may be a significant source of local oestrogen. Cancer-associated aromatase can be written in CAFs, resulting in increased oestrogen production and tumour cell proliferation [5]. Also, distant metastasis is a significant cause of breast cancer death. Metastasis is an ongoing multistage process, including the invasion and growth of tumour cells, ECM degradation, tumour cells infiltrating into the blood and lymphatic systems, and the formation of metastatic clones in distant organs. CAFs activation can affect the invasiveness of breast cancer cells. Studies have demonstrated that CAFs can promote the invasive phenotype of breast ductal [6].

3. Tumour-related macrophages (TAMs) in the tumour microenvironment

TAMs promote tumour cell proliferation and survival with expression and secretion of a large number of factors, such as epidermal growth factor, platelet source growth factor, transform growth factor-β1, liver cell growth factor, etc. In vitro, macrophages and tumour cells were co-cultured, the former can significantly promote the growth of the latter by high secretion of the above factors. The tumour cell growth and development were slowed down or even stopped mice knock out their macrophages, which confirmed the role of macrophages in promoting tumour growth. The results of genetic studies in mice showed that the low rate of tumour growth and low metastasis was strictly related to the smaller number of TAMs. The researchers established the CSF-1 spontaneous breast cancer mouse model to find tumour proliferation. Growth rate and lung metastasis rate were lower than those of the wild-type CSF-1 [7].

Three steps can summarise the role of TAMs in tumour invasion and metastasis: The tumour cells adhere to the extracellular matrix components to release protein hydrolase to degrade extracellular matrix and induce invasion migration with chemokines. The cancer cells are free of charge in the primary lesion after proliferation and adhere to the basement membrane. The enormous number of matrix proteases released by them will have a destructive effect on the extracellular matrix and basement membrane, and then invade the lymphatic vessels or blood vessels to cause damage to the tissue and form a metastatic focus. TAMs secrete a large number of proteolytic enzymes for tumour invasion and metastasis. For example, matrix metalloproteinases, include gelatinase-2, collagen enzyme-1, matrix degradation enzyme-3 and more than 20 kinds of proteins; these TMMPs enzymes can degrade the extracellular matrix and degrade the fibrous collagen. The researchers to establish a breast cancer mouse model and find that lung metastasis decreased the loss of systemic macrophages, indicating that tumour metastasis was affected by TAMs and that macrophages existed in the early stages of lesions, invasion and rupture of the basement membrane. And its proteolytic enzyme expression is increased (such as Cathepsin B), indicating that TAMs are also engaged when tumour cells are in normal tissues around them [8]. Studies have demonstrated that together with tumour cells and macrophages, the latter enhances the dynamic properties of the former by using the form of MMP and TNF-α [9]. The tissue structure and basement membrane can be hit by MMP expression, thus promoting tumour cell growth, diffusion and metastasis. MMP in invasive tumours is generally provided by TAMs [10]. TAMs are synergistic with stomatal tumour cells and epithelial cells to promote tumour metastasis [11]. The destruction of the basement membrane is TAMs, and the proteolytic activity of protease B in the local tissue is increased, indicating that TAMs affect the tumour cells to invade the normal tissues around the tissue [12, 13]. The study showed that TAMs in different tumour tissues synthesised a series of urokinase (urokinase, uPA) involved in tumour invasion, invasion, extracellular matrix degradation and tumour angiogenesis [14]. By separating TAMs from breast cancer cells, it was found that TGF–beta 1 could stimulate the transcription of uPA in TAMs and enhance the stability of uPA Mrna. In addition, TAMs secrete cathepsin to promote tumour development by the expression of cathepsin B, cathepsin D and cathepsin L in breast cancer [15].

4. Exosomes in the tumour microenvironment

The 'seed' cells are situated in the primary site of a tumour. They regulate the 'soil' microenvironment of the target organs so that the scattered 'seed' cells can adapt to the new 'soil' and still survive. In the process of the formation of pre-metastatic niche, exosomes play an essential role in raising the chemokine receptor, changing the expression of cell adhesion molecules and creating an immunosuppressive microenvironment. CHEN and others analyse the proteomics in the serum of patients with colon cancer and normal human serum, they found that the expression of 36 exosomes proteins in colon cancer patients was up-regulated [16]. WANG and others found that a tumour could transfer to the liver by the animal model of subcutaneous colon cancer cells HT-29 in nude mice. The exosomes were secreted by HT-29 cells can collect and express chemokine C-X-C primitives on target organs by CXCR4 [chemokine (C-X-C motif) receptor 4, CXCR4] matrix cells to the tumour cells in this process. The organisation's transfer provides favourable conditions [17]. ZHOU and others found that miR-105 was carried in the exosomes secreted by breast cancer cells, which can specifically lead to the down-regulation of the tight connexin ZO-1 expression in endothelial cells and destroy the vascular endothelial barrier, which plays an important role in the early stage of microenvironment formation [18].

Exosomes promote the development of inflammatory response and create a pure metastatic microenvironment conducive to tumour metastasis. COSTA-SILVA and others found that the exosomes derived from pancreatic cancer cells expressed high expression of macrophage migration inhibitory factor [macrophage migration inhibitory factor (MIF)], and after absorption of these exosomes, the liver macrophages (Kupffer cells) secreted a significant amount of TGF beta, and TGF beta promoted the formation of immunosuppressive microenvironment and thus promoted EMT and blood. The TGF beta secreted by liver macrophages activates the hepatic stellate cells, up-regulated the expression of fibronectin, and then raises bone marrow-derived macrophages in the liver and prepares the microenvironment for the arrival of the tumour cells. The exosomes derived from chronic lymphocytic leukaemia, carrying protein molecules and miRNA can promote the transformation of matrix cells into a tumour-related fibroblasts, release inflammatory response factors, and form a microenvironment to tumour growth [19]. The miRNA (miR-21 and miR-29a) carried by the exosomes can combine the Toll-like receptor [Toll-like receptors (TLRs)] of the immune cells, resulting in the nuclear factor-kappa B [nuclear factor kappa B (NF-kappa)]. The release of tumour necrosis factor–alpha (TNF–a) and IL-6, the activation of the inflammatory response factor to encourage the proliferation and metastasis [20, 21]. Exosomes not only provides a suitable growth environment for migrating tumour cells but also mediates tumour-specific organ metastasis. Hoshino et al. research a variety of exosomes secreted by separate metastatic tumour organs [22]. It is found that these exosomes priorities are combined with their respective present points of receptor cells. The exosomes mediate the tumour's organ-specific transfer through the exosomes related and activate the Src phosphorylation pathway of the receptor cells to up-regulation the gene expression of S100 in order to promote the growth of tumour cells [23].

5. Autophagy associated with cancer metastasis

Autophagy inhibits metastasis of tumour cells by inducing anti-inflammatory effects and lysates can cause inflammation in the surrounding tissues, Degenhardt et al. have proved that the microenvironment of an inflammatory tumour may lead to invasion and metastasis of tumour cells [24]. At the initial stage of primary tumour metastasis, signal stimulation is needed to promote migration and invasion. Tumour cells get into the systemic circulation through vascular infiltration [25]. Hypoxia and oxidative stress usually affect solid tumours, which can lead to cell necrosis and inflammatory reaction and inflammatory cells infiltrate. Although some inflammatory cells, such as cytotoxic T cells and natural killer cells can antitumour immune responses and influence metastasis of tumour. Importantly, inflammatory mediators such as macrophages infiltration are often associated with poor clinical prognosis [25–27]. The PyMT (polyoma middle T) transgenic model of breast cancer metastasis has proved that macrophage infiltration in primary tumours is required for invasion and metastasis [28]. Degenhardt and others find that autophagy can indirectly inhibit the inflammatory response on the metastatic promoter site, by raising the survival rate of tumour cells under hypoxia and metabolic stress [29]. Also, autophagy can also regulate the inflammatory response directly by controlling the release of immunoregulatory factors such as the release of high mobility group protein 1 [high mobility group box protein 1 (HMGB1)]. Once HMGB1 is released, it will activate dendritic cells through the Toll-like receptor–4 (Toll-like) of these cells to play a role in inducing cells to produce potent antitumour immune responses that kill tumour cells and prevent their metastasis [30]. More interestingly, high levels of autophagy could be induced during cell death in malignant glioma cells treated with mycin, resulting in a substantial release of HMBG1 from the dead cells [30, 31].

6. Hypoxia-regulated genes implicated in cancer metastasis

The effect of hypoxia on tumour immunity is another essential influence factor. Under the condition of hypoxia, tumour cells can secrete a variety of immunosuppressive factors, transforming growth factor beta (transforming growth factor-beta) is one of the most critical factors. TGF-beta can make tumour cells acquire immune escape function through the following ways: (1) Inhibit the proliferation of cytotoxic T cells and the expression of cytotoxin genes, which makes T cells unable to play an antitumour effect and induces the production of CD4 + CD25+ regulatory T cells with immunosuppressive function. (2) Inhibit the expression of antigen-presenting molecules, conciliatory factors and chemokine receptors to prevent the dendritic cells from functioning normally and make dendritic cells unable to deliver tumour antigens to T cells [32–35]. (3) Inhibit the activation of natural killer (NK) cells and reduces the expression of multiple surface receptors in NK cells so that they cannot identify and dissolve tumour cells [36]. In addition, hypoxia can also directly activate myeloid-derived suppressor cells (MDSCs), dendritic cells, and programmed cell death receptor ligand 1 [programmed cell death-ligand 1 (PD-L1)] through HIF-1 alpha, which can reduce the expression of MDSCs secreting interleukin -6 and interleukin -10 p to promote activation in T cells [37–39].

7. BMPs effect on tumour microenvironment, migration and invasion

BMPs belong to the transforming growth factor-β (TGF-β) superfamily and were initially identified as obstetrician cytokines that can promote bone and cartilage formation in vivo. Recently, BMPs have turned out to be involved in the regulation of tumorigenesis, development and bone metastases, they have been shown to be involved in the regulation of tumour development and bone metastasis. Clement et al. find BMP2 can enhance the migration and invasion of breast cancer cells, those cells with high expression of BMP2 showed more cell migration than GFP and blank control group. Katsuno et al. find that BMP2 promotes the invasion and migration of MDA-MB-231 through BMPs/SMAD pathway, and the two BMPs receptors play an equally important role. Lack of anyone receptor affects the signalling process [40]. BMP2 can promote oestrogen receptor positive MCF7 to invade migration in vivo and in vitro [41]. Scherberich et al. research show that BMP2 enhances the tumour invasion by regulating the expression of skeleton protein M in the tumour microenvironment. BMP2 induces the expression of skeleton protein M by p38 MAPK and JNK signalling pathway. BMP2 can also promote the invasion and migration of breast cancer by up-regulation the ID1 expression [42]. BMP-4 increases the invasion and migration of breast cancer cell by CCN6, which has been shown directly antagonise the BMP-4 mediated invasiveness and metastases in vitro and in vivo to. Fibroblasts stimulated with BMP-4 enhanced the MCF-7 cell invasion, and these effects were inhibited by DMH1. BMP-4 increased the expression of MMP-3 and IL-6 in conditioned medium from treated mammary fibroblasts, suggesting BMP-4 can impact the tumour microenvironment to promote breast cancer invasion [43]. The latest research has found that BMP6 can inhibit the growth and migration of breast cancer cells. Takahashi finds that BMP6 and estradiol co-work can inhibit the proliferation of MCF-7 cells through p38 MAPK cell signalling, however, it will not play a role only BMP6 exists [24]. Yang et al. also find that BMP6 down-regulates the expression of miR-192 to inhibit the transcription of ZEB1, and the decrease of miR-21 expression to impede the migration ability of MDA-MB-231 and BMP6 could also reduce the proliferation ability of MDA-MB-231 cells [25]. Zeisberg et al. find that TGF-beta can reduce the expression of E-adhering to renal epithelial cells, but BMP7 can increase the expression of E-adhering. Buijs et al. Point out that BMP7 can induce the activity of E-adhering to breast cancer cells and reduce invasiveness. Therefore, BMP7 can induce the expression of E-adhering in normal epithelial cells and maintain the stability of epithelial cells, loss of BMP7 gene will decrease of the expression of E- adhering to lead the epithelial cells to the stomatal cells in the evolution of the tumour [44]. Alamo finds that BMP7 stimulates the growth of two breast cancer cell lines and inhibits the proliferation of four breast cancer cell lines. Exogenous BMP7 can significantly enhance the migration of MDA-MB-231 in vitro. The causes of these two differences are not yet clear, Ye Lin has found that the expression of BMP10 in breast cancer is reduced. It can inhibit the invasion and migration of MDA-MB-231 through the BMPs/SMAD pathway and suggests that BMP10 can serve as a target for molecular therapy of breast cancer [45].

8. BMPs and bone metastasis

There are comparatively few studies on the role of BMPs in bone metastasis of breast cancer. Recently, it has been noted that BMPs is involved in the process of breast cancer bone metastasis. BMP has been involved in the development of bone metastases in up-regulating or down-regulating the corresponding regulatory factors in breast cancer cells. BMPs can increase the expression of Osteoblast bone saliva protein BSP. BSP is related to the formation of new bone, so it can connect to the process of breast cancer with bone metastasis. Runx2 similar to BSP is that the target gene of BMP, which is closely linked to the osteolytic metastasis of breast cancer [46].

The overexpression of BMP7 or exogenous BMP7 can significantly reduce the formation of bone metastasis by reducing the expression of romantic, increasing the expression of E-cadherin and reversing the EMT in the animal model of mouse breast cancer bone metastases. In contrast, additional studies found BMPs could increase the invasion of a tumour and the ability of bone metastases and the active SMAD1/5/8 was detected in primary and metastatic tumours [47].

In conclusion, BMPs involves the growth and invasion of breast cancer. Different types of BMPs have different roles in the same breast cancer cell line, even if the same kind of BMPs has different effects on various breast cancer cell lines. It is believed that this mechanism will be clarified with the research. BMP9 can inhibit the growth of breast cancer cells in vitro and in vivo, BMP-9 is also involved in the inhibition of tumour growth in bone by down-regulation of connective tissue growth factor(CTGF).

9. Conclusions

It has shown that tumour microenvironment plays an essential role in cancer progression. The more recent studies have demonstrated hypoxic and autophagy in both primary tumours and metastases, contributing to angiogenesis, invasion, BMPs can inhibit or promote the growth of breast cancer by different signalling pathway. It detects a promising therapeutic value for BMPs in the management of metastases by influencing the propensity to disseminate to and survive in the bone microenvironment.

Author details

Ke Wang

Address all correspondence to: wk125@126.com

Clinical Laboratory, Yongchuan Hospital of Chongqing Medical University, Chongqing, China

References

[1] Scherz-Shouval R, Santagata S, Mendillo ML, et al. The reprogramming of tumor stroma by HSF1 is a potent enabler of malignancy. Cell. 2014;**158**(3):564-578

[2] Locatelli A, Lofgren KA, Daniel AR, et al. Mechanisms of HGF/met signaling to Brk and Sam68 in breast cancer progression. Hormones and Cancers. 2012;**3**(1-2):14-25

[3] Arrigoni C, De Luca P, Gilardi M, et al. Direct but not indirect co - culture with osteogenically differentiated human bone marrow stromal cells increases RANKL /OPG ratio in human breast cancer cells generating bone etastases. Molecular Cancer. 2014;**13**:238-244

[4] Suda T, Oba H, Takei H, et al. ER-activating ability of breast cancer stromal fibroblasts is regulated independently of alteration of TP53 and PTEN tumor suppressor genes. Biochemical and Biophysical Research Communications. 2012;**428**(2):259-263

[5] Osuala KO, Sameni M, Shah S, et al. IL-6 signaling between ductal carcinoma insitu cells and carcinoma -associated fibroblasts mediates tumor cell growth and migration. BMC Cancer. 2015;**15**:584-597

[6] Tham M, Tan KW, Keeble J, et al. Melanoma - initiating cells exploit M2 macrophage TGFβ and arginase pathway for survival and proliferation. Oncotarget. 2014;**5**(23):12027-12042

[7] Wang R, Lu M, Zhang J, et al. Increased IL - 10 mRNA expression in tumor - associated macrophage correlated with late stage of lung cancer. Journal of Experimental & Clinical Cancer Research. 2011;**30**:62

[8] Deryugina EI, Zajac E, Juncker-Jensen A, et al. Tissue – Infiltrating neutrophils constitute the major in vivo source of angiogenesis-inducing MMP - 9 in the tumor microenvironment. Neoplasia. 2014;**16**(10):771-788

[9] Gocheva V, Wang HW, Gadea BB, et al. IL - 4 induces cathepsin protease activity in tumor -associated macrophages to promotecancer growth and invasion. Genes & Development. 2010;**24**(3):241-255

[10] Hu J, Jo M, Eastman BM, et al. uPAR induces expression of transforming growth factor β and interleukin-4 incancer cells to promote tumor-permissive conditioning of macrophages. The American Journal of Pathology. 2014;**184**(12):3384-3393

[11] Shen Z, Yan Y, Ye C, et al. The effect of Vasohibin - 1 expression and tumor -associated macrophages on theangiogenesis in vitroand in vivo. Tumour Biology. 2016;**37**(6):7267-7276

[12] Ji H, Cao R, Yang Y, et al. TNFR1 mediates TNF—α induced tumour lymphangiogenesis and metastasis by modulating VEGF C—VEGFR3 signalling. Nature Communications. 2014;**5**:4944

[13] Strieter RM, Belperio JA, Phillips RJ, et al. CXC chemokines inangiogenesis of cancer. Seminars in Cancer Biology. 2004;**14**(3):195-200

[14] Ma HC, Shi XL, Ren HZ, et al. Targeted migration of mesenchymal stem cells modified with CXCR4 to acute failing liver improves liver regeneration. World Journal of Gastroenterology. 2014;**20**(40):14884-14894

[15] Zheng SQ, Huang RQ, Zhang YJ. Role of matrix metalloproteinase (MMP) - 2 and - 9 and vascular endothelial growth factor C in lymph node metastasis of breast cancer. Chinese Journal of Pathology. 2010;**39**(4):240-244

[16] Chen Y, Xie Y, Xu L, et al. Protein content and functional characteristics of serum-purified exosomes from patients with colorectal cancerrevealed by quantitative proteomics. International Journal of Cancer. 2017;**140**(4):900-913

[17] Wang X, Ding X, Nan L, et al. Investigation of the roles of exosomes in colorectal cancer liver metastasis. Oncology Reports. 2015;**33**(5):2445-2453

[18] Zhou W, Fong MY, Min Y, et al. Cancer-secreted miR-105 destroys vascular endothelial barriers to promote metastasis. Cancer Cell. 2014;**25**(4):501-515

[19] Costa-Silva B, Aiello NM, Ocean AJ, et al. Pancreatic cancer exosomes initiate pre-metastatic niche formation in the liver. Nature Cell Biology. 2015;**17**(6):816-826

[20] Paggetti J, Haderk F, Seiffert M, et al. Exosomes released by chronic lymphocytic leukemia cells induce the transition of stromal cells into cancerassociated fibroblasts. Blood. 2015;**126**(9):1106-1117

[21] Fabbri M, Paone A, Calore F, et al. MicroRNAs bind to toll-like receptors to induce pro-metastatic inflammatory response. Proceedings of the National Academy of Sciences of the United States of America. 2012;**109**(31):E2110-E2116

[22] Hoshino A, Costa-Silva B, Shen TL, et al. Tumour exosome integrins determine organotropic metastasis. Nature. 2015;**527**(7578):329-335

[23] Lobb RJ, Lima LG, Moller A. Exosomes: Key mediators of metastasis and pre-metastatic niche formation. Seminars in Cell & Developmental Biology. 2017;**67**:3-10

[24] Degenhardt K, Mathew R, Beaudoin B, et al. Autophagy promotes tumor cell survival and restricts necrosis, inflammation, and tumorigenesis. Cancer Cell. 2006;**10**(1):51-64

[25] Tlsty TD, Coussens LM. Tumor stroma and regulation of cancer development. Annual Review of Pathology. 2006;**1**:119-150

[26] DeNardo DG, Johansson M, Coussens LM. Immune cells as mediators of solid tumor metastasis. Cancer Metastasis Reviews. 2008;**27**(1):11-18

[27] DeNardo DG, Barreto JB, Andreu P, et al. CD4 + T cells regulate pulmonary metastasis of mammary carcinomas by enhancing protumor properties of macrophages. Cancer Cell. 2009;**16**(2):91-102

[28] Bingle L, Brown NJ, Lewis CE. The role of tumour- associated macrophages in tumour progression: Implications for new anticancer therapies. The Journal of Pathology. 2002;**196**(3):254-265

[29] Lin EY, Nguyen AV, Russell RG, et al. Colony - stimulating Factor1 promotes progression of mammary tumors to malignancy. The Journal of Experimental Medicine. 2001; **193**(6):727-740

[30] Apetoh L, Ghiringhelli F, Tesniere A, et al. Toll like receptor 4- dependent contribution of the immune system to anticancer chemotherapy and radiotherapy. Nature Medicine. 2007;**13**(9):1050-1059

[31] Yu Y, Tang D, Kang R. Oxidative stress mediated HMGB1 biology. Frontiers in Physiology. 2015;**6**:93

[32] Chang L, Lin Y, Mahalingam J, et al. Tumor-derived chemokine CCL5 enhances TGF-β–mediated killing of CD8+ T cells in colon cancer by T-regulatory cells. Cancer Research. 2012;**72**(5):1092-1102

[33] Conroy H, Galvin KC, Higgins SC, et al. Gene silencing of TGF-beta1 enhances antitumor immunity induced with a dendritic cell vaccine by reducing tumor-associated regulatory T cells. Cancer Immunology, Immunotherapy. 2012;**61**(3):425-431

[34] Noman MZ, Desantis G, Janji B, et al. PD-L1 is a novel direct target of HIF-1alpha, and its blockade under hypoxia enhanced MDSC-mediated T cell activation. The Journal of Experimental Medicine. 2014;**211**(5):781-790

[35] Wiktorowska-Owczarek A, Owczarek J. The effect of hypoxia on PGE2-stimulated cAMP generation in HMEC-1. Cellular & Molecular Biology Letters. 2015;**20**(2):213-221

[36] Yaqub S, Tasken K. Role for the cAMPprotein kinase A signaling pathwayin suppression of antitumor immune responses by regulatory T cells. Critical Reviews in Oncogenesis. 2008;**14**(1):57-77

[37] Whiteside TL, Mandapathil M, Schuler P. The role of the adenosinergic pathway in immunosuppression mediated by human regulatory T cells (Treg). Current Medicinal Chemistry. 2011;**18**(34):5217-5223

[38] Baginska J, Viry E, Paggetti J, et al. The critical role of the tumor microenvironment in shaping natural killer cell-mediated anti-tumor immunity. Frontiers in Immunology. 2013;**4**:490

[39] Viry E, Baginska J, Berchem G, et al. Autophagic degradation of GZMB/granzyme B: A new mechanism of hypoxic tumor cell escape from natural killer cell-mediated lysis. Autophagy. 2014;**10**(1):173-175

[40] Katsuno Y, Hanyu A, Kanda H, et al. Bone morphogenetic protein signaling enhances invasion and bone metastasis of breast cancer cells through Smad pathway. Oncogene. 2008;**27**(49):6322-6333

[41] Clement JH, Raida M, Sänger J, et al. Bone morphogenetic protein 2 (BMP-2) induces in vitro invasion and in vivo hormone independent growth of breast carcinoma cells. International Journal of Oncology. 2005;**27**(2):401-407

[42] Scherberich A, Tucker RP, Degen M, et al. Tenascin-W is found in malignant mammary tumors, promotes alpha8 integrin-dependent motility and requires p38MAPK activity for BMP-2 and TNF-alpha induced expression in vitro. Oncogene. 2005;**24**(9):1525-1532

[43] Zabkiewicz C, Resaul J, Hargest R, Jiang WG, Ye L. Bone morphogenetic proteins, breast cancer, and bone metastases: Striking the right balance. Endocrine-Related Cancer. 2017;**24**(10):R349-R366

[44] Sapkota G, Alarcón C, Spagnoli FM, et al. Balancing BMP signaling through integrated inputs into the Smad1 linker. Molecular Cell. 2007;**25**(3):441-454

[45] Ye L, Bokobza S, Li J. Bone morphogenetic protein-10 (BMP-10) inhibits aggressiveness of breast cancer cells and correlates with poor prognosis in breast cancer. Cancer Science. 2010;**101**(10):2137-2144

[46] Awolaran O, Brooks SA, Lavender V. Breast cancer osteomimicry and its role in bone specific metastasis; an integrative, systematic review of preclinical evidence. Breast. 2016;**375**(30):156-171

[47] Allison SE, Chen Y, Petrovic N, et al. Activation of the pro-migratory bone morphogenetic protein receptor 1B gene in human MDA-MB-468 triple-negative breast cancer cells that over-express CYP2J2. International Journal of Biochemistry and Cell Biology. 2016;**80**:173-178

14

What's New Among Cancer Etiology Horizon?

Trinanjan Basu

Abstract

The commonest saying goes as "cancer has no answer," we have really come a long way in that aspect. From being able to detect and diagnose the disease early, effective treatment modalities, improvement in therapeutic outcome and even effective palliative measures. The research focus emphasized upon detecting preventable risk factors. Tobacco a Global culprit is often discussed as the most important risk factor for cancer. Modern day life and with its so-called stress measures are the ones often been blamed without a concrete scientific evidences. Psychological makeup of a person, emotional stress and cellular phones are intricately associated with a modern lifestyle. In this chapter we would be focusing upon the causal relationship between these factors and malignancy with available scientific literature. At the end we would present possible measures to avoid them and any future research areas to be looked upon.

Keywords: cancer, emotional stress, psychological factors, cellular phones, modern lifestyle, habituation, modifiable risk factors

1. Introduction

Cancer is a term coined by the great Greek physician Hippocrates (460–370 BC). He is considered the "Father of Medicine." Hippocrates used the terms carcinos and carcinoma to describe non-ulcer forming and ulcer-forming tumors. Later on Galen (130–200 AD), another Roman physician used the term oncos (Greek for swelling) to describe tumors. Oncos is the root word for oncology or study of cancers.

It has been described in ancient mummies and over several years it has awakened a sense of fear and loss among the Human race. However technology also progressed at a rapid rate and main therapeutic modalities to treat cancer become a triad of surgery, chemotherapy and radiotherapy.

Parallel to these early diagnosis and preventive measures have also been researched in a large scale. This brings us to a domain called etiological factors for cancer. Tobacco has been linked to all head and neck cancers, esophageal cancers, bladder cancer especially, whereas dietary factors are predominant in breast and colon malignancies [1–5]. Interestingly few of the literature dates even more than 50 years back and current data also includes personal sexual behavior, Human papilloma virus infection (HPV) and tobacco in smokers as known risk factors.

These are often mentioned and often discussed issues. Effective strategies in cases of known risk factors have also been developed. Cancer vaccine is one such preventive step. In the case of cervical cancer a preventable vaccine is also been developed and shows promising outcome [6, 7].

Modern day lifestyle also brings along stress in terms if not only physical factors but also emotional issues. Low mood, depression and chronic anhedonia are household terns these days. There have been infrequent reports regarding emotional stress being causative factor for cancer [8–10]. Till date this is an important issue which lacks concrete evidence.

The other modern day risk being cellular phones aka mobile phones. Childhood brain tumors have been linked to it in several reports and it might have some significance. But again a large database and definite evidence is still to come out [11–13].

In this section we would elaborate the available literature related to these two less discussed etiologies of cancer viz. emotional/psychological stress and cellular phones. We would try and find if at all any link exists between them and related issues as per different sites of cancers.

2. Emotional stress

2.1. Introduction

Emotional stress, psychological factors or stressful life events these terms are often used interchangeably. Whatever may be the definition it has long been speculated to be linked to cancer development? The assumption of an association between stress and cancer is popular in the lay public [14]. Long back in 1992 Baghurst et al. described preventable issues but most of them were diet related. There was however a mention about environmental factors but emotional stress was not highlighted. Doll and Peto in 1985 also elaborate the dietary risk factors in different cancers and incidentally stress was highlighted to be a major contributory factor in colon, lung and breast cancers [15].

2.2. Definition

World Health Organization (WHO) defined health as "a state of complete physical, mental and social well-being and not merely the absence of disease or infirmity" [16]. With over half a decade and World witnessing several changes the WHO definition also should focus on the ability to adapt and self-manage in face of social, physical, and emotional challenges [17]. With the change in socio-cultural and demographic profile across world social support and emotional stress were linked to chronic diseases. As per American Psychosomatic Society social support is defined as "information leading the subject to believe that he is cared for and loved, esteemed, and a member of a network of mutual obligations [18]." The article enumerates that social support can protect people during crisis from a wide variety of pathological states like low birth weight to death, from arthritis through tuberculosis to depression, alcoholism, and the social breakdown syndrome. It has bigger implications like reduction in the amount of medication required, acceleration of recovery and compliance to medical regimens prescribed. These data never actually stated development of cancer related to social stress.

2.3. Pathophysiology

Psychological health itself is a difficult domain to assess. Aspects of psychological well-being like self-acceptance, positive relations with others, autonomy, environmental mastery, purpose in life and personal growth were mainly analyzed [19]. All these give a hint of link to chronic disorder and may be malignancy but without much evidence. Long back Evans suggested that the death of a spouse or other close relation could be an important cause of cancer. It was stated that "cancer is a miscarriage of this driving force, under the influence of the collective unconscious which is unrestrained after the patient has given up hope and interest in life (when the objective attachment is broken), that is, after the conscious has given up the struggle with the unconscious" [20]. However the study also could not establish a direct link. There is also no physiological mechanism to account for an increase in the incidence of or mortality from cancer after stressful events has yet to be specified in detail [8]. Loss of an important emotional relationship has been identified in several studies as an event with a high risk of subsequent illness [20–22]. Psychological stress activates the nervous system and the hypothalamic-pituitary-adrenal axis, leading to release of hormones such as glucocorticoids and norepinephrine. It has been shown that stress and the subsequent hormonal dysfunction can cause impairment of DNA repair and hence can suppress the immune system. Additionally, stress may lead to epigenetic silencing: altering DNA methylation and histone acetylation and all these are important in tumor development [23–25].

There is a separate discipline which studies these factors and called as psychoneuroimmunology. The multistep immune reactions are either inhibited or enhanced as a result of previous or parallel stress experiences, depending on the type and intensity of the stressor. As a rule both stressors and depression are associated with the decreased cytotoxic T-cell and natural-killer-cell activities. This further affect processes such as immune surveillance of tumors. This will lead to the events that modulate development and accumulation of somatic mutations and genomic instability [24].

From the time of the ancient Greeks, there has been an interest in the relationship between psychological states and cancer. Epidemiologic evidences have supported the role of biobehavioral risk factors in cancer progression. These are namely social adversity, depression, and stress. This is important both in initiation and progression phases [26, 27].

Early research on central nervous system (CNS) effects on cancer predominantly focused on the following:

a. Down-regulation of the immune response as a potential mediator of impaired surveillance for metastatic spread [27–31].

b. Stress effects on DNA repair [32, 33].

It is to be understood that there is no singular system available in explaining the biological effects of stress pathways on cancer progression. Over the last 10 years, the focus of mechanistic biobehavioral oncology research has broadened and it includes examination of the effects of stress on (a) tumor angiogenesis; (b) invasion and anoikis; (c) stromal cells in the tumor microenvironment, and (d) inflammation [27].

The salient features and how they affect immune system and cancer development or progression is enumerated in **Table 1**.

Biobehavioral factors	Main cause	Pathophysiology	Implications
Cellular immune response in cancer progression [34, 35]	Negative psychosocial states, such as chronic stress, depression, and social isolation	Down-regulation of the cellular immune response, mediated largely by adrenergic and glucocorticoid signaling	1. Depression has also been associated with a poorer cellular immune response to specific antigens in breast cancer 2. One study reported that depressed patients with hepatobiliary carcinoma had lower NK cell numbers and shorter survival compared to their non-depressed counterparts [36]
Angiogenesis and invasion [37–40].	Cancer-related mortality largely results from the spread of cancer cells from the primary tumor to other sites in the body, a process called metastasis. Successful metastatic spread requires several sequential steps, including angiogenesis, proliferation, invasion, embolization, and colonization of a new secondary site	Angiogenesis: this process is tightly controlled by a variety of positive and negative factors secreted by both tumor and host cells in the tumor microenvironment	Stress hormones such as norepinephrine (NE) have been shown to induce production of IL-6 and IL-8 by ovarian cancer and melanoma cells demonstrating effects of stress response pathways on tumor signaling mechanisms
Stress effects on anoikis [41–44]	Anoikis is the normal process of programmed cell death (apoptosis) occurring when anchorage-dependent cells become separated from the ECM. Cancer cells acquire the ability to resist anoikis, thus enhancing their ability to migrate, re-attach, and establish themselves in secondary sites	Catecholamines were found to protect ovarian cancer cells from anoikis, both in vitro and in vivo. These effects were mediated by focal adhesion kinase (FAK), a tyrosine kinase that promotes cell adhesion, which demonstrated increased activation (phosphorylation of pFAKY397) in response to NE. Clinically, elevated levels of pFAKY397 were observed in the tumor tissue of ovarian cancer patients reporting depression and those with higher levels of tumor NE	Ovarian cancer progression

Biobehavioral factors	Main cause	Pathophysiology	Implications
Stromal cells in the tumor microenvironment [43–46]	Tumor growth is to a large extent shaped and promoted or inhibited by signaling between tumor cells and the cells of the microenvironment. In addition to effects of stress hormones on tumor cells, there are marked effects on host cells such as macrophages in the tumor microenvironment	Monocytes are drawn to the tumor microenvironment by tumor-derived chemotactic factors and then differentiate into macrophages. However, under the influence of the pro-inflammatory microenvironment, macrophages are induced to shift from their phagocytic phenotype to a pro-tumor phenotype that produces tumor promoting factors such as VEGF and MMPs, while simultaneously down-regulating the cellular immune response by production of immunosuppressive cytokines such as IL-10 and TGFβ (75–78). TAMs are thus directly involved in promoting angiogenesis, tumor proliferation, invasion, metastases, and down-regulation of adaptive immunity. TAM infiltration is also associated with poorer survival	In ovarian cancer patients, biobehavioral risk factors that have been associated with higher NE levels, such as depression and stress
Glucocorticoid dynamics and cancer progression [47–49]		Glucocorticoids can directly mediate processes promoting tumor growth as well. Cortisol has been shown to stimulate growth of prostate cancer cells (85) and to enhance proliferation of human mammary cancer cells by nearly two-fold	In a murine breast cancer model, social isolation induced an elevated corticosterone stress response, greater tumor burden and alterations in gene expression in metabolic pathways that are known to contribute to increased tumor growth

Table 1. Stress and different pathophysiology.

2.4. Childhood cancers

It is altogether a different entity. Investigators have tried to assess the link between early life stress and development of childhood cancers. It is a unique scenario and in developed countries it is a leading cause of child deaths. Almost half of childhood cancers are diagnosed before 5 years of age and thus the importance of identifying early life risk factors for developing prevention strategies [50–53]. There is a certain physiological aspect also but like in adults the pathways are not very clear.

Large population-based cohort studies from Denmark and Sweden showed a small but statistically significant overall increased risk of childhood cancer was observed among children exposed to bereavement owing to the death of a family member. Exposure was also associated with CNS tumors and leukemia [53].

2.5. Conclusion

There is a definite correlation between stress and immunologic pathways for development of cancer and also for progression. In the clinical literature, lack of perceived social support is a factor that emerges repeatedly in associations with biological variables related to cancer progression, and social isolation has shown similar effects in the preclinical literature. Understanding what it is about social relationships that underlie these associations will be important in future research. Additional questions include the following: How much stress, in terms of thresholds or chronicity, is needed to modulate tumor-related pathways?

Many clinical studies even if prospective have failed to highlight life time stress as causative factor for cancer. The results of a large, prospective, population-based study therefore do not support the hypothesis that life stress, when defined as stressful life events, increases the risk for developing cancer [10].

3. Cellular phones

3.1. Introduction

There are three main reasons why people are concerned that cell phones (also known as "mobile" or "wireless" telephones) might have the potential to cause certain types of cancer or other health problems. Various literature reviews actually gives a very conflicting results. The exposure among pediatric and adult population is different and so as the outcome. As a potential etiology for cancer, cellular phones are yet to be regarded as common pathogens. As Munshi et al. describes "Centuries ago, we advanced from pigeons to postal services as a more modern means to communicate. Since then, communication has made quantum leaps, buoyed by the successes in physics and technology. From crude telephone sets to modern landline, cordless phones and finally cellular phones" [11].

3.2. Background knowledge

Mobile phones first came to use in the early 1990s for professional work-related reasons, and henceforth have attained tremendous growth, becoming able symbols for consumer status and needs. At present, nearly 5 billion people worldwide own cellular phones. India herself can boast of 800 million cellular phone users [54].

Another review by Munshi and Jalali highlighted how the fear of cellular phones and cancer develop. A decade ago a man in Florida, US sued a cell phone company alleging it lead to brain tumor in his wife [55]. The scientific evidence shows that mobile phones emit electromagnetic radiation (radiofrequency, RF) that is essentially non-ionizing. (frequencies between 300 MHz and 300 GHZ) [56–58]. The specific absorption rate (SAR) measures the energy dose that subjects exposed to RF absorb and is expressed in power (watts) by tissue mass (kilograms) [W/kg]. Effects of this dose deposition by use of cellular phones, however, take long to manifest. In some cases, this duration may be 10 years or more.

In general public there can be 3 reasons of concern:

a. Cell phones emit radiofrequency energy (radio waves), a form of non-ionizing radiation, from their antennas. Tissues nearest to the antenna can absorb this energy.

b. The number of cell phone users has increased rapidly. As of December 2014, there were more than 327.5 million cell phone subscribers in the United States, according to the Cellular Telecommunications and Internet Association. This is a nearly threefold increase from the 110 million users in 2000. Globally, the number of subscriptions is estimated by the International Telecommunications Union to be 5 billion.

c. Over time, the number of cell phone calls per day, the length of each call, and the amount of time people use cell phones have increased. However, improvements in cell phone technology have resulted in devices that have lower power outputs than earlier models [59].

It is to be noted that cell phones are often held tightly against the head. Electromagnetic radiation is governed by an interesting law known as the inverse square law. This essentially means that if we increase distance from the source by a factor of 2, the exposure gets reduced by 1/4th. It is for this reason, that distance from the device is a critical factor which decides the exposure received from a particular device. It is for the same reason that, if indeed a true risk exists, children would be at particular risk because their skulls are thinner. Also the cumulative lifetime exposure of children to cell phones would likely be greater than the exposure of current adults [11].

3.3. Clinical studies

Most of the work in cancer etiology and cellular phones has been based on brain tumors and parotid/salivary gland tumors because of the vicinity between these structures and cellular phone when used by an individual. Among brain tumors also most studies linked to glioma, meningioma and acoustic neuroma/schwannomas [11, 55].

There has been a meta-analysis published in JCO in 2009 about cellular phones and cancer risk. Myung et al. have selected initial 465 articles meeting their criteria and finally 23 case-control studies, which involved 37,916 participants were chosen. They found that a significant positive association (harmful effect) was observed in a random effects meta-analysis of eight studies using blinding, whereas a significant negative association (protective effect) was observed in a fixed-effects meta-analysis of 15 studies not using blinding. Mobile phone use of 10 years or longer was associated with a risk of tumors in 13 studies reporting this association (odds ratio = 1.18; 95% CI, 1.04–1.34) [60].

In reply to the above Stang et al. Criticized these random effects and have pointed out flaws related to the methodology. They have also highlighted their own data from uveal melanoma. After their initial case report they carried out case-control study on uveal melanoma focusing on mobile phone use and used the same detailed exposure assessment as the Interphone study used. The authors could not corroborate their previous results that showed an increased risk of uveal melanoma among regular mobile phone users. They accepted that probabilistic multiple error sensitivity analyses to evaluate the potential of exposure misclassification bias and selection bias did not explain the null result [61, 62].

The Interphone study group published the outcomes of an interview-based, case-control study with 2708 glioma and 2409 meningioma cases and matched controls. The study was conducted in 13 countries using a common protocol. The result of the study suggested that no increase in risk of glioma or meningioma was observed with use of mobile phones [63]. The cell phone companies faced these challenges and as of now they claim that Cell phone technology too is rapidly advancing and the electromagnetic exposure is progressively less with newer phones [64].

The World Health Organization (WHO) set up an expert panel to evaluate the effect of cell phones on the human body. On May 31, 2011 the expert panel said that cell phones might possibly cause side effects. The International Agency for research on Cancer (IARC) panel found cell phones to be "possibly carcinogenic," and stated that heavy cell phone use might or might not cause glioma [65]. Further in 2015 it was declared in a multicentric study that cell phone radiation can cause brain tumors and this to be categorized as probable human carcinogen category 2A. This study stated that previous IARC classification of Group 2B (possible) carcinogen in 2011 should be reclassified as a Group 2A (probable) carcinogen [12].

The basis of the above was another large scale epidemiologic study called CERENAT study which was a French case-control study of cases ≥16 years of age diagnosed between June 2004 and May 2006 included 253 glioma and 194 meningioma cases with two age- and gender-matched controls per case selected between 2005 and 2008. They included Potential confounders such as the level of education, smoking, alcohol consumption, and occupational exposures to pesticides, extremely low frequency electromagnetic fields (ELF-EMF), radiofrequency electromagnetic fields (RF-EMFs), and ionizing radiation. Risks of glioma were reported for heavy mobile phone use (≥896 cumulative hours of use). When heavy mobile phone use was examined by years since first use, glioma risk increased from >1 year since first use, to >2 years and to >5 years, OR 2.89, [95% confidence interval (CI) 1.41–5.93], OR 3.03, (95% CI 1.47–6.26), and OR 5.30, (95% CI 2.12–13.23), respectively. There was a borderline significant risk for glioma in the temporal lobe. This study also suggested risk for meningioma but lesser than glioma [66].

Interestingly these EM radiations can both initiate and promote tumor progression. In an Australian study of regional hospital-based data for the years 2000–2008, Dobes et al. stated, a significant increasing incidence in glioblastoma multiforme (GBM) was observed in the study period particularly after 2006 [67]. An increasing incidence of brain tumors during 2003–2012, 41.2% among men and 46.1% in women has been noted in Denmark, cases of GBM nearly doubled in the previous 10 years [68].

3.4. Precautions

Munshi and Jalali have beautifully highlighted how we can take few precautions. (1) Use the cell phone whenever it is really needed. For most routine work and casual talks, use the regular landline connection. (2) Discourage children from excessive use of cell phones.

(3) Whenever possible, use a wired ear piece connected to the cell phone. (4) Avoid cell phone use when the signal is weak. (5) Consider alternating between left and right ear while talking on cell phone. (6) Use texting (SMS) instead of calling when possible [55]. Morgan et al. also stated that until further evidence is available, it is prudent to follow the ALARA standard used in pediatric radiology. The ALARA approach would require hardware and software designers to create proximity sensors and embed flash notices regarding simple advisories about safer use within devices [12].

3.5. Conclusion

The data regarding cellular phone usage and cancer risk is ever emerging. We have some progress towards stronger association as IARC classification changed. As time advances newer and more mature results will come up. At the same time it is also true that a billionaire cellular phone Industry will also come up with safer devices. We will also need prospective data as the major limitation of epidemiological studies addressing the health effects of mobile phone use is related to exposure assessment. These limitations are inherent in case-control studies [69]. Borrowing the lines from Munshi et al. "it may be some time before we know if the friendly gizmos in our hands have the ability to cause aggressive tumors, for the time being, you have the free choice—to talk or not to talk" [11].

Acknowledgements

This was a unique opportunity. I would like to thank my parents (Mrs. Karabi Basu and Mr. PM Basu) for always supporting and not forcing me in all my decisions and my wife (Reshmi Ghosh) who has been my friend, philosopher, counselor and motivator. I always draw inspiration from daily patients in my practice and several thoughts have actually originated from their sufferings. I would take this opportunity to thank my MD guide Prof. Anup Majumdar, my teachers at Tata Memorial Hospital, Mumbai (Dr. Siddhartha Laskar, Dr. Sarbani G Laskar, Dr. JP Agarwal and all other teachers and friends). A personal thank you to my seniors Dr. Shikha Goyal, Dr. Deepak Gupta and Dr. Susovan Banerjee who always encouraged me to perform better, and to my childhood friend Dr. Shirshendu Sinha, a practicing psychiatrist at Mayo College, USA, for believing in me. Last but never the least, thank you for everything to the Almighty.

Author details

Trinanjan Basu

Address all correspondence to: trinanjan.doctor@gmail.com

HCG Apex Cancer Centre, Borivali West, Mumbai, India

References

[1] Armstrong B, Doll R. Environmental factors and cancer incidence and mortality in different countries, with special reference to dietary practices. International Journal of Cancer. 1975;**15**:617-631

[2] Wynder EL, Bross IJ, Feldman RM. A study of the etiological factors in cancer of the mouth. Cancer. 1957;**10**:1300-1323

[3] Wynder EL, Bross IJ. A study of etiological factors in cancer of the esophagus. Cancer. 1961;**14**:389-413

[4] Gandhi AK, Kumar P, Bhandari M, Devnani B, Rath GK. Burden of preventable cancers in India: Time to strike the cancer epidemic. Journal of the Egyptian National Cancer Institute. 2017;**29**:11-18

[5] Shah A, Malik A, Garg A, Mair M, Nair S, Chaturvedi P. Oral sex and human papilloma virus-related head and neck squamous cell cancer: A review of the literature. Postgraduate Medical Journal. 2017 Aug 4 pii: postgradmedj-2016-134603

[6] Jindal HA, Kaur A, Murugan S. Human Papilloma Virus vaccine for low and middle income countries: A step too soon? Human Vaccines & Immunotherapeutics. 2017 Aug 28:1-3. DOI: 10.1080/21645515.2017.1358837 [Epub ahead of print]

[7] Huh WK, Joura EA, Giuliano AR, Iversen OE, de Andrade RP, Ault KA. Final efficacy, immunogenicity, and safety analyses of a nine-valent human papillomavirus vaccine in women aged 16-26 years: A randomised, double-blind trial. Lancet. 2017 Sep 5. pii: S0140-6736(17)31821-4. DOI: 10.1016/S0140-6736(17)31821-4 [Epub ahead of print]

[8] Jones DR, Goldblatt PO, Leon DA. Bereavement and cancer: Some data on deaths of spouses from the longitudinal study of Office of Population Censuses and Surveys. British Medical Journal (Clinical Research Ed.). 1984;**289**:461-464

[9] Taylor C, Trowbridge P, Chilvers C. Stress and cancer surveys: Attitudes of participants in a case-control study. Journal of Epidemiology and Community Health. 1991;**45**:317-320

[10] Bergelt C, Prescott E, Grønbaek M, Koch U, Johansen C. Stressful life events and cancer risk. British Journal of Cancer. 2006;**95**:1579-1581

[11] Munshi A. Cellular phones: To talk or not to talk. Journal of Cancer Research and Therapeutics. 2011;**7**:476-477

[12] Morgan LL, Miller AB, Sasco A, Davis DL. Mobile phone radiation causes brain tumors and should be classified as a probable human carcinogen (2A) (review). International Journal of Oncology. 2015;**46**:1865-1871

[13] McKinney PA. Brain tumours: Incidence, survival, and aetiology. Journal of Neurology, Neurosurgery, and Psychiatry. 2004;**75**(Suppl 2):ii12-17

[14] Baghurst KI, Baghurst PA, Record SJ. Public perceptions of the role of dietary and other environmental factors in cancer causation or prevention. Journal of Epidemiology and Community Health. 1992;**46**:120-126

[15] Doll R, Peto R. The causes of cancer: Quantitative estimates of avoidable risk of cancer in the United States today. Journal of the National Cancer Institute. 1981;**66**:1193-1265

[16] Callahan D. The WHO definition of 'health'. Studies—Hastings Center. 1973;**1**:77-88

[17] Nobile M. The WHO definition of health: A critical reading. Medicine and Law. 2014; **33**:33-40

[18] Cobb S. Presidential Address-1976. Social support as a moderator of life stress. Psychosomatic Medicine. 1976;**38**:300-314

[19] Ryff CD. Happiness is everything, or is it? Explorations on the meaning of psychological well-being. Journal of Personality and Social Psychology. 1989;**57**:1069-1081

[20] Evans E. A Psychological Study of Cancer. New York: Dodd Mead and Co; 1926

[21] LeShan L. An emotional life history pattern associated with neoplastic disease. Annals of the New York Academy of Sciences. 1966;**125**:780-793

[22] Muslin HL, Gyarfas K, Pieper WJ. Separation experience and cancer of the breast. Annals of the New York Academy of Sciences. 1966;**125**:802-806

[23] Kiecolt-Glaser JK, Glaser R, Williger D, et al. Psychosocial enhancement of immunocompetence in a geriatric population. Health Psychology. 1985;**4**:25-41

[24] Reiche EM, Nunes SO, Morimoto HK. Stress, depression, the immune system, and cancer. The Lancet Oncology. 2004;**5**:617-625

[25] Hunter RG. Epigenetic effects of stress and corticosteroids in the brain. Frontiers in Cellular Neuroscience. 2012;**6**:18

[26] Brock AJ. Greek Medicine: Being Extracts Illustrative of Medical Writers from Hippocrates to Galen. London, England: JM Dent and Sons; 1929

[27] Lutgendorf SK, Sood AK. Biobehavioral factors and cancer progression: Physiological pathways and mechanisms. Psychosomatic Medicine. 2011;**73**:724-730

[28] Levy S, Herberman R, Lee J, Whiteside T, Kirkwood J, McFeeley S. Estrogen receptor concentration and social factors as predictors of natural killer cell activity in early-stage breast cancer patients. Natural Immunity and Cell Growth Regulation. 1990;**9**:313-324

[29] Levy S, Herberman R, Lippman M, D'Angelo T, Lee J. Immunological and psychosocial predictors of disease recurrence in patients with early-stage breast cancer. Behavioral Medicine. 1991;**17**:67-75

[30] Levy S, Herberman R, Maluish A, Schlein B, Lippman M. Prognostic risk assessment in primary breast cancer by behavioral and immunological parameters. Health Psychology. 1985;**4**:99-113

[31] Levy SM, McCabe PM, Schneiderman N, Field TM, Skyler JS, editors. Stress, Coping and Disease: Behavioral and Immunological Host Factors in Cancer Risk. Hillsdale, NJ: Lawrence Erlbaum Associates; 1991. p. 237-253

[32] Glaser R, Thorn B, Tarr K, Kiecolt-Glaser J, D'Ambrosio S. Effects of stress on methy-transferase synthesis: An important DNA repair enzyme. Health Psychology. 1985;**4**:403-412

[33] Kiecolt-Glaser JK, Stephens RE, Lipetz PD, Speicher CE, Glaser R. Distress and DNA repair in human lymphocytes. Journal of Behavioral Medicine. 1985;**8**:311

[34] Blomberg BB, Alvarez JP, Diaz A, Romero MG, Lechner SC, Carver CS, Holley H, Antoni MH. Psychosocial adaptation and cellular immunity in breast cancer patients in the weeks after surgery: An exploratory study. Journal of Psychosomatic Research. 2009;**67**:369-376

[35] Sephton SE, Dhabhar FS, Keuroghlian AS, Giese-Davis J, McEwen BS, Ionan AC, Spiegel D. Depression, cortisol, and suppressed cell-mediated immunity in metastatic breast cancer. Brain, Behavior, and Immunity. 2009;**23**:1148-1155

[36] JL GDA, Gamblin TC, Olek MC, Carr BI. Depression, immunity, and survival in patients with hepatobiliary carcinoma. Journal of Clinical Oncology. 2007;**25**:2397-2405

[37] Fidler IJ. The pathogenesis of cancer metastasis: The 'seed and soil' hypothesis revisited. Nature Reviews. Cancer. 2003;**3**:453-458

[38] Folkman J. What is the evidence that tumors are angiogenesis dependant? Journal of the National Cancer Institute. 1990;**82**:4-6

[39] Folkman J, Klagsbrun M. Angiogenic factors. Science. 1987;**235**:442-447

[40] Senger DR, Galli SJ, Dvorak AM, Perruzzi CA, Harvey VS, Dvorak HF. Tumor cells secrete a vascular permeability factor that promotes accumulation of ascites fluid. Science. 1983; **219**:983-985

[41] Shanmugathasan M, Jothy S. Apoptosis, anoikis and their relevance to the pathobiology of colon cancer. Pathol Int. Apr 2000;**50**(4):273-279

[42] Yawata A, Adachi M, Okuda H, et al. Prolonged cell survival enhances peritoneal dissemination of gastric cancer cells. Oncogene. 1998;**16**:2681-2686

[43] Pollard JW. Tumour-educated macrophages promote tumour progression and metastasis. Nature Reviews. Cancer. 2004;**4**:71-78

[44] Sica A, Allavena P, Mantovani A. Cancer related inflammation: The macrophage connection. Cancer Letters. 2008;**267**:204-215

[45] Sica A, Rubino L, Mancino A, et al. Targeting tumour-associated macrophages. Expert Opinion on Therapeutic Targets. 2007;**11**:1219-1229

[46] Sica A, Schioppa T, Mantovani A, Allavena P. Tumour-associated macrophages are a distinct M2 polarised population promoting tumour. European Journal of Cancer. 2006;**42**:717-727

[47] Zhao XY, Malloy PJ, Krishnan AV, et al. Glucocorticoids can promote androgen-independent growth of prostate cancer cells through a mutated androgen receptor. Nature Medicine. 2000;**6**:703-706

[48] Simon WE, Albrecht M, Trams G, Dietel M, Holzel F. In vitro growth promotion of human mammary carcinoma cells by steroid hormones, tamoxifen, and prolactin. Journal of the National Cancer Institute. 1984;**73**:313-321

[49] Elenkov IJ. Glucocorticoids and the Th1/Th2 balance. Annals of the New York Academy of Sciences. 2004;**1024**:138-146

[50] Anderson LM. Environmental genotoxicants/carcinogens and childhood cancer: Bridgeable gaps in scientific knowledge. Mutation Research. 2006;**608**:136-156

[51] Kaatsch P. Epidemiology of childhood cancer. Cancer Treatment Reviews. 2010;**36**:277-285

[52] Parkin DM, Whelan S, Ferlay J, et al. Cancer Incidence in Five Continents VIII. Vol. 155. Lyon, France: IARC Scientific Publications (IARC); 2002

[53] Momen NC, Olsen J, Gissler M, Cnattingius S, Li J. Early life bereavement and childhood cancer: A nationwide follow-up study in two countries. BMJ Open. 2013;**3**(5):e002864. DOI: 10.1136/bmjopen-2013-002864

[54] Hoskote SS, Kapdi M, Joshi SR. An epidemiological review of mobile telephones and cancer. The Journal of the Association of Physicians of India. 2008;**56**:980-984

[55] Munshi A, Jalali R. Cellular phones and their hazards: The current evidence. National Medical Journal of India. 2002;**15**:275-277

[56] Heynick LN, Johnston SA, Mason PA. Radio frequency electromagnetic fields: Cancer, mutagenesis, and genotoxicity. Bioelectromagnetics. 2003;**6**:S74-100

[57] Chang SK, Choi JS, Gil HW, Yang JO, Lee EY, Jeon YS, et al. Genotoxicity evaluation of electromagnetic fields generated by 835-MHz mobile phone frequency band. European Journal of Cancer Prevention. 2005;**14**:175-179

[58] Hardell L, Sage C. Biological effects from electromagnetic field exposure and public exposure standards. Biomedicine & Pharmacotherapy. 2008;**62**:104-109

[59] Available from: https://www.cancer.gov/about-cancer/causes-prevention/risk/radiation/cell-phones-fact-sheet. [Accessed: May 2017]

[60] Myung SK, Ju W, McDonnell DD, Lee YJ, Kazinets G, Cheng CT, et al. Mobile phone use and risk of tumors: A meta-analysis. Journal of Clinical Oncology. 2009;**27**:5565-5572

[61] Stang A, Anastassiou G, Ahrens W, et al. The possible role of radiofrequency radiation in the development of uveal melanoma. Epidemiology. 2001;**12**:7-12

[62] Stang A, Schmidt-Pokrzywniak A, Lash TL, et al. Mobile phone use and risk of uveal melanoma: Results of the risk factors for uveal melanoma case-control study. Journal of the National Cancer Institute. 2009;**101**:120-123

[63] Interphone Study Group. Brain tumour risk in relation to mobile telephone use: Results of the INTERPHONE international case-control study. International Journal of Epidemiology. 2010;**39**:675-694

[64] Pope L, Silva P, Almeyda R. Phone applications for the modern day otolaryngologist. Clinical Otolaryngology. 2010;**35**:350-354

[65] Available from: http://www.iarc.fr/en/media-centre/pr/2011/pdfs/pr208_E.pdf [Accessed: 2011 Aug 2]

[66] Coureau G, Bouvier G, Lebailly P, et al. Mobile phone use and brain tumours in the CERENAT case-control study. Occupational and Environmental Medicine. 2014;**71**:514-522

[67] Dobes M, Khurana VG, Shadbolt B, Jain S, Smith SF ea. Increasing incidence of glioblastoma multiforme and meningioma, and decreasing incidence of Schwannoma (2000-2008): Findings of a multicenter Australian study. Surgical Neurology International. 2011;**2**:176

[68] The Danish Cancer Society. The Increase in New Cases of Aggressive Brain Cancer. http://www.cancer.dk/Nyheder/nyhedsartikler/2012kv4/Kraftigstigningihjernesvulster.html. [Accessed: 22-09-2014]

[69] Auvinen A, Toivo T, Tokola K. Epidemiological risk assessment of mobile phones and cancer: Where can we improve? European Journal of Cancer Prevention. 2006;**15**:516-523

Permissions

All chapters in this book were first published in CM, by InTech Open; hereby published with permission under the Creative Commons Attribution License or equivalent. Every chapter published in this book has been scrutinized by our experts. Their significance has been extensively debated. The topics covered herein carry significant findings which will fuel the growth of the discipline. They may even be implemented as practical applications or may be referred to as a beginning point for another development.

The contributors of this book come from diverse backgrounds, making this book a truly international effort. This book will bring forth new frontiers with its revolutionizing research information and detailed analysis of the nascent developments around the world.

We would like to thank all the contributing authors for lending their expertise to make the book truly unique. They have played a crucial role in the development of this book. Without their invaluable contributions this book wouldn't have been possible. They have made vital efforts to compile up to date information on the varied aspects of this subject to make this book a valuable addition to the collection of many professionals and students.

This book was conceptualized with the vision of imparting up-to-date information and advanced data in this field. To ensure the same, a matchless editorial board was set up. Every individual on the board went through rigorous rounds of assessment to prove their worth. After which they invested a large part of their time researching and compiling the most relevant data for our readers.

The editorial board has been involved in producing this book since its inception. They have spent rigorous hours researching and exploring the diverse topics which have resulted in the successful publishing of this book. They have passed on their knowledge of decades through this book. To expedite this challenging task, the publisher supported the team at every step. A small team of assistant editors was also appointed to further simplify the editing procedure and attain best results for the readers.

Apart from the editorial board, the designing team has also invested a significant amount of their time in understanding the subject and creating the most relevant covers. They scrutinized every image to scout for the most suitable representation of the subject and create an appropriate cover for the book.

The publishing team has been an ardent support to the editorial, designing and production team. Their endless efforts to recruit the best for this project, has resulted in the accomplishment of this book. They are a veteran in the field of academics and their pool of knowledge is as vast as their experience in printing. Their expertise and guidance has proved useful at every step. Their uncompromising quality standards have made this book an exceptional effort. Their encouragement from time to time has been an inspiration for everyone.

The publisher and the editorial board hope that this book will prove to be a valuable piece of knowledge for researchers, students, practitioners and scholars across the globe.

List of Contributors

Paulo C.M. Lyra-Junior, Nayara G. Tessarollo, Isabella S. Guimarães, Taciane B. Henriques, Diandra Z. dos Santos, Marcele L.M. de Souza and Leticia B.A. Rangel
Laboratory of Cellular and Molecular Biology of Human Cancer, Department of Pharmaceutical Sciences and Biotechnology Program, Federal University of Espirito Santo State, Vitória, Brazil

Hugo M. Victor Marques, Laura F.R.L. de Oliveira, Krislayne V. Siqueira and Alan T. Branco
Laboratory of Cellular and Molecular Biology of Human Cancer, Department of Pharmaceutical Sciences, Vitória, Brazil

Ian V. Silva
Department of Morphology, Health Sciences Center, Federal University of Espirito Santo State, Vitória, Brazil

Diana Linhares, and Armindo Rodrigues
Faculty of Sciences and Technology, University of the Azores, Ponta Delgada, Portugal
IVAR, Institute of Volcanology and Risks Assessment, University of the Azores, Ponta Delgada, Portugal

Patrícia Garcia
Faculty of Sciences and Technology, University of the Azores, Ponta Delgada, Portugal
cE3c, Centre for Ecology, Evolution and Environmental Changes, and Azorean Biodiversity Group, University of the Azores, Ponta Delgada, Portugal

Maher Soliman
Oncology Department, Faculty of Medicine, Alexandria University, Alexandria, Egypt

Hassan Adwan, Dina Elharouni, Danira Habashy and Nadine Banna
Department of Pharmacology and Toxicology, Faculty of Pharmacy and Biotechnology, The German University in Cairo, Cairo, New Cairo City, Egypt

Rania Georges and Martin R. Berger
Toxicology and Chemotherapy Unit, German Cancer Research Center, Heidelberg, Germany

Asim Pervaiz
Department of Allied Health Sciences, University of Health Sciences, Lahore, Pakistan

Görkem Eskiizmir
Department of Otorhinolaryngology, Head and Neck Surgery, Celal Bayar University, School of Medicine, Manisa, Turkey

Erdoğan Özgür
Department of Otorhinolaryngology, Head and Neck Surgery, Muğla Sıtkı Koçman University, School of Medicine, Muğla, Turkey

Jianhai Sun, Chunxiu Liu and Jingjing Zhang
State Key Laboratory of Transducer Technology, Institute of Electronics, Chinese Academy of Sciences, Beijing, China

Jinhua Liu, Yanni Zhang, Xiaofeng Zhu and Zhanwu Ning
Beijing Municipal Institute of Labour Protection, Beijing, China

Chrisostomos Sofoudis
Department of Obstetrics and Gynecology, Konstandopoulio General Hospital, Athens, Greece

Austin Carver and Vincent S. Gallicchio
Department of Biological Sciences, College of Science, Clemson University, Clemson, South Carolina, United States of America

Anushka Dikshit and Jennifer Zhang
Department of Dermatology, Duke University Medical Center, Durham, NC, USA

Zhaoping Qiu, Jianlin Wang and Yadi Wu
Department of Pharmacology and Nutritional Sciences, University of Kentucky School of Medicine, Lexington, KY, USA
Department of Markey Cancer Center, University of Kentucky School of Medicine, Lexington, KY, USA

Kwok Kin Lee
Cancer Science Institute of Singapore, National University of Singapore, Singapore

Wee Joo Chng
Cancer Science Institute of Singapore, National University of Singapore, Singapore
Department of Medicine, Yong Loo Lin School of Medicine, National University of Singapore, Singapore
Department of Haematology-Oncology, National University Cancer Institute of Singapore, National University Health System, Singapore

Sudhakar Jha
Cancer Science Institute of Singapore, National University of Singapore, Singapore
Department of Biochemistry, Yong Loo Lin School of Medicine, National University of Singapore, Singapore
Michael Higgins, Ismael Obaidi and Tara McMorrow
School of Biomolecular and Biomedical Sciences, Conway Institute, University College Dublin, Dublin, Ireland

Ke Wang
Clinical Laboratory, Yongchuan Hospital of Chongqing Medical University, Chongqing, China

Trinanjan Basu
HCG Apex Cancer Centre, Borivali West, Mumbai, India

Index

www.ingramcontent.com/pod-product-compliance
Lightning Source LLC
LaVergne TN
LVHW081034210926
848485LV00004B/1020